The Comprehensive Guide
to Equine
Veterinary
Medicine

Barb Crabbe, DVM

Illustrations by Kip Carter, MS, CMI

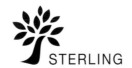
STERLING

New York / London
www.sterlingpublishing.com

STERLING and the distinctive Sterling logo are trademarks of the Sterling Publishing Co., Inc.

Library of Congress Cataloging-in-Publication Data

Crabbe, Barb.
  The comprehensive guide to equine veterinary medicine / Barb Crabbe.
    p. cm.
  ISBN-13: 978-1-4027-1053-7
  ISBN-10: 1-4027-1053-4
  1. Horses—Health. I. Title.
SF951.C82 2007
636.1'089—dc   222006101861

1 0 9 8 7 6 5 4 3 2 1

Published by Sterling Publishing Co., Inc.
387 Park Avenue South, New York, NY 10016
© 2007 by Barb Crabbe, DVM
Distributed in Canada by Sterling Publishing
c/o Canadian Manda Group, 165 Dufferin Street
Toronto, Ontario, Canada M6K 3H6
Distributed in the United Kingdom by GMC Distribution Services
Castle Place, 166 High Street, Lewes, East Sussex, England BN7 1XU
Distributed in Australia by Capricorn Link (Australia) Pty. Ltd.
P.O. Box 704, Windsor, NSW 2756, Australia

Design and layout by Carol Petro
Unless otherwise noted, all photographs are by Jim Bortvedt.

Printed in China
All rights reserved

Sterling ISBN-13: 978-1-4027-1053-7
        ISBN-10: 1-4027-1053-4

For information about custom editions, special sales, premium and
corporate purchases, please contact Sterling Special Sales Department at 800-805-5489 or
specialsales@sterlingpub.com.

To my Mom. Because she always told me I could.

CONTENTS

ACKNOWLEDGMENTS

◆

It is amazing how many people it takes to make a project like this happen, and to all of those who helped me I will be forever grateful.

My staff Nikki James, Jeni Cline, Selma Kendrick, and Charlotte Haines who supported every part of this book's development. Especially Nikki ("the typist"), who spent countless hours editing text, looking up details, and working with all of that digital artwork.

My associate, Dr. Jennifer Posey, who took on our whole caseload single-handedly for days at a time, always with a smile. And who knows how to find amazing bits of information with a stroke of the keyboard.

Kip Carter for your amazing artwork, and Jim Bortvedt for being the most efficient photographer and friend who can always get that perfect shot.

My mentor and friend Jennifer Forsberg Meyer. Because you're always there when I need you.

My agent and editor Madelyn Larsen. You must have had your doubts, but when the chips were down, you made me believe it could really happen. Paula Schlosser and John Woodside admirably contributed to the production aspects of my book. And Steven Magnuson, who must be the most patient man in publishing.

Most of all, my family—Katie, Jamie, and Bob. Even though you wished I'd said "No," you never wavered in your support. The next five years are all yours.

INTRODUCTION

◆

WHEN SOMETHING IS WRONG with your horse, it's agonizing. I know; I've been there. I recall one time when my gelding, Snuff, was so lame he refused to put any weight on his foot at all. As I attempted to move him from his stall to the barn aisle, he held his left front foot in the air and hopped. Weeping, I called the vet and described the problem.

"Help!—It's an emergency. My horse has broken his leg." Like a knight in shining armor, she arrived in her Dodge truck. With a simple stroke of her hoof knife, the abscess exploded in the barn aisle, and Snuff could walk again. She was my hero. I was 12 years old.

Just the other day, I pulled up in my own Dodge truck and relieved another horse's discomfort with a stroke of the knife. In many ways, not all that much has changed in the practice of horse doctoring. In other ways, it's a whole new world.

Less than 100 years ago, general anesthesia wasn't even available, and surgical procedures were limited by the veterinarian's ability to forcibly restrain the horse. These days, surgery to correct a displaced intestine in a colicky horse or to repair a fractured bone is commonplace.

Back then, medical treatments were limited to the concoctions mixed up in the vet's buggy—and often included substances such as warm ox urine and pitch. Now, medications are carefully researched to establish safety and efficacy—as well as appropriate dosing strategies. Of course, that doesn't mean a sharp hoof knife has lost its place, or that the occasional old-time remedy won't do the trick. In fact, I still listen carefully whenever I hear a health-care tip from an old-time horseman.

In the chapters that follow, I've included all of the tidbits I've learned along the road to becoming a "seasoned" horse vet. My knowledge comes from many sources—old cowboys who've forgotten more about horses than most of us will ever know, and state-of-the-art veterinary lectures presented at national and international meetings. More than from anyone, I've learned from my clients, who so often make incredibly insightful observations about their equine companions, and from the horses themselves, who always have something more to teach.

I think you'll enjoy the historical treatments outlined at the beginning of each chapter; I know I had fun researching them. In the chapters themselves, you'll find helpful current information about most of your horse's health-care concerns. My hope is that it helps to make those difficult times when something is wrong with your horse a little less agonizing.

PART ONE

Basic Horse Care

CHAPTER 1

Getting to Know You

THEN AND NOW

Accounts of surgical procedures performed on horses
are found as far back as the
13th century, with restraint of
the patient requiring stocks,
ropes, and straps. Often,
in order to perform a procedure, horses were cast, or
thrown to the ground and tied
in restraints. One account
describes how sponges
soaked in anesthetic sub-
stances were packed in
the nostrils of the horse to
induce unconsciousness and
analgesia before surgery.

These days, the equine surgical patient is anesthetized
with intravenous administration of medications that
quickly and easily drop him
to the ground. For longer procedures, the horse is intu-
bated and maintained in a
sleeping state through inhala-
tion of gas anesthetics—
accompanied by intensive
monitoring of his vital signs
and depth of consciousness
to ensure he's safe.

THE HERD GRAZES PEACEFULLY, moving slowly across the open
fields. An occasional skirmish erupts as junior members approach
their more dominant herd mates. Pinned ears warn them away, and
the occasional kick of the hind leg emphasizes the message. A coyote call
in the distance leads to suddenly raised heads and pricked ears. Unexpected movement in the nearby bushes causes a few stragglers who've
become separated from the herd to hightail it back to the group. And then
it's quiet again. Just another day in the life of a wild horse herd.

Shift to reality. Your horse looks up when you walk into the barn. He's
standing in his 12×12' box stall, waiting for breakfast. As you open the
feed-room door, he starts to paw, banging on the door with his front foot
with such force you think the boards are sure to break. "Knock it off," you
holler at him. He stops momentarily, then he resumes pawing. When you
finally throw him his flake of hay he pins his ears in your direction, then
quiets down to eat.

Basic Behavior

To understand your horse's health and behavior, you must first take a look
at how he would be living in his natural environment. He is a herd animal,
living in a structured social setting. He is well aware of his place within the
herd hierarchy, either as a dominant member of the group or as a more
submissive follower. His herd provides protection from danger, which is
especially important because your horse is a prey animal who must flee
from predators that threaten his safety. His flight instinct is very strong.
He must act first and think later if he's going to survive. When nothing
threatens the herd, your horse spends his time slowly walking and grazing.
Sometimes he naps, but rarely lying down. Instead, he sleeps on his feet
in a semi-alert state, always on the lookout for anything that might
threaten him.

When we domesticate the horse, we ask him to make a complete change of lifestyle. We put him in a stall, isolated from other horses. We feed him 2 or 3 times a day. If he's lucky, we may turn him out in a pasture or paddock every day. Oftentimes, his only exercise consists of an hour with a rider on his back. In his mind, a predator climbs on board. When you work with your horse, keep all of this in mind. It will help you to understand and work with his behavior, and keep you safe.

Your domesticated horse's behavior is strongly linked to the instincts that allow him to survive in the wild. Once you understand these natural behaviors and instincts, it's easy to see how behavior problems arise, and easier to understand how they can be managed.

Life in the Wild

In the wild, the horse must be constantly alert to danger. To accomplish this, he's acquired a number of behavior patterns that allow him to stay safe:

- ADOPTING A HERD LIFESTYLE: There's safety in numbers, and a wild horse follows this principle by living in a herd. The herd lives and travels as a group, and has a complicated social structure. Certain individuals establish themselves as dominant, while others are content to exist at the bottom of the social scale. An occasional social climber may challenge his position, resulting in a skirmish that might either keep him in his place or allow him to move up the ladder. These skirmishes involve a number of behaviors that are used to assert dominance and range from something as simple as a pinned ear and grouchy face to a full-blown bite or kick.

- CONSTANT MOVEMENT: The herd is always "on the move," a strategy that prevents horses from becoming a still target for a predator. They move throughout their home range, foraging all day long for food. The wild horse's small stomach and the need to graze constantly to get adequate nutrition is an adaptation that suits this lifestyle well. He's never weighed down by a full meal and is always prepared to flee if necessary.

- ACT FIRST, THINK LATER: When a threat does suddenly appear, the wild horse doesn't pause to think—he just gets out of there, and fast! Because of his vulnerability as a prey animal, his best survival strategy is to escape, then analyze the situation once he's safe.

If we consider these basics of natural equine behavior, it's easy to see why your horse may find his domesticated lifestyle difficult. When he lives in a stall, he's no longer part of a herd, but lives a life of isolation. His need to move is limited to a few hours of turnout or riding. He's fed on an intermittent schedule instead of foraging all day long, and he's expected to react predictably to whatever you ask him to do.

Let's first examine the most common categories of behavior problems. Then we'll see how these behaviors derive from the natural herd environment and what basic solution strategies you can use to keep your horse happy and keep you safe.

Stereotypical Behaviors

Equine stereotypies are defined as behavior patterns that are repeated time and time again without variation—and with no apparent function. A comparison in humans would be obsessive-compulsive type disorders. In the horse, such behaviors typically occur in response to confinement and isolation from other horses—environmental factors that completely contradict the free-ranging herd existence of a horse in the wild. Once your horse begins to exhibit a stereotypical behavior it can be very difficult to extinguish, even when environmental factors are adjusted. The likely reason is that your horse comforts himself with the behavior, and with this reward he learns to repeat it over and over again.

Examples: Cribbing, weaving, stall walking, self mutilation.

Solution strategies

- Minimize confinement by increasing turnout time and exercise level. As a general rule, turnout should be a minimum of 1 to 2 hours every day, and exercise should be 45 to 60 minutes at least 5 days a week.

- Reduce feelings of isolation by providing companionship. Other horses should be kept within eye- and earshot of your horse. In some situations, a stall mate like a goat or small pony can be a great companion. If none of this is possible, put an unbreakable mirror on the wall of your horse's stall. It might fool him into thinking he has a friend.

- Find ways to help him occupy his time when he's in his stall. Feeding free-choice grass hay throughout the day can be a helpful option because it mimics the full-time grazing lifestyle of a horse in the wild. (Be careful to watch his weight, and choose a low-calorie "filler" hay if your horse gets fat easily.) If you spread the hay out in the four corners of the stall, it may offer the additional advantage of breaking up the movement pattern of a stall walker.

- In some cases, medications that help regulate chemical alterations associated with the behaviors can be successful in treatment, including the antidepressant amitriptyline and the opiate blocker naloxone. Unfortunately, these medications are expensive and generally not practical for routine use.

Dominance Behaviors

Your horse uses dominance behavior to "tell you who's boss." In general, he mimics behaviors he'd exhibit toward his herd mates to deliver the same message within the herd hierarchy. You may not realize that you could be encouraging his or her dominance behavior if your body language conveys a message of submission. Not only that, if you're not careful your horse's aggressive attitude can escalate until these behavior problems become more and more severe. Although most of these behaviors are more "bark than bite," you should always take them very seriously. Stay safe by never turning your back on your aggressive horse, avoid standing in a corner of the stall that's closed off from a quick escape route, handle your horse from the safety zone around the shoulder area, and never work alone in the barn.

Examples: Ear pinning, kicking handlers (offensive—your horse turns his hindquarters in your direction in a planned effort to kick), biting.

Solution strategies

- Reward nonaggression. Try to take an affirmative approach by rewarding your horse either with a treat or praise and a pat every time he greets you with an ears-up positive demeanor.

- Establish yourself in the dominant position. When you enter your horse's stall, immediately make eye contact and don't back down if your horse threatens you with pinned ears or bared teeth. If your horse does begin to threaten you, immediately respond by "threatening back." Try stamping your foot and lunging in your horse's direction. Be careful when you make this move and watch your horse's reaction closely. It's a good idea to carry a crop in your hand when you do enter the stall. If your horse meets you aggressively, you can smack him across the chest or neck (not in the direction of his face) and back out of the stall. Whatever you do, don't lose eye contact, and don't turn and run away. It's important that you don't relay a message of intimidation as you retreat, because that would only reinforce your horse's position of dominance.

- Try standing over your horse's hay, and not allowing him to eat until you move. You can wave your hands, raise the whip, or "growl" if he attempts to approach you. This works because it mimics the way that dominance is established between horses in the wild. Once again, be sure to maintain eye contact as you make this challenge.

- Teach your horse to back on command by pairing the word "back" with pressure on his shoulder or a light tap on his chest with a whip. Reward him with a treat and a pat for this behavior, and then ask him to back whenever you enter the stall. This will prevent him from approaching you aggressively, and will help overcome his dominant behavior.

Territorial Behaviors

In the wild, the herd has a defined home range. If the home range is small, or has only one side to defend, horses in the wild will defend their territory. When a horse exists in domestication, his territory is his stall, which only has one side to defend. He'll exhibit "stay away" behaviors to protect it. In part, territorial behaviors can be related to dominance behavior. For example, your horse may pin his ears or snap his teeth to tell you, "Stay away and I mean business because I'm the boss."
Examples: Stall kicking, ear pinning.

Solution strategies

- See solutions above for dominance behaviors. By taking steps to establish dominance, you may be successful in reducing some of your horse's territorial aggression as well.

- Help your horse feel "safe" by reducing threats to his territory. If his stall has open sides where he can see the horse next door, consider constructing a solid wall to remove the threat.

- Provide well-separated feeding locations, either on opposite sides of the stall or in separate areas in a paddock or pasture. Dominance is a dispute over a scarce resource, and for most horses that resource is food. Minimizing competition at feeding time is critical.

Flight Behaviors

In the wild, the horse depends on flight to protect himself from predators. And as the potential victim of an attack, his reaction is to run. When this response carries over to his domesticated lifestyle, it leads to self-protective behavior problems such as spooking. Simply, whenever he perceives a threat, he wants to flee from it. A horse that's had limited exposure or minimal handling is very likely to exhibit defensive behaviors because he hasn't had the opportunity to learn what things aren't really threatening. A horse that's been at the "bottom of the pile" in a former herd situation may also be more flighty because he's learned just how important self-protection is, both against predators and members of his own herd.
Examples: Spooking, kicking handlers (defensive—your horse kicks out suddenly when startled)

Solution strategies

- Desensitization is the best strategy, and it can be performed with a variety of stimuli, beginning with something as simple as a towel. Stand just next to your horse's shoulder, and begin stroking him with the towel. As your horse accepts the stroking of his shoulder, gradually work your way over his entire body, taking care to stay out of kicking range. When he's relaxed and accepts the stroking, you can begin to make sudden movements with the towel closer to his face, until he

TABLE 1.1

Common Behavior Problems

BEHAVIOR	WHAT IT IS	CLASSIFICATION	CAUSE	RELATIONSHIP TO NATURAL BEHAVIOR	POTENTIAL COMPLICATIONS	FIXABLE?	SPECIFIC SOLUTION
Cribbing	Grabs solid object with front teeth, pulls back, and sucks air. If no appropriate surface is available to grab, horse may suck in air with head and neck extended.	Stereotypical behavior.	Induced by confinement and stress. May have a genetic component. May be related to high-carbohydrate diets, especially those that contain molasses.	None. An abnormal behavior that does not occur in the wild.	Wears down front teeth. Develops strong muscles on underside of neck. Destructive to stalls or fencing.	Difficult.	See stereotypical behaviors. Cribbing collars can be effective. Minimize or eliminate carbohydrates, especially containing molasses.
Weaving	Shifts weight back and forth between front legs, actually walks in place and swings head from side to side.	Stereotypical behavior.	Induced by confinement. Becomes more frequent when horse is anticipating something, such as feeding or turnout.	None. An abnormal behavior that does not occur in the wild.	Stresses lower legs and feet and can lead to soundness problems. May cause weight loss due to energy expenditure and decreased eating time.	Difficult.	See stereotypical behaviors. Increase his stall size or pasture him. Remove bars from doors or between stalls so he won't feel so confined.
Stall walking	Circles continuously in stall.	Stereotypical behavior.	Induced by confinement and isolation.	Natural lifestyle involves constant movement as horses roam free and graze. Stall walking exaggerates this behavior.	Stress to lower legs and feet can lead to soundness problems. May cause weight loss due to energy expenditure and decreased eating time.	Difficult.	None.

BEHAVIOR	WHAT IT IS	CLASSIFICATION	CAUSE	RELATIONSHIP TO NATURAL BEHAVIOR	POTENTIAL COMPLICATIONS	FIXABLE?	SPECIFIC SOLUTION
Pawing	Paws ground with front feet. Occurs commonly at feeding time or prior to riding or other activity.	Frustration behavior.	Induced by anticipation of an upcoming event such as feeding or exercise.	In the wild, horses paw to access snow-covered forage. This pawing can carry over as an expression of anticipation and frustration in stall-bound horses.	Injury to front feet or lower legs, especially if pawing occurs in stall and is accompanied by banging against stall door or wall.	Yes.	See frustration behaviors.
Self-mutilation	Bites at flank, chest, or front legs. Occurs most commonly in stallions and very rarely in mares.	Stereo-typical behavior.	Induced by frustration, often related to sexual frustration.	None.	May cause serious injuries, including skin lacerations or chronic, deep sores.	Difficult.	See stereotypical behaviors. Castration is often curative for stallions. Minimize exposure of stallions to mares in heat so that sexual frustration is reduced.
Kicking handlers	Kicks with hind legs when hind-quarters are approached.	Flight behavior when defensive. Dominance behavior when offensive.	Often a startle response and protective mechanism if a horse is surprised by a sudden approach. May be an aggressive "stay away" behavior if threatened.	Horses in the wild kick to protect them-selves and their herd from predators. May also come into play in herd dynamics to help protect position in the herd.	Dangerous for handlers.	Yes.	See flight behaviors, dominance behaviors.

Chart continues on page 10

Continued from page 9

BEHAVIOR	WHAT IT IS	CLASSIFICATION	CAUSE	RELATIONSHIP TO NATURAL BEHAVIOR	POTENTIAL COMPLICATIONS	FIXABLE?	SPECIFIC SOLUTION
Stall kicking	Repeatedly kicking stall walls.	Dominance behavior.	Induced by confinement and close proximity of other horses.	Horses in the wild can approach or avoid other horses at will. These options are not available when confined. Kicking asserts horse's "rights."	Injury to hind legs. Destructive to stall walls.	Yes.	See dominance behaviors and territorial behaviors. Negative reinforcement using kick chains may work in severe cases.
Spooking	Startles, jumps, or spins in response to sudden stimuli.	Flight behavior.	A protective mechanism in response to threat.	In a herd, horses react first and think later when faced with potential dangers. This natural behavior allows horses to survive as prey animals in the wild.	Can be dangerous for handlers and riders if horse spooks excessively. May predispose to trauma if environment has dangerous objects present.	Yes.	See flight behaviors.
Biting	Bites at handlers or other horses.	Dominance behavior.	A means of asserting dominant position.	In the wild, horses will bite at herd mates to establish dominant position. Biting is common during ritualistic fighting between stallions.	Dangerous for handlers and can cause injuries to other horses.	Yes for handlers. May be difficult for other horses.	See dominance behavior. Immediate punishment with a whip applied to the chest can be effective.
Ear pinning	Pins ears at handlers or other horses. May also scrape teeth against grates or stall doors.	Dominance behavior, territorial behavior.	Aggressive stance that indicates dominance and a position of power.	In the wild, ear pinning is acceptable, instinctive behavior that's used to establish dominance in herd.	Can escalate to biting or other more serious aggressive behavior if unchallenged. If accompanied by teeth scraping, damage to incisors (front teeth) and dental imbalances can result.	Yes—in some situations. Difficult in turn-out with other horses.	See dominance behaviors, territorial behaviors.

accepts its being flipped or even thrown in his direction without flinching. Be very patient during these sessions. It may take 20 or 30 minutes before you can even move the towel toward his hindquarters. If you take the time you need, you can accustom your horse to almost every stimulus you can think of using this very gradual approach.

- Reward good behavior and avoid punishment. Because these types of behavior are related to a lack of confidence, it's especially important that you take a positive approach. Reward a quiet response to anything that might be frightening with pats and words of praise, and avoid punishing your horse for overreacting. If you punish his flight response (for example, you smack him with the whip when he spooks), you simply reconfirm his belief that there's a reason to be frightened, and the behavior will become more and more ingrained.

Frustration Behavior

Your horse knows something's coming, such as food or exercise, and he's ready, now! His anticipation and frustration lead to pawing or dancing around, which are undesirable behaviors. In the wild, the horse is not forced to wait for anyone. If he wants to eat, he simply drops his head to take a bite. It is probably not coincidental that pawing is the one behavior he sometimes has to use in a natural environment to access food through snow or ice—and pawing is the most commonly observed frustration behavior we see in domesticated horses.

Examples: Pawing, self-mutilation (stereotypical behavior) may have a component of sexual frustration.

Solution strategies

- Many of the solution strategies described above for stereotypical behaviors can help reduce the frustration associated with isolation and confinement.

- Avoid rewarding the behavior. Often frustration behaviors are rewarded unintentionally. For example, if your horse bangs on his stall door at feeding time, you feed him and he stops. You've just success-fully reinforced his stall banging with the reward of feeding. Instead, wait until a moment when he stops banging to feed him, and withhold his feed as long as he's still banging. That way you'll be rewarding good behavior (not banging) instead of bad behavior (banging).

- Minimize frustration. If your horse exhibits anticipation at feeding time, feed him first to alleviate his frustration. If he paws while on the cross-ties prior to an exercise session, try tacking him up in his stall instead. Anything you can do to minimize his frustration will help to extinguish the behavior over time.

- Counter-condition your horse by teaching him a desirable behavior that's incompatible with the behavior you want him to stop. For example, if your horse paws when you're waiting on the trail, ask him to walk in a small circle—using the opportunity to ask him to bend correctly and soften to the contact. He can't paw when he's walking, and you'll be teaching him something positive instead.

Physical Restraint

At times you'll need to restrain your horse, either for basic handling or in order to perform a procedure he may not appreciate—such as getting oral medication or an injection. The following restraint techniques will come in handy.

Basic Tie   FIGURES 1.1–1.6

What it does
Restrains you horse's head so he'll stand still for basic handling procedures such as grooming, picking feet, or saddling.

Rules to remember for safety's sake

- Always use a quick-release knot when tying your horse. This allows you to untie him in an instant if he should spook or pull back.

- Always tie high enough, and with a short enough rope to prevent your horse from putting his head down to the ground. A rope tied at or above your horse's wither level is ideal. This will prevent accidents that might occur if your horse were to get his foot over the rope when tied.

- Untie your horse prior to performing any procedure he might object to, such as administering an injection or an oral medication. This will prevent injury if he should pull back against the rope.

- Never walk underneath the rope or your horse's head when he is tied. Walk around behind him instead. This will protect you from injury should your horse pull back or lunge forward when you are underneath the rope.

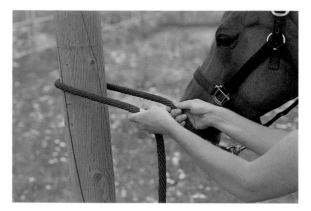

FIGURE 1.1 **To tie a safety release knot, first hold the rope with the horse end in your right hand, and the free end in your left hand. Pass the free end of the rope around or through the object to which you'll be tying it.**

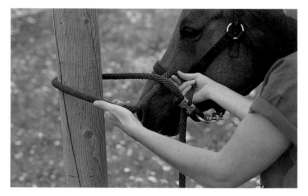

FIGURE 1.2. **Take the free end in your right hand, and pass it under the horse end. Use your left hand to hold the other side in a bend. This will form a triangle shape with the rope, the post, and your two hands as the three corners.**

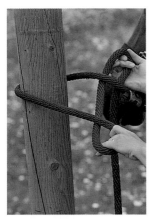

FIGURE 1.3. **Rotate your left hand toward you to form a loop in the corner of the rope.**

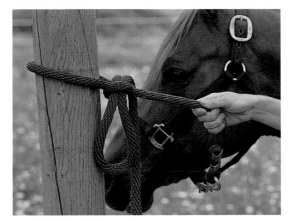

FIGURE 1.5. **Pull on the horse end of the rope to tighten your tie against the post.**

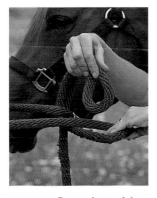

FIGURE 1.4. **Form a loop of the free end of the rope in your right hand, and pass it down through the loop of rope in your left hand.**

FIGURE 1.6. **The horse is safely tied with approximately 1 foot of rope between his head and the post, and the knot placed above wither level. To release the safety knot, simply pull on the free end of the rope.**

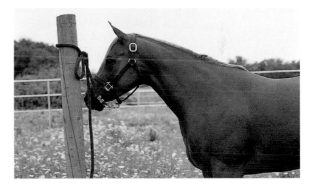

Cross-Tie

What it does

Restrains your horse's head on two sides so he'll stand still for basic handling procedures. Cross-ties are commonly used in confined grooming or tack-up areas to keep the horse's body centered, making it easier to work on both sides of him.

Rules to remember

- Never crosstie a horse that hasn't been trained to tie. Horses may be less predictable and more easily injured if they pull back on cross-ties than on a conventional tie.

- Use only quick-release snaps on both sides of the cross-ties so your horse will be freed easily if he does become frightened or pulls back.

- Adjust the length of the ties so that they can be snapped together when pulled tightly across the cross-tie area. This will leave just enough room to snap them to your horse's halter. Cross-ties that are too long allow your horse too much freedom to move around, and increase the risk of injury.

Twitch FIGURES 1.7–1.10

What it does

At minimum, a twitch will direct your horse's attention away from an unpleasant procedure. Many experts believe that the use of a twitch actually has a tranquilizing effect by stimulating the release of endorphins (the body's natural painkillers).

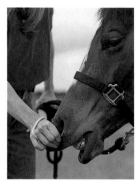

FIGURE 1.8. **Quickly and firmly grasp your horse's muzzle in your hand.**

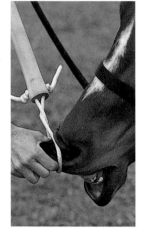

FIGURE 1.9. **Slide the rope loop of the twitch over your hand until it circles his muzzle. Begin twisting the twitch handle until the rope tightens around his muzzle.**

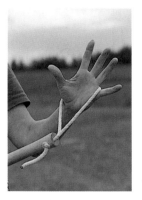

FIGURE 1.7. **To apply a twitch, stand to the side of your horse's neck, as close to his shoulder as possible. Place the loop of the twitch over your strongest hand, with the rope between your ring and little fingers to prevent the loop from sliding down your arm.**

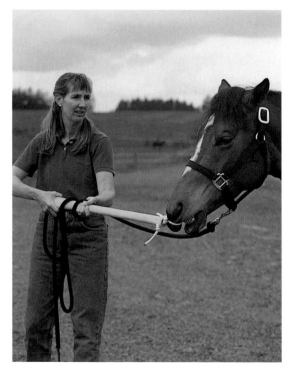

FIGURE 1.10. **Once the twitch is secure, stand back and to the side, and gauge your horse's reaction. If it's working well, your horse's eyes may appear to glaze over and he'll stand quietly for the necessary procedure.**

Rules to remember

- Horses can respond unpredictably to twitches. If you are inexperienced with horse behavior, it would be wise to seek help from your veterinarian or a knowledgeable friend the first time you attempt to apply a twitch to your horse.

- Always stand to the side or by your horse's shoulder when applying or holding a twitch. Some horses react to twitches by striking out with a front leg, which puts you in a dangerous position if you stand directly in front of your horse.

- Pay very close attention to your horse's reaction when applying a twitch for the first time. Some horses will react adversely to a twitch and may rear or blow-up when it's applied. In such cases, a different form of restraint will be necessary.

Shoulder Roll (Skin Twitch) FIGURE 1.11

What it does
Directs your horse's attention away from an unpleasant procedure. Like the twitch, a shoulder roll may have a mild tranquilizing effect by stimulating the release of endorphins.

FIGURE 1.11. **To apply a shoulder roll or skin twitch, place your hand with your fingers pointing toward your horse's head, just in front of the junction between his neck and shoulder. Firmly grasp the skin and underlying tissues with your fingers, and roll your hand in toward your horse's neck.**

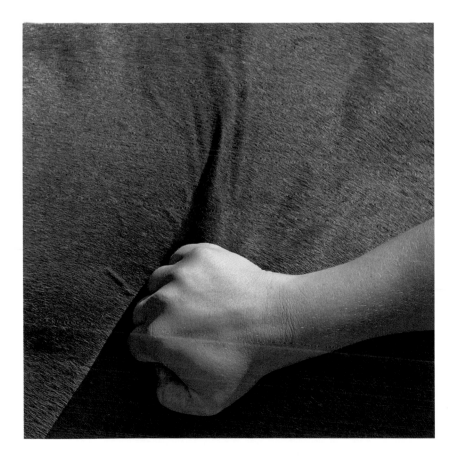

Rules to remember

- Your horse may rapidly back away as you begin to apply this restraint technique. Pay attention so you don't get injured.

- When using this technique, stand next to your horse's shoulder, not directly in front of him, to avoid being struck with a front leg.

Nose or Lip Chain   FIGURES 1.12–1.14

What it does

Gives you a stronger restraint for controlling your horse's head than a simple halter and leadline. Different configurations of the chain can be used depending on the individual horse's behavior. A chain over the nose is useful for controlling horses that flip their heads in the air, rear, or try to barge forward as you're leading them. A chain under the chin can be helpful for horses that lag behind as you're leading them. And a chain over the mucous membranes of the upper teeth (lip chain) is a strong method of controlling a very unruly horse.

Rules to remember

Whenever you apply pressure to a chain, do it rapidly followed immediately by a release. If you maintain constant pressure on a chain, your horse is likely to react strongly, and may be injured in the process.

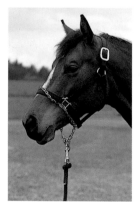

FIGURE 1.12. **To apply a chain over your horse's nose, pass the snap through the bottom ring on the halter. Pass the chain through the ring on the left side of the halter, over and around the nosepiece of the halter, through the ring on the right side of the halter, and back to the bottom ring.**

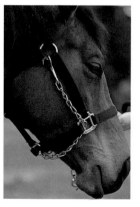

FIGURE 1.13. **To apply a chain under your horse's chin, pass the snap through the ring on the left side of the halter, through the bottom ring on the halter, and snap it to the ring on the right side of the halter.**

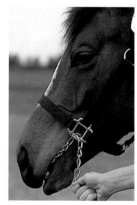

FIGURE 1.14. **To use the chain as a lip chain, run the snap through the ring on the left side of the halter, pass it under your horse's upper lip against his gums, and snap it to the ring on the right side of the halter. This is a severe, but extremely effective, restraint device that should only be used if you are comfortable with the technique. When using a lip chain, it is particularly important that you immediately release pressure once you apply it.**

Chemical Restraint FIGURES 1.15–1.16

If the restraint techniques described above aren't successful, your horse may require chemical restraint in the form of a sedative. Your vet may administer a sedative intravenously (directly in the vein, or IV), or you may obtain these medications from your vet for intramuscular (into the muscle, or IM) or oral administration. The following are the most commonly prescribed sedatives:

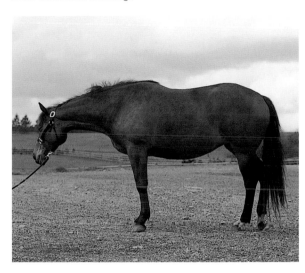

FIGURE 1.15. **This sedated horse is demonstrating typical signs of a dropped head and rested hind leg.**

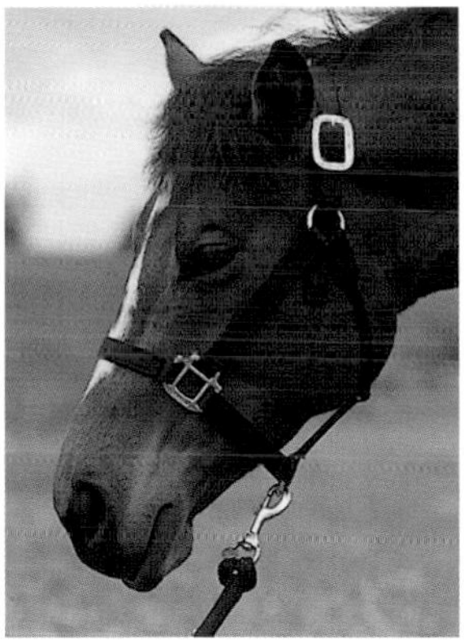

FIGURE 1.16. **A look at her face shows floppy ears, partially closed eyes, and a drooping lower lip.**

Xylazine

DRUG CLASS. Alpha-2 agonist.

EFFECT. Mild sedative with pain-relieving properties. Xylazine lowers your horse's heart rate and may cause a change in heart rhythm, including dropped beats. Through its effect on his central nervous system (brain and spinal cord), it also causes overall muscle relaxation, leading to a loss of coordination.

USED FOR. Xylazine is used as a mild sedative for routine procedures. It may also be administered as a first line of defense against abdominal pain from colic. This drug is often used in combination with other drugs, such as butorphanol (see below).

DOSAGE. 0.2–1.1 mg/kg given either IV or IM.

WARNINGS. Horses may react unpredictably when given xylazine. Most notably, they can kick out suddenly and unexpectedly. In rare cases, xylazine produces a severe aggressive response.

Detomidine

DRUG CLASS. Alpha-2 agonist.

EFFECT. Profound sedative with pain-relieving properties. Detomidine belongs to the same class of medications as xylazine and has very similar effects.

USED FOR. Detomidine is used as a sedative for routine procedures requiring deep sedation, such as dentistry, joint injections, or other veterinary procedures. It may also be used to control pain during a colic episode.

DOSAGE. 0.005–0.02 mg/kg IV or IM.

WARNINGS. Same as xylazine. Horses may be unpredictable, may kick unexpectedly, and can become aggressive. Detomidine also causes a more profound loss of coordination, which can make handling difficult.

Acepromazine

DRUG CLASS. Phenothiazine tranquilizer.

EFFECT. Mild sedative. Acepromazine dilates small blood vessels, leading to a drop in blood pressure. This medication will also cause the penis of a gelding or stallion to relax and drop.

USED FOR. Acepromazine is used as a mild tranquilizer for common procedures including clipping, hauling, and routine veterinary care. In small doses, it can be useful for calming horses for riding, during and after long layups, and for calming competition horses. (*Note: Rules regarding tranquilizer use in competition horses vary widely, depending on the sport and geographic location. Be sure to check rules carefully for your individual situation whenever tranquilizing medications are to be administered before or during competition.*) Because this medication has the effect of dilating small blood vessels, it is also used to improve circulation in certain medical conditions such as laminitis or tying up.

DOSAGE. 0.03–0.10 mg/kg IV, IM, or given orally.

WARNINGS. Acepromazine can result in permanent penile paralysis, and should not be used in breeding stallions. Because of its effect on small blood vessels and the resulting drop in blood pressure, it is often not given to horses that are dehydrated or in shock. Always ask your veterinarian before administering this medication to your sick horse. Individual horses will respond very differently to acepromazine depending on their own metabolism and the environment. For example, if a horse is already excited before acepromazine is administered, it may have very little noticeable effect. Don't assume your horse will act sedated just because you've administered this drug.

Butorphanol

DRUG CLASS. Narcotic.

EFFECT. Sedation and pain relief.

USED FOR: Sedation and pain control. Butorphanol is often used in combination with xylazine or detomidine to sedate for routine procedures. This medication can reduce the incidence of kicking or aggression seen with these other medications. Its potent pain-relieving properties make it a useful drug for controlling colic symptoms.

DOSAGE. 0.02–0.05 mg/kg IV or IM.

WARNINGS. Butorphanol is a controlled substance, meaning its use is carefully monitored by the Federal Drug Administration (FDA). It may cause muscle twitching and a profound loss of coordination.

CHAPTER 2

Preventative Health Care

I N THIS CHAPTER, WE'RE GOING to learn about the basics of a preventative health-care program. To keep the horse healthy and safe, he needs the following:

- A safe place to live
- Food and water
- Protection against infectious diseases
- Protection against internal and external parasites
- Regular foot care
- Regular dental care

Basic Facility Requirements

In his natural environment, the horse lives in a wide open space, with room to roam wherever he pleases, as he grazes continuously throughout the day. He looks for trees or other natural barriers to protect him from adverse weather conditions, and grows a shaggy winter coat to keep him warm. His water comes from streams, ponds, or lakes.

When we domesticate the horse, our goal is to provide an environment and management plan that mimics his natural lifestyle as closely as possible.

Barn Basics

The barn environment should be clean, well ventilated, and free from any hazards that could cause injury. Stalls should be a minimum of 12×12' for the average 1000-pound horse, allowing him room to move and lie down safely. Flooring in stalls should be constructed to allow for drainage. For example, stall mats over a packed gravel base are a good choice. Ventilation is another important concern. A good barn would be constructed with good cross-ventilation and open stalls that allow air to flow freely through the horse's living space.

To take care of intestinal worms, horsemen in times past were advised to gather the roots of small black walnut trees, cut up the roots, and boil them. The mixture would then be poured into the animal. According to the experts of the time, this treatment would cause the worms to leave.

Of course, now we know that black walnut is more likely to kill the horse than the worms. Bedding containing black walnut shavings is a well-known cause of laminitis, and additional toxic effects such as colic, respiratory distress, and even death are possible when portions of the black walnut tree are ingested. Instead, there are many highly effective, safe medications available to keep intestinal parasites at bay.

Turnout

The horse will be healthiest if he can spend as much time outside as possible. Turnout into pasture or, at minimum, a paddock attached to his stall will allow him freedom to move and graze, and will help to minimize his exposure to dust and other irritants that occur in a closed barn environment. FIGURE 2.1

Of course, safety must be an utmost consideration. Shelter from adverse weather should be available, fences must be properly constructed, and any debris that could cause injury should be removed from the environment. FIGURES 2.2–2.3

In addition, if a horse has problems with excessive weight gain, free access to pasture may not be the healthiest alternative. In these situations, a dry lot, where calories can be controlled, may be necessary.

Feeding

Management of Food and Water

In order to mimic the natural environment, it's best if the horse has access to forage as much as possible throughout the day. If grazing isn't possible, that means frequent feedings (3 to 4 times daily) are the ideal. Hay is best fed on the ground. This greatly decreases the impact of dust and other respiratory irritants the horse is exposed to while eating.

Fresh, clean water should be available at all times. During cold winter months, warm water provided daily will increase the horse's water consumption by as much as 40 percent. This can significantly decrease the risk of certain types of colic. Most horsemen (including veterinarians) prefer buckets to provide water in a stall rather than automatic waterers. Buckets can be cleaned daily, and the horse's daily water consumption can be monitored. However, automatic waterers are a convenient alternative. The water source in a pasture should be a large, safe tub that can be easily monitored and cleaned regularly.

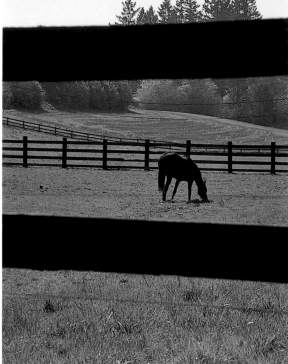

FIGURE 2.1. **Daily turnout into a pasture allows the horse freedom to move and graze. This is ideal for maintaining optimal health.**

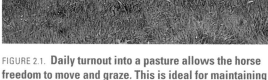

FIGURE 2.3. **A simple plastic cap will protect the horse, and is a good example of a commonsense safety precaution.**

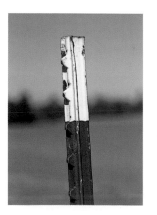

FIGURE 2.2. **Safety should be first and foremost when considering the horse's environment. Although commonly used for horse fencing, T-posts such as this can cause serious injury.**

Basic Horse Care

Nutrition Basics

The horse's basic nutritional requirements can be broken down into five major categories: energy, fiber, protein, vitamins and minerals.

Energy

Energy is the most basic of the horse's requirements, and the simplest to understand. It simply means the number of calories he needs to keep his body working. Too much energy in the horse's ration means "fat," too little means "thin." An inappropriate amount of energy is one of the most common feeding mistakes.

How are the horse's energy needs met? Through pasture, hay, and grain, the basic building blocks of his daily diet. A rule of thumb that you can use for meeting daily energy needs is: 1.5–2 pounds of hay per 100 pounds of body weight. To evaluate the horse's condition, firmly run your hand along his side. You should just barely be able to feel his ribs if you apply 1–2 pounds of pressure. If his ribs are easily visible, he needs more energy! If you can't feel them no matter how hard you push, it may be time to cut back his ration. Commercially available weight tapes can also be used to estimate your horse's weight and monitor gains or losses. FIGURE 2.4

If you're wondering about your hay, just keep this in mind: in general, legume hays like alfalfa have a higher energy content than do grasses. If your horse is a "hard keeper" (difficult to keep weight on) and can't get enough energy from the hay you're feeding, consider feeding more of a high-energy variety. If he's fat and needs something to do, emphasize low-caloric grass. FIGURE 2.5

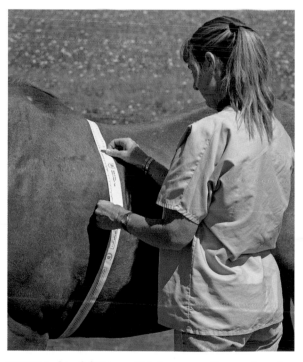

FIGURE 2.4. **A weight tape will help you monitor your horse's weight with a simple measurement performed around his girth.**

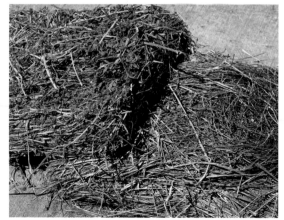

FIGURE 2.5. **In general, a legume hay such as the alfalfa pictured on the left is higher in energy than the grass hay pictured on the right.**

As your horse's energy demands increase in a variety of situations—like pregnancy or hard training—the additional requirements can be met by adding something other than forage to his ration such as a high-fat supplement or concentrate (grain) ration.

Fiber

The horse's fiber requirement is extremely important, and easy to forget. Not only is an adequate amount of fiber critical for proper functioning of the gastrointestinal tract, a high-fiber diet can help control behavior problems that arise in stall-kept horses frustrated by confinement. Remember, the horse's natural lifestyle involves a full-time commitment to walking and grazing. This is a need best met with fiber.

Fiber needs are met with good-quality hay or pasture, which should make up at a minimum 70 percent of the horse's diet. Feeding oats as the concentrate portion of the horse's ration also helps meet fiber needs, as oats are higher in fiber and lower in energy than other grain choices, such as corn or barley. Keep in mind that grain feeding should be kept to a minimum. Most of the recent research done in equine nutrition shows that high-carbohydrate diets are unhealthy.

Protein

Protein is essential in your horse's diet to keep his body functioning properly. While your mature horse's protein requirement of 8–10 percent may be less than you realize, this requirement does increase with pregnancy, growth, or increased exercise. You can always find out the protein content in the hay you buy. Most legumes (like alfalfa) are as high as 18 percent protein, while grass or oat hay is generally closer to 8–10 percent. The concentrate (grain) ration should have the protein content listed on the bag. Cereal grains like oats, barley, and corn typically contain 9–10 percent protein.

Another important consideration when it comes to protein is that it's often *quality* not *quantity* that makes the difference. The amino acid lysine (a building block of protein) is most important for meeting protein needs. A soybean meal–based protein source is the most reliable source of lysine; look for soybean meal on the label of your higher protein concentrate sources to check for quality. (Lysine is also present in high quantities in alfalfa hay.)

Vitamins

The B-complex vitamins are produced by the horse's digestive tract, and vitamin C is produced by his liver, making it unlikely that he'll fall short of either of these important vitamins.

Most of your horse's basic vitamin needs are met through hay and grain. Vitamin A is present in large quantities in fresh green hay or grass, but can become a problem if you're feeding poorly cured or stored hay. If your hay or pasture isn't green your horse might be lacking vitamin A.

In fact, as a general rule, if you're concerned about the quality of feed that makes up your horse's ration, a good, balanced vitamin supplement can't hurt.

Minerals

Calcium, phosphorus, magnesium, sodium, chloride, potassium, iron, copper, zinc, iodine and selenium are the most important minerals in the horse's diet. Most are provided in the horse's hay, and you should *always* have a trace mineral block available. Research shows that horses have an excellent ability to self-regulate their mineral intake according to their needs.

Selenium is the one mineral that can require special consideration in certain areas of the country. Ask your vet whether your hay comes from selenium-deficient soil. If it does you'll need to make sure selenium is included in your horse's diet at a dose of approximately 3.0–5.0 mg/day for a typical 1000-pound horse. Well-balanced, selenium-containing vitamin mixes are usually available in selenium-deficient areas. The vet can also run a simple blood test to determine whether your horse's selenium levels are adequate.

Supplements

BASIC VITAMIN/MINERAL. An all-around basic vitamin and mineral supplement may not be necessary if you're feeding good-quality hay. In general, however, it can't hurt to feed one, and it will help to ensure your horse is getting all of the vitamins and minerals he needs.

BIOTIN. This protein has been scientifically documented to help improve hoof wall strength and stimulate growth. It is warranted for horses with shelly, weak hooves, a history of abscesses, or other hoof problems at a dose of 20 milligrams a day. (Note that other hoof supplements, including methionine, have no scientific documentation of efficacy. They may help, and anecdotal reports support their use, but there is no proof.)

CHONDROITIN SULFATE/GLUCOSAMINE. These large polysaccharide (sugar) molecules are purported to help lubricate and provide nutrients to joints. There is little clinical evidence to support their use, although anecdotal reports indicate that they are likely to be helpful for the athletic horse. Correct dosages aren't really established, and quality control of different products is questionable at best, making decisions about how much of which supplement to use extremely difficult.

METHYLSULFONYLMETHANE (MSM). This sulfur-containing substance is a metabolite of dimethyl sulfoxide (DMSO), and is known to have both anti-inflammatory and antioxidant properties. It can be helpful for managing degenerative joint disease or other inflammatory conditions. Specifically, many owners report improvement in comfort levels of their older horses when MSM is given. The recommended dosage for this supplement is between 10 and 30 grams per day.

SELENIUM. The basic vitamin/mineral supplement should contain adequate selenium for the average horse. Blood selenium levels can be measured, and additional selenium supplementation may be recommended based on these results. However, because of a low margin of safety with this mineral it's critical that you don't supplement too much. Selenium requires adequate vitamin E for proper absorption.

VITAMIN E. This vitamin has antioxidant properties and can help support the immune system. It is often recommended for horses with muscle problems such as a history of tying up. It may also be useful for horses that seem to have weakened immune systems and are more prone to respiratory viruses passing through the barn. A dose as high as 6000 IU of vitamin E per day may be recommended.

Vaccination

Vaccine Technology: How Does It Work?

Vaccination helps protect the horse against infectious diseases by stimulating his own immune system to fight back when he's exposed to a virus or bacteria. When the horse is vaccinated, he's administered a dose of antigen, which usually consists of an inactivated portion of a disease-producing organism. The specific antigen is injected into his muscle and stimulates his immune system to produce antibodies against that organism. These antibodies are the body's disease-fighting defenders. After vaccination, the antibodies then circulate in the horse's bloodstream, attacking and killing invading organisms—so he's less likely to get sick.

The most exciting new technology introduced in recent years has been intranasal vaccines for respiratory diseases. These are administered through a spray up the horse's nose, where they stimulate local immune system functions that are the horse's first line of defense against organisms causing respiratory diseases. Now widely available for both influenza and strangles (a respiratory disease), they've proven to be more effective and have fewer side effects than the older intramuscular vaccines.

FIGURE 2.6

As technology becomes more and more sophisticated, vaccines become more and more effective. The horse's immune system is extremely complex and involves much more than just the production of antibodies for the prevention of disease. In the future, more effective carriers for vaccines (called adjuvents) that have immune-stimulating effects on other branches of the immune system beyond simple antibody production will improve vaccine efficacy. Another advance on the horizon is DNA vaccines, which work by injecting segments of genetic material of the disease-producing organism rather than killed or attenuated organisms. These vaccinations are likely to give better, longer-lasting immunity with fewer side effects compared with conventional vaccines.

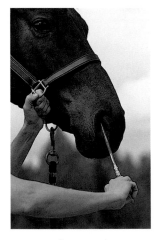

FIGURE 2.6. **Intranasal vaccines administered through a spray up the horse's nose are now available for several different respiratory diseases.**

Do Vaccines Really Work?

Most vaccinations are effective to a certain degree. They will usually either prevent the horse from getting sick or will reduce the severity and duration of his signs if he does get sick. However, vaccination won't completely protect the horse against disease in every situation. The following facts about vaccine testing will explain what we do know about vaccine efficacy, and what the pitfalls are:

Approval requirements: In order to be approved and licensed by the USDA, a vaccination must demonstrate a certain increase in the number of antibodies (called a rise in antibody titer) following administration. Unfortunately we don't always know that an increase in the number of antibodies will effectively fight disease.

Challenge studies: In some cases, challenge studies are also performed. During a challenge study, both vaccinated and unvaccinated horses are exposed to a specific disease, and the difference in the number of horses that get sick and the severity of their signs is recorded. Challenge studies are believed to be a more effective indicator of a vaccine's effectiveness than a simple rise in antibody titer. Challenge studies are difficult and expensive to carry out and are therefore often not performed.

All of this means that even with USDA approval, we don't always know whether a given vaccination will actually provide complete protection against the disease in question—or if it does, just how complete that protection will be. There are a number of reasons why the horse can still get sick, even though he's been vaccinated. These include:

- His ability to fight off the disease is dependent on more than just antibodies in his system. And although those antibodies may help, he can still get sick.

- He may have been exposed to a virus or strain of virus different from what was included in the vaccination administered. This is especially a problem with respiratory diseases, where the viruses in the environment are changing faster than vaccine manufacturers can keep up.

- He may have been exposed to a particularly strong or virulent virus that was able to overwhelm the antibodies circulating in his system and still cause disease.

- He may have been under a lot of stress at the time he was exposed to the virus (for example, at a horse show). Stress can suppress his immune system, allowing him to succumb to disease even if he does have a good level of antibodies in his system.

- He may have been receiving medications that suppress his immune system at the time of vaccination, causing a lowered response to the vaccination. For example, corticosteroids such as dexamethasone administered for an allergy can have a negative impact on the horse's response to vaccination.

- He may simply be a poor responder to vaccination in general. The effectiveness of a specific vaccination will vary with the individual horse's response. If two horses are vaccinated using the same vaccine, one may respond well and be unlikely to get sick if faced with the disease, while the other may not respond at all. Regrettably, there's no good method for determining a horse's individual level of response to a specific vaccine.

Making the Most of Vaccinations

The following steps will help to ensure vaccinations will be as effective as possible:

- Maintain all horses in a group on the same vaccination schedule. This strategy takes advantage of the concept of "herd immunity." This means that if the majority of horses in a group respond effectively to a vaccination, the remainder of the horses will also be protected and an epidemic is less likely. This strategy is particularly helpful for the "nonresponders" in a barn, that is, those horses that don't respond well to vaccination.

- Be sure that vaccines are properly administered. If you choose to vaccinate your horse yourself, ask your veterinarian to teach you how. This will not only ensure that the vaccinations will be as effective as possible but also reduce the chances that the horse will have an adverse reaction.

- Make sure you obtain your vaccines from a reliable source where they've been kept in a clean, refrigerated environment. They'll lose their effectiveness if they become warm, and you'll have an increased risk for problems such as injection-site reactions if they become contaminated.

A Word about Adverse Reactions

Even if everything is done correctly, there's always a chance that an adverse reaction could occur. These include:

- ACUTE ALLERGIC REACTIONS (CALLED ANAPHYLAXIS). In this situation, the horse's immune system responds too strongly to the antigen that's administered. This leads to a cascade of events that can result in collapse or even death. Anaphylactic reactions, although frightening, are extremely rare.

- LOCAL INJECTION-SITE REACTIONS. These range from sore spots in the muscle to the formation of an abscess. Abscesses can occur if bacteria enter the skin during the vaccination process. It's also possible for the horse to develop a "sterile abscess"—one that contains no bacteria—simply because of the way his body responds to the vaccine.

Beat the Bugs

With all of that said, what vaccinations should you administer to your horse? The following is a summary of the diseases and commonly available vaccines.

Tetanus

Protects the horse against the bacteria *Clostridium tetani,* which invades open wounds or punctures and can cause potentially life-threatening paralysis.

DOES HE NEED IT? Every horse should be vaccinated against tetanus because of the seriousness of the disease and prevalence of the organism in the environment.

HOW OFTEN? Annually. It should be re-administered if the horse suffers a wound and has not been vaccinated during the preceeding 6 months.

(Note: When you vaccinate, be sure to administer a tetanus toxoid designed to prime your horse's immune system. A second type of tetanus vaccine, called tetanus antitoxin, also exists and is a direct source of antibodies for use if an injured horse has no history of vaccination.)

Eastern and Western encephalomyelitis (sleeping sickness)

Protects the horse against two viruses—Eastern (EEE) and Western (WEE). A third form of sleeping sickness, Venezuelan (VEE), also exists but is only a concern for horses living on or near the Mexican border of the United States. These viruses are transmitted by bloodsucking insects and can cause life-threatening neurological disease.

DOES HE NEED IT? All horses should be vaccinated against EEE and WEE because of the seriousness of the disease. Horses living within 40 miles of the Mexican border should be vaccinated against VEE.

HOW OFTEN? Annually, or twice annually in areas where mosquitoes are especially prevalent or the disease is common.

Influenza (flu)

This vaccine protects the horse against one of the most common viral causes of respiratory diseases. The influenza virus is spread through particles in the air or carried on solid objects.

DOES HE NEED IT? Although influenza is rarely fatal, it can take the horse out of action for several weeks or more. Young horses (under 3 years) are most susceptible and should definitely be vaccinated. Show horses exposed to many different horses, or horses with other respiratory problems (like heaves), should be vaccinated.

HOW OFTEN? The new intranasal vaccines have demonstrated effectiveness for 6 months and have been tested using challenge studies. They also have a very low incidence of side effects. Intramuscular vaccines have some effectiveness for 3 to 4 months. Horses should be vaccinated quarterly for best results with the intramuscular vaccine.

Equine viral rhinopneumonitis
(rhino, also called equine herpes virus, or EHV)

The rhino virus can have several different forms and cause a variety of problems, including neurological disease, respiratory disease, and abortion in pregnant mares. It's passed through the air from horse to horse. The rhino vaccination will reduce the horse's chance of becoming ill with respiratory disease, although it's not 100 percent effective and has no efficacy at all against the neurological form. Immunity is also short-lived, lasting only 2 to 3 months. A large percentage (as high as 80 percent) of horses are carriers of the virus, meaning they harbor the virus in their system without becoming ill. Vaccination will have minimal benefit for these carriers.

DOES HE NEED IT? Rhino has historically been a component of many horses' routine vaccination schedules. But, because of its limited effectiveness, short duration of immunity, and the fact that carrier horses won't benefit from the vaccine, some veterinarians are now opting to forego routine rhino vaccinations except in pregnant or pre-foaling mares. Although the vaccine is not labeled for protection against the neurological form of the disease, there is some recent evidence that the modified live type of the vaccine may provide a small degree of protection against this form of the disease. That would be the most compelling reason to opt for routine vaccination, specifically using a modified live type vaccine.

HOW OFTEN? To ensure maximum protection, the horse would require vaccination every 2 to 3 months. Vaccination every 6 months with the modified live vaccine may be advised.

West Nile virus

This virus attacks your horse's nervous system. It was first identified in the U.S. in 1999 and spread rapidly across the country. It's carried by birds, and transmitted to horses and humans by mosquitoes. There is no evidence that infected horses can transmit the disease to healthy horses or other animals. Signs in horses include stumbling, lack of coordination, weakness, paralysis, and muscle twitching. Mortality rates in horses are reported to be as high as 30 percent.

DOES HE NEED IT? The vaccination has demonstrated good efficacy and has very few side effects. Vaccination is recommended throughout the U.S.

HOW OFTEN? Although it's labeled for annual administration, most experts recommend biannual vaccinations in areas where the disease has been identified.

Potomac Horse Fever (PHF)

This severe diarrheal disease is caused by a bacterial organism called *Ehrlichia risticii* and is carried by ticks. Fresh-water snails have recently been identified as part of the PHF transmission cycle. The vaccination will reduce the horse's chances of getting sick, and will help keep symptoms to a minimum if he does contract the disease.

DOES HE NEED IT? The horse's requirement depends on his geographic location and his exposure to other horses. If PHF is in the area, he should be vaccinated.

HOW OFTEN? Annually, or twice a year in high-risk geographic areas. The best time to vaccinate is just before summer, when snails will emerge.

Rabies

Rabies is a 100 percent fatal viral disease that's transmitted by a wild animal bite. The vaccine is safe and effective.

DOES HE NEED IT? Geographic location and the horse's lifestyle will determine his need for a rabies vaccination. If he lives on a big pasture where he has the potential to come in contact with wild animals, a rabies vaccination should be a part of your plan.

HOW OFTEN? Annually.

Strangles

This respiratory disease, caused by a bacterial organism called *Streptococcus equi*, is characterized by large abscesses that form in the horse's lymph nodes. It is passed from horse to horse, and flies may play a role in its transmission.

DOES HE NEED IT? The vaccination can result in serious side effects, including an immune system reaction called purpura hemorrhagica, which can be fatal. Many veterinarians only recommend it in the face of high exposure risk. The newer intranasal vaccine may have a reduced chance for side effects, although they're still possible. If the horse will be in a barn where strangles has been diagnosed, vaccination is a good idea, but *not* if there's a chance he's already been exposed. Vaccination risks are significantly increased if the horse already has a large number of antibodies circulating in his system. The vet may recommend measuring antibodies against the strangles organism in your horse's blood before proceeding with the vaccination.

HOW OFTEN? Annually. Best given just before fly season begins, or at least 2 weeks prior to anticipated exposure.

Equine protozoal myeloencephalitis (EPM)

This disease affects your horse's spinal cord, causing a wide range of signs including ataxia (loss of coordination), lameness, difficulty chewing, and seizures. It's carried by possums, and exposure to the organism is very prevalent in some locations. As many as 70 to 80 percent of horses in some areas have antibodies in their blood against the EPM organism, yet never show signs of the disease.

DOES HE NEED IT? There's a lot of controversy surrounding this vaccine. Effectiveness has not been well established, and vaccinating the horse will complicate diagnosis if he should ever actually contract the disease. Antibodies in the blood and fluid that surrounds the spinal cord are used to diagnose EPM, and diagnosis of the disease is already difficult and confusing. The vaccination stimulates these antibodies as well, which makes diagnosis even more complex.

HOW OFTEN? Annually, if you decide to vaccinate at all.

Botulism

This disease, caused by the soil-dwelling organism *Clostridium botulinum*, causes a progressive muscle weakness and eventual paralysis. It is prevalent in Kentucky and in areas along the East Coast.

DOES HE NEED IT? If the horse lives in an area where botulism is known to be a problem, vaccination is recommended. Ask your vet.

HOW OFTEN? Annually in high-risk areas.

Parasites

All horses are exposed to parasites—both internal and external. When the horse grazes on pasture, he ingests larvae or eggs from a variety of different worms that travel throughout his body, wreaking havoc wherever they go. At the same time, he's tormented by various species of insects that bite his skin, cling to his face, or lay eggs on his body. It's a never-ending battle that we must help him fight by establishing an effective parasite control program.

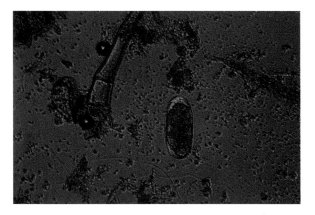

FIGURE 2.7. **Fecal examination can be performed to count parasite eggs such as this egg from a large strongyle. However, this test can be negative even if the horse does have a significant parasite burden, making careful interpretation of results essential.** (Author photo)

Parasite infestation causes a wide variety of health problems for the horse, ranging from something as simple as a skin welt from a fly bite to something as serious as a life-threatening colic. Perhaps most significant are the subclinical effects of parasitism. The horse appears thin, potbellied, has a rough hair-coat, or lacks energy for performance because parasites feeding from his intestinal tract or bloodsucking insects are robbing him of essential nutrients.

Diagnosis of parasitism is more difficult than it might seem. Fecal examination can be performed to count parasite eggs and assess the number of eggs being shed in the feces. Unfortunately, this test is an inaccurate assessment of the horse's overall parasite burden. Eggs won't be detected during certain stages of the parasite's life cycle, such as larval migration or the period when larvae are encysted in the horse's intestinal walls. This means the horse's fecal egg counts can be negative even when his parasite burden is high. Other tests are also available, including blood tests to test for exposure to tapeworms and endoscopic examination of the stomach to observe larvae of the botfly. None of these tests, however, are completely accurate or practical for routine use. Given that parasites are everywhere, the best strategy is to develop an effective parasite control program as a regular part of the horse's preventative health care plan.

In order to learn how to best protect the horse, it helps to understand the basics about the most common types of equine parasites, including nematodes (roundworms), cestodes (tapeworms) and arthropods (flies and gnats). (For details about specific species of internal and external parasites, refer to the charts on pages 34–35.)

Nematodes FIGURES 2.7–2.12

Nematodes comprise the largest group of internal parasites in the horse and include large and small strongyles as well as ascarids, commonly referred to as roundworms. They are highly prevalent in his environment. In general, adult roundworms live in the horse's intestinal tract, where they feed either from ingesta within the intestines or by sucking blood from the intestinal walls. In both cases, they rob the horse of nutrients and may impair his ability to digest and absorb his food. Adult nematodes

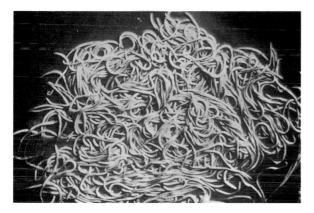

FIGURE 2.8. **A large number of ascarids or "roundworms" such as these can result in an obstruction of the intestinal tract. This is most common in younger horses.** (Photo courtesy of Jan Palmer, DVM, Diplomate ACVS)

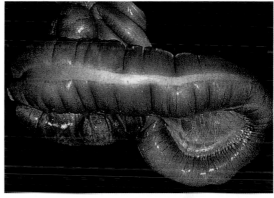

FIGURE 2.10 **Large strongyles are one of the most damaging types of parasites. Damage to the blood vessels supplying the intestine has resulted in the blackened, dead segments of intestine visible here.** (Author photo)

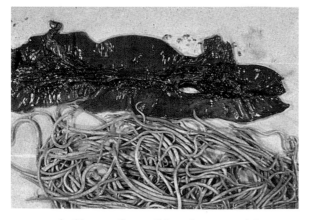

FIGURE 2.9. **In this case the small intestine ruptured due to a heavy load of ascarids.** (Author photo)

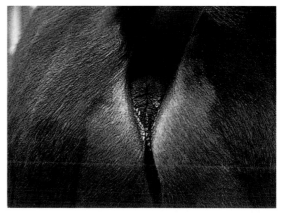

FIGURE 2.11. **Pinworms lay eggs around the horse's anus, and will cause him to attempt to scratch his tail.** (Author photo)

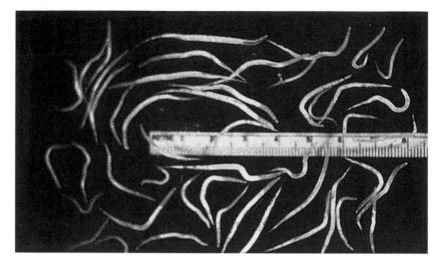

FIGURE 2.12. **These small white worms are pinworms that can live within the intestine, robbing the horse of vital nutrients.** (Author photo)

lay eggs, which are passed in the horse's feces to hatch in the pasture and develop into larvae. The horse ingests different larval stages as he grazes, which then proceed to migrate through his system on their way to his intestinal tract, causing damage to various body organs along the way.

Cestodes   FIGURE 2.13

Cestodes, or tapeworms, have only recently been recognized as a significant cause of parasite problems in horses. Their prevalence varies widely, depending on geographic location. Incidence of tapeworm infestation has been shown to be as high as 96 percent in the Upper Midwest states of the U.S. and as low as 13 percent on the West Coast. Youngsters (under 2 years) and older horses (over 15 years) are most susceptible to tapeworm infestations.

These parasites differ from roundworms in that they involve a mite in their life cycle. The forage, or "oribatid," mite is very prevalent in the horse's environment and lives in the hay or pasture. The mite eats tapeworm eggs from the pasture, which then develop into immature forms of the tapeworm, called cysticercoids, within the body of the mite. The horse ingests the mite from the pasture or hay, tapeworm cysticercoids emerge and then develop into mature worms that take up residence in the horse's intestinal tract. Tapeworm eggs are passed out in the feces when body segments of the worm containing eggs break off of the adult worm. Adult tapeworms live at the junction between the ileum (the end of the small intestine) and the cecum (the blind sac at the beginning of the large intestine) of the horse. Their physical presence can lead to colic, the result of either impactions in this area or spasms of the intestines.

FIGURE 2.13. **Tapeworms are flat, yellowish segmented worms that live in the horse's small intestine and can cause obstruction.** (Author photo)

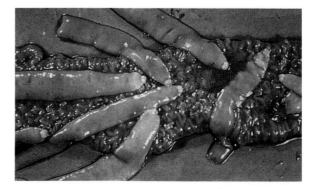

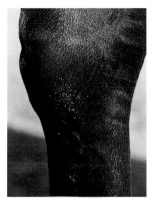

FIGURE 2.14. **These tiny yellow eggs on the horse's legs are laid by botflies.**

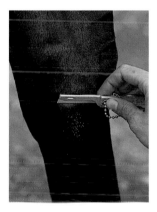

FIGURE 2.15. **The botfly eggs can be removed using a bot knife or block, which prevents the larvae from entering the horse's intestinal tract upon hatching.**

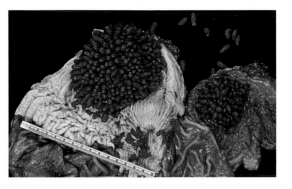

FIGURE 2.16. **Once inside the stomach, bot larvae continue to develop and accumulate. They will cause stomach ulceration that can lead to diarrhea and unthriftiness.**

(Author photo)

Arthropods   FIGURES 2.14–2.16

The arthropod group of parasites includes the botfly, considered an internal parasite of the horse, and a wide variety of flies and gnats that comprise a large number of external parasites.

Botflies are considered an internal parasite because a major portion of their life cycle takes place within the body of the horse, causing significant damage and disruption within the gastrointestinal tract. Adult botflies lay eggs on the horse's legs or face. The horse licks these eggs. The eggs then hatch and migrate through the horse's mouth and esophagus to take up residence in his stomach. There, they attach to the stomach lining and mature, until they are passed out in the feces to mature and hatch.

Other significant arthropod species include the stable fly, horsefly, and culicoides gnats. These are all external parasites that can irritate your horse's skin or eyes, spread infectious diseases, and generally damage his health. Control of these external parasites should include regular application of fly sprays or lotions as well as use of physical barriers such as fly masks or sheets. (For more information on fly related health issues, refer to the chapter on skin diseases.)   FIGURES 2.17–2.19

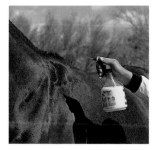

FIGURE 2.17. **Fly control, including regular application of a repellent spray, can help minimize skin irritation and other diseases resulting from insect bites.**

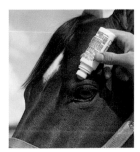

FIGURE 2.18. **Special attention should be paid to the eyes to help minimize conjunctivitis that occurs when flies congregate.**

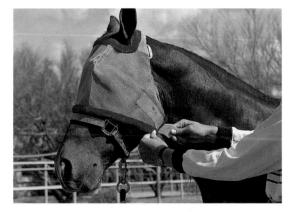

FIGURE 2.19. **A well-fitted fly mask is a good way to protect the horse's face and eyes from flies.**

TABLE 2.1

Common Equine Parasites: Internal Parasites

PARASITE	CLASS	LOOKS LIKE	LIFE CYCLE DETAILS	SPECIFIC DAMAGE DONE	EFFECTIVE DEWORMING MEDICATIONS	COMMENTS
Large strongyles (*Strongylus vulgaris*)	Nematode.	Dark red and round, ½ – 1 inch long. Large mouth with teeth.	Larvae migrate through blood vessels supplying intestines. Adults live in large intestine.	Affect blood supply to intestines, resulting in intestinal death.	Ivermectin. Moxidectin. Benzimidazoles. Pyrantel.	Causes thrombo-embolic colic due to intestinal death.
Small strongyles (*Cyanthostominae*)	Nematode.	Similar to large strongyles, but smaller: ¼ inch long or less.	Larvae encyst in intestinal walls during winter months to carry over infection to following year. Adults live in large intestine.	Larvae emerge from intestinal walls in spring, resulting in diarrhea, dehydration, and colic.	Fenbendazole. (5-day larvicidal treatment). Moxidectin.	Encysted stage not affected by routine deworming. Requires specific larvicidal treat-ment. Can develop resist-ance to deworm-ing medications.
Roundworms (Also referred to as ascarids.) (*Parascaris equorum*)	Nematode.	White and round. Up to 15 inches long.	Eggs hatch in the intestine. Larvae migrate through liver and lungs. Adults live in large intestine.	Damage to liver and lungs from larval migration. Large size of adults can result in obstruction and impaction colic.	Ivermectin. Moxidectin. Benzimidazoles. Pyrantel.	Young horses are particularly susceptible due to undeveloped immunity.
Pinworms (*Oxyuris equi*)	Nematode.	White and round with a pointed tail. Females up to 4 inches long, males as small as 1/8 inch.	Spend entire life cycle in intestinal lumen, with no larval migration. Adults lay eggs on rectum.	Minimal damage. Ingest material from the intestines.	Ivermectin. Moxidectin. Benzimidazoles. Pyrantel.	Pinworms are often blamed for tail rubbing as they lay their eggs on the horse's rectum. Rarely are they the actual cause of tail rubbing, however.
Threadworms (*Strongyloides westeri*)	Nematode.	Tiny (less than ¼ inch long), thin white worms.	Larvae can gain access either through ingestion or skin penetration. Most commonly transmitted to foals through mare's mammary secretions.	Irritation to the foal's gastro-intestinal tract results in diarrhea.	Ivermectin. Moxidectin. Benzimidazoles. Pyrantel.	Common underlying cause of foal diarrhea.

PARASITE	CLASS	LOOKS LIKE	LIFE CYCLE DETAILS	SPECIFIC DAMAGE DONE	EFFECTIVE DEWORMING MEDICATIONS	COMMENTS
Lungworms (*Dictyocaulus arnfieldi*)	Nematode.	White worms approximately 2–5 inches long.	Adults live in large airways of the lungs. Ingested larvae enter the bloodstream from the intestines to travel to the lungs for maturation.	Lung damage, resulting in respiratory symptoms such as a cough.	Ivermectin. Moxidectin.	Larvae mature only in donkeys. Horses must share pasture with donkeys to become infected.
Habronema muscae	Nematode.	Adult worms up to 1 inch long.	Adults live in stomach. Eggs passed in feces are ingested by flies, and develop into larval stages which are deposited on skin by the fly.	Minimal or no damage from adults in stomach. Larvae deposited on wounds or around the face cause skin lesions called "summer sores."	Ivermectin. Moxidectin.	None.
Onchocerca spp	Nematode.	Very long (up to 10 inches). Adults live under the horse's skin.	Larvae injected into the horse's skin when flies carrying the parasite feed.	Larvae in skin cause dermatitis.	Ivermectin. Moxidectin.	None.
Bots (*Gasterophilus* spp)	Arthropod.	Adult flies approximately ½ to 1 inch long. Larvae in stomach approximately ½ inch, cylindrical, and red. Tiny yellow eggs visible on hair of legs or face.	Horse licks eggs on skin, stimulating larvae to hatch and enter stomach via the mouth. Larvae attach to stomach lining, mature, and are passed out in feces where they develop into mature botflies.	Damage and ulceration of mouth due to larval migration. Larvae attached to stomach cause damage resulting in gastric ulceration and subsequent gastritis diarrhea and unthriftiness.	Ivermectin. Moxidectin. Control flies in environment with sprays and barriers. Remove eggs from horse's legs and face before larvae can be ingested.	Different species distinguished by location where they lay eggs on the horse's body.
Tapeworms (*Anaplocephala* spp)	Cestode.	Flat, white segmented worms up to 3 inches long and ½ inch wide.	Mites carrying the parasite are ingested. Parasite is released into the intestines and develops into a mature worm.	Physical presence of worm can cause obstructions or spasms of the intestines.	Praziquantel. Pyrantel pamoate (high dose). Pyrantel tartrate.	None.

Parasite Control

There are two basic strategies used for parasite control in horses: daily deworming and interval deworming. Both strategies must also incorporate a number of special considerations that should be part of every effective internal parasite control program.

Daily deworming

The horse is administered a daily dose of the deworming agent pyrantel tartrate in his feed. This kills parasite larvae within the intestines on a daily basis prior to migration, thus preventing any damage from occurring. It's effective against all of the major horse parasites except for bots. Although it has some efficacy against tapeworms it's not complete, and these parasites should still be considered separately. When daily deworming was first introduced it was thought that resistance would develop to this medication due to constant exposure of the parasites to low levels of the drug. This problem has been reported in certain geographical locations. Consult with your veterinarian if you are considering a daily dewormer for your horse.

Interval deworming

The horse is administered a dose of liquid or paste dewormer every 6 to 8 weeks. Depending on the product used, only parasites at certain stages of the life cycle will be killed, therefore damage from migrating larvae can occur between dewormings. If you choose to use an avermectin-based anthelmintic (ivermectin or moxidectin), migrating larvae will be killed with each administration, minimizing damage.

Three sub-strategies are suggested for horses on interval deworming programs, taking into account concerns about parasite resistance. These include fast rotation (using a different class of medication at each deworming), slow rotation (changing medication class on a yearly basis), and no rotation (using an ivermectin or moxidectin deworming medication at each scheduled deworming). In fact, the only class of parasites that have shown significant resistance to known anthelmintics are the cyathostomes, which have developed resistance to some classes of benzimidazoles and pyrantel. To date, there has been no significant reported resistance to ivermectin or moxidectin in horse parasites when properly administered. These facts mean a no-rotation strategy for interval deworming may actually be the most effective option, especially given the better efficacy of avermectins against most classes of parasites. It is important to keep in mind, however, that development of resistance to these dewormers is still possible in the future.

Special considerations

BOTS. The horse should be dewormed twice a year, after the first winter freeze and after the first spring thaw, with a product that's effective against bots. Dewormers effective against these parasites include avermectins. With an interval deworming program, this can simply be done as part of the regular schedule. With daily deworming, ivermectin or moxidectin should be administered twice a year.

TAPEWORMS. Tapeworms can be controlled with a dose of praziquantel or a double dose of pyrantel pamoate (Strongid® paste) every year or every other year, depending on the prevalence of these parasites in your area. Although not as common as some other equine parasites, tapeworms are now believed to be a parasite worth taking into account, especially because they're not controlled with most standard deworming medications.

ENCYSTED SMALL STRONGYLES. To control the encysted larval stage of these parasites a larvicidal treatment consisting of a double dose of fenbendazole dewormer daily for a period of 5 days should be administered annually, ideally during winter months when larvae are most likely to be encysted in the intestinal wall. This treatment can replace one of a regular-interval dewormings, or be given as an add-on to a daily deworming program.

Foot Care

No foot, no horse. It's no secret that care of the horse's feet is one of the most critical components of a complete health-care plan. Foot care involves two primary elements:

- Daily cleaning. The horse's feet should be picked clean daily to remove packed dirt or mud from the sole and crevices around the frog. Regular twice-weekly treatment with a "thrush" medication applied to the soles and area surrounding the frog will help prevent this common infection from developing. Many commercial medications are available (such as Koppertox® or Thrush Buster®). A mixture of 50 percent bleach and water is also effective. This preventative step is especially important if the horse is living in a wet environment.

- Regular farriery. The farrier should trim or reshoe the horse every 4 to 10 weeks, depending on the individual horse's foot structure and exercise requirements and the time of year. It is extremely important that the horse's visits from the farrier are frequent enough to maintain proper balance of the horse's feet, and strength and integrity of the hoof wall.

Dental Care

In order to support his grazing lifestyle, the horse's teeth erupt continuously throughout his lifetime. This, and the fact that grinding of forage causes heavy wear and tear, means his teeth require regular care. The veterinarian helps maintain the horse's ability to chew effectively with routine procedures that involve grinding, filing, and cutting the teeth to ensure they stay balanced. Basic dental maintenance should include an examination by the veterinarian twice each year and dental balancing at least annually. (For more detailed information about routine dental maintenance see chapter 14.)

TABLE 2.2

Preventative Health-Care Calendar

This calendar is a sample of a preventative health-care plan.

MONTH	VACCINATIONS	DEWORMING*	DENTISTRY	FARRIER
January				
February		Fenbendazole larvicidal Rx.		Trim/shoe.
March	Tetanus, EWEE, IN flu, WNV.		Dental check. Balance if needed.	
April		Ivermectin.		Trim/shoe.
May				
June	PHF, rabies.	Moxidectin with praziquantel.		Trim/shoe.
July				
August		Ivermectin.		Trim/shoe.
September	IN flu, WNV.		Dental check. Balance if needed.	
October		Moxidectin.		Trim/shoe.
November				
December		Ivermectin.		Trim/shoe.

* If a daily deworming option is chosen, a weight-appropriate dose of dewormer will be administered daily. February larvicidal deworming and May/November ivermectin dosing should still be scheduled.

CHAPTER 3

Horse First Aid

I F YOU OWN OR WORK AROUND HORSES, emergencies are sure to happen. If you're prepared, however, you can turn a potential disaster into a minor inconvenience. In this chapter, we're going to discuss basic emergency preparedness so you'll know what to do and how to do it if an emergency should strike at your barn. First, you'll learn how to assess your horse's condition by taking his vital signs. Then, we'll discuss basic first-aid techniques such as bandaging and administering medications. Finally, we'll review what can happen and what steps you should take when faced with the most common equine emergencies you're likely to encounter, including colic, cuts, and sudden lameness.

Taking Vital Signs

Whenever your horse is sick or injured, your first priority should be to assess his overall health status by taking his vital signs. The following is a guide to gathering this important information.

Heart Rate   FIGURE 3.1

WHAT IT IS. Your horse's heart rate is a measure of how fast his heart is beating, measured in beats per minute (bpm).

HOW TO MEASURE. To take your horse's heart rate, place the stethoscope against his chest up under his left elbow. Count the number of beats in 15 seconds, then multiply by 4 to determine heartbeats per minute.

(Note: If you hear absolutely nothing, first check your stethoscope by tapping lightly on the flat surface that you hold against your horse's side. When you do so, the tapping sound should be amplified in your ears. If you can't hear the taps, try rotating the head of the stethoscope. This device is often designed to amplify from either side of the head, depending on the way it's turned.)

NORMAL RANGE. 28 to 36 beats per minute.

WHAT IT MEANS. A rapid heart rate may indicate pain, stress, exertion, or a fever. A slower than normal heart rate may indicate shock. Your horse's heart rate will rise rapidly if he's nervous or just been exercised, so be sure to measure it when he's calm and relaxed.

Respiratory Rate

WHAT IT IS. Your horse's respiratory rate is a measure of how fast he is breathing, measured in breaths per minute (bpm).

HOW TO MEASURE. Observe the rise and fall of your horse's chest or the flaring of his nostrils as he breathes. Count the number of breaths he takes in a 30-second period, and multiply by 2 to determine the breaths per minute.

NORMAL RANGE. 12 to 18 breaths per minute.

WHAT IT MEANS. A faster than normal respiratory rate may mean your horse has a fever, is in pain, or is having difficulty breathing because of an abnormality in his lungs or airways. His respiratory rate will also increase if he's nervous or has just been exercised, so make sure he's in a rested state when you take this measurement. A lower than normal respiratory rate isn't usually cause for concern.

Rectal Temperature   FIGURES 3.2–3.3

WHAT IT IS. A measure of your horse's body temperature. Be aware that his rectal temperature is lower than his "core temperature," the temperature at the center of his body. However, it's still meaningful as an indicator of how warm or cold his body is.

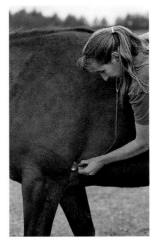

FIGURE 3.1. **The horse's heart can be most easily heard with the stethoscope placed against his chest, under his left elbow.**

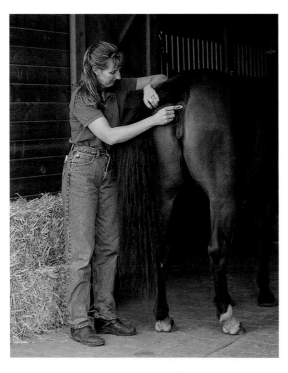

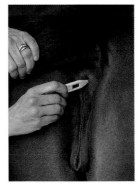

FIGURE 3.2. **Stand to the side of your horse where you'll be out of kicking range in order to insert the thermometer into his rectum.**

FIGURE 3.3. **Wait until the indicator beep tells you that the digital thermometer is ready, then read the result.**

Basic Horse Care

HOW TO MEASURE. Lubricate the tip of a glass or digital thermometer with a water-soluble lubricant (such as KY®) or petroleum jelly (such as Vaseline®). Stand to the side of his hindquarters, and insert the thermometer into his rectum. Wait 2 minutes for a glass thermometer, or until the indicator beep tells you your digital thermometer is ready. Read the result.

NORMAL RANGE. 99.5 to 101.5 degrees F (approximately 37.5 to 38.5 degrees C).

WHAT IT MEANS. A lower than normal temperature may indicate that your horse is in shock, or simply cold, due to exposure to cold weather. A higher than normal temperature may indicate pain or infection. Your horse's rectal temperature will increase significantly with exercise, so make sure to take this measurement when he's resting.

Mucous Membrane Color   FIGURE 3.4

WHAT IT IS. The color of your horse's gums.

HOW TO MEASURE. Raise your horse's muzzle, or upper lip, in order to observe the gum tissue just above his teeth.

NORMAL RANGE. Your horse's mucous membranes should be pale pink.

WHAT IT MEANS. Mucous membrane color is a quick check of your horse's circulatory status—whether blood is being effectively pumped through his body. White or very pale mucous membranes may indicate shock (his heart isn't pumping effectively) or anemia (he has a low red blood cell count). Very dark or purple mucous membranes may indicate even more severe shock or toxemia (his heart isn't pumping effectively, and blood is pooling in these distant capillaries or small blood vessels).

Capillary Refill Time

WHAT IT IS. The amount of time it takes for blood to return to small blood vessels after it has been squeezed out. Like mucous membrane color, this measurement is an evaluation of your horse's circulatory status.

HOW TO MEASURE. Use your finger to press firmly against your horse's gums. Take your finger away, and observe the blanched or pale area you create. Count the number of seconds it takes for the area to refill with blood and return to its normal pink color.

NORMAL RANGE. Blood should return to the area within 1 to 3 seconds.

WHAT IT MEANS. A very slow capillary refill time indicates that your horse may be in shock (his circulation isn't functioning as it should). If the capillary refill time seems very fast, it's most likely normal.

Gut Sounds   FIGURE 3.5

WHAT IT IS. Gurgles and bubbles in your horse's intestines, indicating that the food he's eaten is moving through. These sounds are an important indicator of the well-being of his digestive tract.

HOW TO MEASURE. Take your stethoscope and hold the head (the round end) flat against your horse's flank—the depressed area between his ribs and

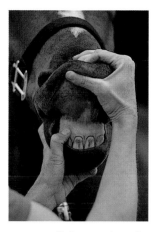

FIGURE 3.4. **Raise your horse's muzzle with one hand to observe the color of his mucous membranes (the gum tissue just above his teeth). Then, to measure capillary refill time, apply pressure with your thumb and time how long it takes for the normal pink color to return to the blanched area you create.**

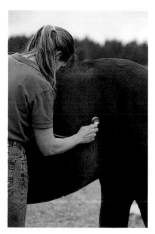

FIGURE 3.5. **Listen at two locations (high and low) on the flank on each side of your horse to assess his gut sounds.**

his hindquarters. Listen for at least one minute at each of four different locations on his flank, one high and one low on each side.

NORMAL RANGE. On average, you should hear 2 to 4 low sounds (bubbles and gurgles) every minute, and a loud sound (a rumble) every 2 to 3 minutes. These guidelines will vary from horse to horse and may depend on the time of day. They'll be louder, for example, just before feeding time. If you practice listening to a number of horses in your barn you will learn to recognize the range of normal gut sounds and be better prepared to interpret what you hear.

WHAT IT MEANS. If gut sounds are louder and more frequent than normal, your horse may be experiencing a mild colic due to intestinal spasms or gas accumulation. If there are no gut sounds it means there's no gut movement. He may be in shock or experiencing a severe colic episode with a shutdown of his digestive tract.

Digital Pulse   FIGURE 3.6

WHAT IT IS. The pulse in the arteries that supply blood to his feet.

HOW TO MEASURE. Squat next to your horse's front foot. Place three fingers of your hand on the inside of his fetlock joint, and rest your thumb on the outside of the joint to stabilize your hand. Apply gentle pressure with your fingers, and slide them around the side of the joint toward the back, until you feel a small cord-like structure slip beneath your fingers. This structure is the medial (inside) digital artery. Once you've located the artery, place your fingers over it and apply gentle pressure. Within several seconds, you should feel a very soft pulse. If you don't, adjust the amount of pressure you're applying and try again. If you apply too much pressure you'll cut off the blood flow. If you apply too little you won't create enough resistance to feel the pulse. A normal digital pulse is very soft, so be patient. You may have to adjust your finger position slightly and change the pressure several times before you feel it.

NORMAL RANGE. It's strength rather than pulse rate that you're evaluating. The rate of the digital pulse will correspond to your horse's heart rate. If the pulse feels strong or "throbby," it indicates there's inflammation or a disruption in blood flow to your horse's foot. He may have a foot bruise, sole abscess, laminitis, or another foot-related abnormality. If the pulse is very weak or you can barely find it, it's most likely normal.

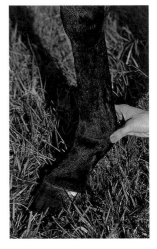

FIGURE 3.6: **Locate the arteries on either side of your horse's fetlock to feel the strength of his digital pulse.**

Basic First-Aid Techniques

In order to care for your horse when a health disaster strikes, you'll need to know basic first aid, including cleaning and managing wounds, applying bandages, and administering medications. The following information will help you.

Basic Horse Care

Wound Cleaning/Flushing

Wounds should be cleaned not only to reduce chances of contamination and infection, but also to allow complete examination of the injured area. For basic wound cleaning, you'll need an antiseptic scrub (such as betadine or chlorhexadine), an antiseptic solution, a sharp pair of clippers or a safety razor, and a syringe. Take the following steps:

- Gently clean the wound using an antiseptic scrub. Use the clippers or safety razor to remove hair surrounding the wound site.

- Dilute a betadine or chlorhexadine solution with water into a weak tea-colored solution (approximately 1 part antiseptic to 10 parts water).

- Fill the syringe with the diluted antiseptic solution, and gently flush the wound area to remove dirt, foreign objects, or other debris.

- If the wound is very dirty, or located on a lower leg where it's associated with swelling, cleanse the wound by cold-hosing the area for 15 to 20 minutes. This will not only help to clean and remove debris but will also minimize inflammation and swelling in the area.

Bandaging   FIGURES 3.7–3.24

If your horse has a laceration, swollen leg, or tendon injury of a lower leg, you may need to apply a bandage. A bandage will protect a wound to help keep it clean, prevent excessive swelling, and help support structures of the lower leg. A number of different types of bandages might be required, including the following:

- BASIC BANDAGE: A basic bandage covers the area between the coronary band and just below the knee (front) or hock (hind). It would be needed for wounds or swelling in this area, or simply to provide support for structures of the lower legs.   FIGURES 3.8–3.11

FIGURE 3.7. **To apply a basic bandage, you'll need a pair of bandage scissors, a roll of sheet cotton (2 to 3 layers), one or two rolls of 6-inch brown gauze, a roll of 3M™ Vetrap™, and a roll of self-adhesive tape (such as Elastikon®).**

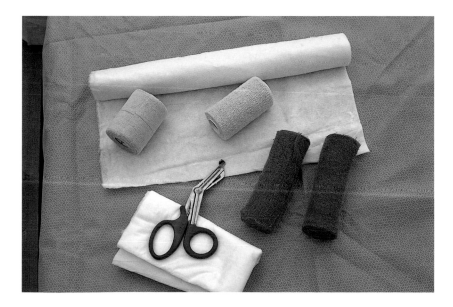

- SWEAT BANDAGE: A sweat bandage creates heat to help draw out fluid and reduce swelling. Examples of when it might be needed include if the horse develops an infection under the skin from a small wound (cellulites) or if a skin condition causes excessive swelling due to inflammation. FIGURES 3.12–3.14

- FULL OR "STACK" BANDAGE: A full or "stack" bandage covers the leg from the coronary band to above the knee (front) or hock (hind). It would be used for wounds or swelling above the knees and hocks that require protection. FIGURES 3.15–3.18

- FOOT BANDAGE: A foot bandage covers the entire hoof, and has extra layers underneath the foot to help keep it intact. It would be used for wounds of the coronary band, hoof, or lower pastern area.
  FIGURES 3.19–3.24

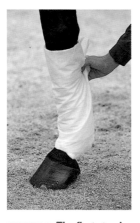

FIGURE 3.8. **The first step in applying a basic bandage is to wrap a roll of 2 to 3 sheet cottons around the horse's leg, extending from the coronary band to just under the knee. The wraps should be smooth and snug to ensure there are no wrinkles underneath your final bandage.**

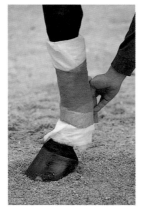

FIGURE 3.9. **Beginning at the middle of the cannon bone, wrap with brown gauze in a spiral fashion, first down toward the coronary band and then back up toward the top. Your wrap should be smooth and snug. As a rule, you should be able to slide two fingers underneath the sheet cottons when you're finished. Always leave approximately ½ to 1 inch of sheet cotton exposed at the top and bottom of the wrap. By doing so, you'll protect your horse against injuries to soft tissues that can occur if gauze or Vetrap™ is applied directly to the skin.**

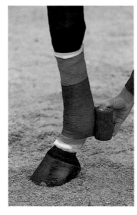

FIGURE 3.10. **Next, follow the same sequence with the Vetrap™ as for the brown gauze. For a basic pressure bandage, you can wrap tight enough to take approximately 50 percent of the stretch out of the wrap material. Again, proper snugness of the bandage should allow you to slide two fingers underneath the sheet cotton when you are finished.**

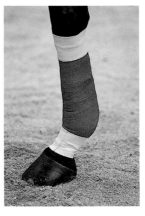

FIGURE 3.11. **Seal the top and bottom of your bandage with several loops of self-adhesive elastic bandage. This helps prevent debris from getting under the wrap and contaminating a wound, and helps hold the wrap in place.**

Basic Horse Care

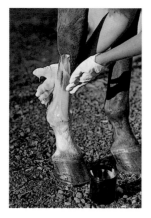

FIGURE 3.12. **To apply a nitrofurazone sweat wrap, begin by applying a thick layer of nitrofurazone ointment to the skin.**

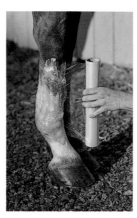

FIGURE 3.13. **Cover the ointment with a loosely applied sheet of plastic wrap.**

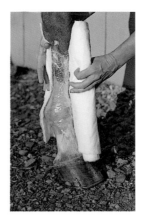

FIGURE 3.14. **To complete the sweat wrap, apply a basic bandage over the top of the plastic.**

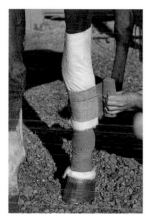

FIGURE 3.15. **To bandage the upper leg (above the knee in front, or above the hock in back), it's best to apply an upper bandage that overlaps a bandage on the lower leg. This prevents slippage. Use the same materials in the sequence described for the basic bandage.**

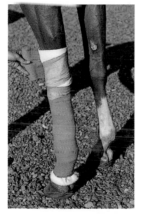

FIGURE 3.16. **After you've placed the sheet cottons, spiral around the leg with brown gauze, using a figure-8 pattern over the joint. Avoid covering the bone that protrudes from the back of the knee (the accessory carpal bone). This will help to avoid pressure sores in that sensitive area.**

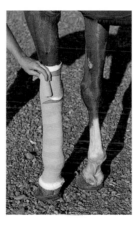

FIGURE 3.17. **Follow the same pattern with the Vetrap™, using a figure-8 over the knee to minimize pressure over the protruding accessory carpal bone.**

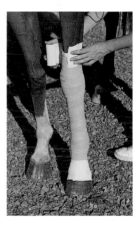

FIGURE 3.18. **Complete your bandage with several loops of self-adhesive elastic bandage, just like you did for the basic bandage.**

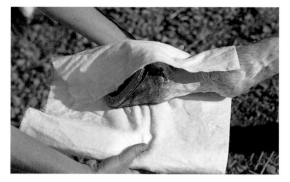

FIGURE 3.19. **To apply a bandage over a wound on the foot or coronary band area, hold the foot off the ground, and wrap 2 to 3 layers of sheet cottons around the hoof and lower leg. Begin just below the fetlock joint and extend 5 to 6 inches beyond the bottom of the foot.**

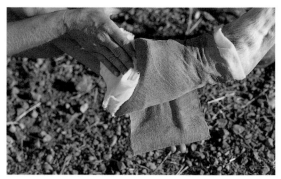

FIGURE 3.20. **Beginning at the pastern, spiral around the leg and foot with 6-inch brown gauze. As you are wrapping, fold the excess sheet cottons over the bottom of the foot and include them under the brown gauze layers.**

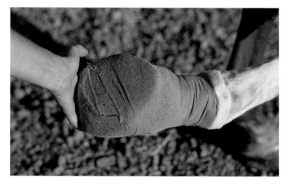

FIGURE 3.21. **When you are through, the entire foot should be encased in brown gauze, and there will be several extra layers padding the sole to help prevent the horse from walking through the bandage.**

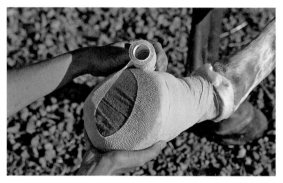

FIGURE 3.22. **Use a spiral pattern to completely cover the pastern and foot with Vetrap™.**

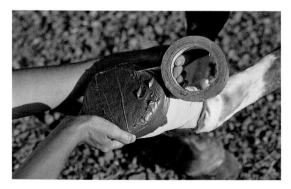

FIGURE 3.23. **Cover the bottom of the foot with duct tape to provide an extra layer that will help keep the bandage moisture proof.**

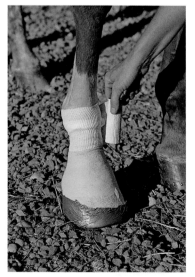

FIGURE 3.24. **Finally, seal the top of the bandage with several layers of self-adhesive tape.**

Administer Oral Medications   FIGURE 3.25

Your veterinarian may recommend an oral medication for your horse such as antibiotics to treat an infection, or an anti-inflammatory to help manage an injury. Although your horse may eat some medications mixed in grain or a bran mash, direct administration using an oral dosing syringe is the most reliable method to use. To administer oral medications, you'll need an oral dosing (catheter-tipped) syringe.

Administer Intramuscular Injection   FIGURES 3.26–3.28

Your veterinarian may recommend an injectable medication if your horse is ill. Additionally, you might opt to self-administer vaccinations or other preventative health care, such as joint treatments. Before you can do so, you must know both where and how to give your horse an intramuscular injection. To administer an intramuscular injection, you'll need a syringe containing medication and an appropriately sized needle. (*Note: The size of the needle will vary with the medication being administered, and should be obtained from your veterinarian.*)

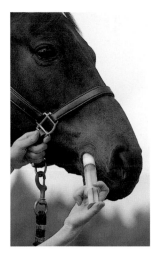

FIGURE 3.25. **To give your horse an oral medication, you'll first need to mix crushed- up tablets or powder with water, honey, or molasses to create a paste if it's not already in paste form. Stand next to the horse's shoulder, with your hand on his halter or over his nose to control his head movement. With your other hand, place the tip of the dosing syringe full of medication in the corner of his mouth. Rapidly depress the plunger to administer the medication into his mouth. It's best if the horse's mouth is empty prior to administering oral medications so he won't be able to spit out the medicine with a chunk of chewed grass or hay. Plan to medicate before feeding, or at least 30 minutes after he's come in from the pasture.**

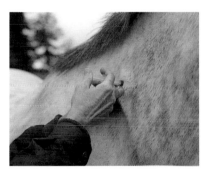

FIGURE 3.26. **To administer an intramuscular injection, firmly and smoothly insert the needle into the muscle at a 90-degree angle to the skin. Secure the needle hub with your free hand, and attach the syringe. Then draw back on the plunger to ensure you haven't entered a vein or artery. If you see blood, remove the needle and begin again using a fresh needle. If you don't see blood, depress the plunger to administer the injection. Then remove the needle and attached syringe.**

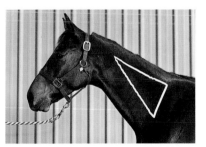

FIGURE 3.27. **The neck is the most common location for intramuscular injection. To identify the proper injection site, draw an imaginary triangle on your horse's neck with a line extending along your horse's spinal column, a line extending below the nuchal ligament, and a line extending along his shoulder. The proper neck injection site is in the flat muscle at the center of this triangle.**

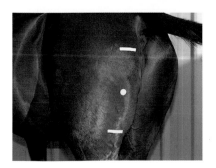

FIGURE 3.28. **The hamstring muscles on the horse's hindquarters are an excellent location for administering an intramuscular injection. To identify the proper location, identify the bony lump at the top, just below the level of his rectum, and the stringy ligaments at the bottom, just opposite the level of his stifle joint. The proper hamstring injection site is between these two landmarks, directly in the middle of this large muscle group.**

Ice or Cold-Hose FIGURE 3.29

If your horse experiences any kind of injury, application of cold (ice or cold-hosing) will help minimize inflammation and reduce swelling. In general, cold therapy will be recommended in several daily sessions of 15 to 20 minutes each during the first 48 hours following any injury.

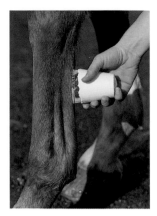

FIGURE 3.29. **A Styrofoam cup filled with water in the freezer makes a handy icing device for an injury. Simply peel the Styrofoam away to expose the ice, and apply it directly to the injured area.**

Common Equine Emergencies

Nightmare or nuisance? That's the question you'll be asking if your horse becomes sick or injured. Is it just a little scratch? Or something more serious? The following guide to the most common equine emergencies will help you determine when to call the vet and what home treatment options you can safely apply.

Colic FIGURE 3.30

The horse experiences abdominal discomfort and shows signs that include pawing, rolling, sweating, or looking back at his sides. Many acute colic situations are simply due to accumulation of gas within the intestinal tract and will resolve within 15 or 20 minutes. However, if a colic becomes more serious, veterinary care is necessary. (See the chapter on the gastrointestinal system for a full review of colic.)

When to call the vet

- The horse exhibits any signs of GI pain for longer than 30 minutes.
- Signs of pain are violent or severe enough that the horse can't be controlled.
- The horse has not passed feces within 12 hours prior to the colic episode.
- The horse refuses feed for an hour or longer.

Home treatment advice

- Walk the horse to encourage gut movement and to prevent him from injuring himself if he goes down to roll. If the horse goes down and will lie quietly, allow him to do so.
- Withold all feed until instructed otherwise by the vet.
- DO NOT administer any medications without direct instructions from your veterinarian.

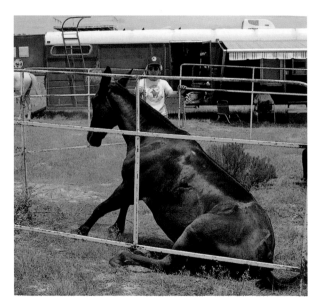

FIGURE 3.30. **This horse is exhibiting typical signs of colic as he sweats and rolls with discomfort. Signs such as these should prompt an emergency call to the veterinarian.** (Photo courtesy of Jan Palmer, DVM, Diplomate ACVS)

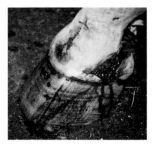

FIGURE 3.31. **The gaping edges on this heel bulb laceration make it an emergency that should be seen by the vet immediately. It will need sutures and immobilization to heal properly.** (Photo courtesy of Jan Palmer, DVM Diplomate ACVS)

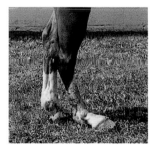

FIGURE 3.32. **This cut is complicated by the fact that vital supporting structures have been damaged. It will require immediate, aggressive repair.** (Photo courtesy of Jan Palmer, DVM Diplomate ACVS)

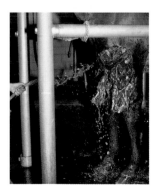

FIGURE 3.33. **Cold-hosing wound before the vet arrives will minimize inflammation and swelling, and flush away contamination and debris.** (Author photo)

Wounds

The horse experiences an abrasion (an injury that doesn't completely penetrate the full thickness of the skin), a laceration (an injury that penetrates the full thickness of the skin and may involve deeper tissues), or a puncture wound (a deep wound with a small skin opening).

When to call the vet   FIGURES 3.31–3.32

- The wound has gaping skin edges that can be easily separated, indicating that sutures are needed.
- The wound is directly over a joint, where healing will be complicated by movement.
- The horse is very lame.
- Thick, yellowish fluid (synovial fluid) is present, indicating that a joint, bursae, or other critical structure may have been penetrated.
- The wound is associated with bleeding that does not stop on its own or is difficult to control.
- The wound appears to be very deep, is swollen, or is associated with a large amount of drainage, indicating either a puncture or infection could be involved.

Home treatment advice

- Apply direct pressure or a pressure bandage if necessary, to control bleeding.
- Cold-hose or ice the injury.   FIGURE 3.33
- Clean the wound with a dilute antiseptic solution (1 part antiseptic to 10 parts water).
- Apply a bandage if possible, to contain swelling and protect tissues.
- Administer a nonsteroidal anti-inflammatory medication such as phenylbutazone to control swelling and inflammation.

Lameness

The horse becomes suddenly lame and is reluctant or refuses to bear weight on one leg. An acute lameness may be associated with other signs of trauma such as a wound or noticeable swelling.

When to call the vet

- The horse has a wound associated with the lameness.
- The horse is unable to bear weight and shows other signs of distress such as refusing to eat, a heart rate higher than 60 beats per minute, or rapid, shallow respiration, indicating extreme pain.
- There is any sign of instability of a bone or joint, indicating possible fracture.

- A nail is detected in the horse's foot. In this case, it's best to leave the nail in position until the veterinarian arrives. A radiograph with the nail still in the foot will help determine whether critical structures have been penetrated and will help guide treatment.

Home treatment advice

- Check for a strong digital pulse in the lame leg. If a strong pulse is present, soak the foot in warm water with Epsom salts to draw out a possible sole abscess. DO NOT administer an anti-inflammatory such as phenylbutazone if an abscess is suspected. In this situation, reducing inflammation may drive the abscess "underground," making it less likely to open and drain.
- Ice or cold-hose swelling associated with the lameness.
- Apply a support bandage if swelling is present below the knees or hocks.

Eye Injuries

The horse's eye is swollen, red, or weepy. To further evaluate, use a penlight to examine the horse's cornea (the clear outer layer of the eye) and check for a possible foreign body.

When to call the vet

It's best to call the vet whenever your horse experiences an eye injury. The vet can help you to determine whether an emergency visit would be advisable. The following signs indicate a serious eye problem that requires immediate veterinary care.

- A whitish/bluish tinge to the cornea, indicating edema or fluid accumulation that might accompany a corneal scratch or ulcer.
- Squinting or swelling so severe that the cornea cannot be evaluated.
- A visible foreign body that requires removal.
- A laceration to an eyelid that should be sutured back in place to preserve the normal architecture of the eye.

Home treatment advice

- Rinse the eye with saline solution to clean away discharge, dust, or other irrititants and relieve discomfort.
- Ice or cold compresses to control swelling.
- DO NOT administer any ophthalmic ointment containing cortisone (includes dexamethasone and hydrocortisone). If your horse has scratched or ulcerated his cornea, cortisone will delay healing and increase risk of infection. An ophthalmic ointment containing only antibiotic is generally safe to administer for any eye injury.
- Administer a nonsteroidal anti-inflammatory such as phenylbutazone or flunixin meglumine to relieve pain.

Your First-Aid Kit

FIGURE 3.34

Every barn and horse trailer should have a first-aid kit available for handling emergencies. This kit should contain the following items:

- **STETHOSCOPE.** Used for taking heart rates and listening to gut sounds.
- **WATCH WITH SECOND HAND.** Used to measure heart and respiratory rates.
- **THERMOMETER.** Used to take rectal temperature.
- **PENLIGHT OR FLASHLIGHT.** Helps in poor or dim light to evaluate capillary refill time. Can help examine an eye or a wound in inadequate light.
- **BETADINE SCRUB.** Used to cleanse and shave wounds.
- **BETADINE SOLUTION.** Used to clean and flush wounds. Betadine solution should be diluted with water to a weak-tea color for flushing wounds (no stronger than 1 part betadine to 10 parts water).
- **SALINE SOLUTION.** Used to flush an injured or irritated eye. May also be used to flush or clean a wound.
- **DOSING SYRINGE.** Can be used to administer oral medications or for flushing a wound.
- **ANTIBIOTIC WOUND OINTMENT.** Used to dress a wound or treat superficial abrasions.
- **BANDAGE MATERIAL.** Used to apply a wrap to a wound or swollen leg. Include 3 to 4 sheet cottons, 6-inch brown gauze, Vetrap™, self-adhesive tape, and several nonstick wound dressings.
- **BANDAGE SCISSORS.**
- **NAIL PULLER.** Used to remove a shoe.
- **DUCT TAPE.** Used for just about everything.

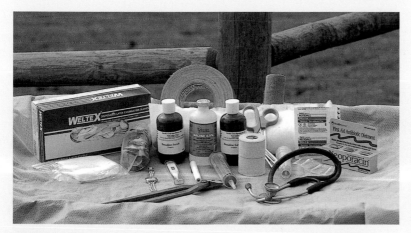

FIGURE 3.34. **Every barn and horse trailer should have a fully stocked first-aid kit such as the one pictured here.**

(Note: Your veterinarian may suggest that you have on hand certain prescription medications such as phenylbutazone [an anti-inflammatory], antibiotics, or tranquilizers, particularly if you travel extensively with your horse or trail ride in remote locations. Ask your vet for recommendations and advice.)

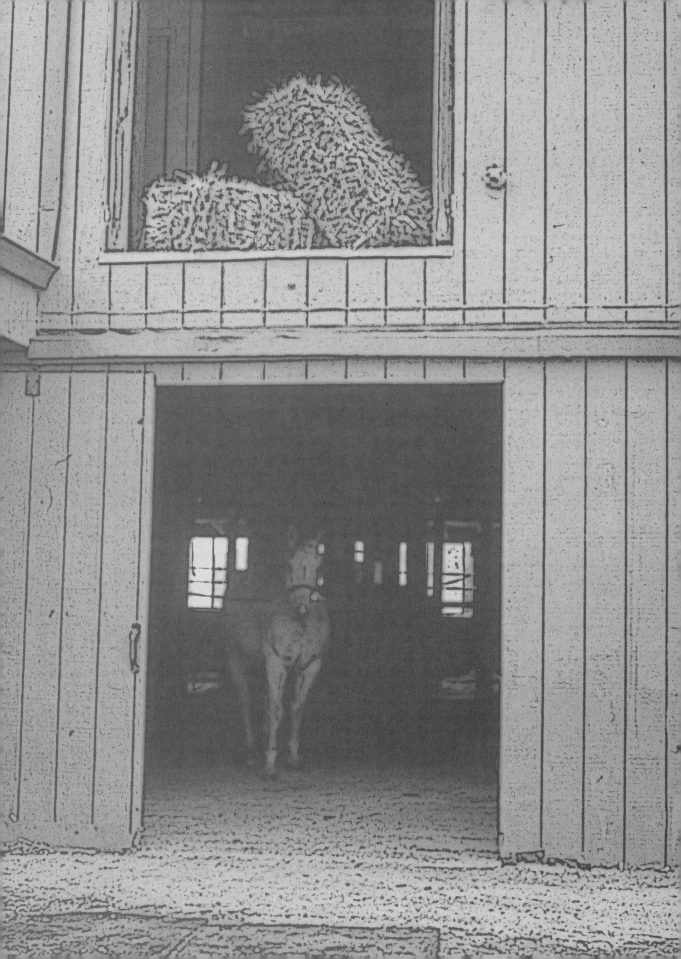

PART TWO

The Horse's Body: Health and Disease

CHAPTER 4

The Musculoskeletal System

THE HORSE'S MUSCULOSKELETAL SYSTEM is the framework of structures that support his internal organs, allow him to stand, graze, and flee from predators, and make it possible for him to perform all of the activities such as galloping, jumping, and working cows that define his relationship with humans.

Knowledge of the basic structure of the horse's bones, joints, and soft tissues is one of those things that distinguish the true horseman from the hobbyist. Not only is that knowledge critical for understanding the huge range of musculoskeletal problems the horse can experience; a true horsewoman familiar with the structures of the lower legs will recognize swelling, heat, or other abnormalities immediately as she checks her horse's legs each day. Because of this, she might identify small problems before they become severe.

The following is an overview of the basic structures that make up the musculoskeletal system of the horse, followed by a detailed description of the anatomy of specific regions of the horse's body.

Basic Structures

Bones

Bones comprise the framework of the body. The skeleton provides a support structure for the other organ systems as well as the basis for all movement. In general, bones are composed of two types of tissue. The spongy or "cancellous" bone at the center of each bone is covered by the compact or "cortical" bone. The outermost layer of the bones, the periosteum, is a tough, fibrous tissue that primarily provides strength for the attachment of tendons and ligaments.

Joints

Joints are the connections between bones that allow for movement. Basic joint structure consists of these layers:

- JOINT CAPSULE: A fibrous layer that encloses the entire joint, it contains blood vessels and nerves that help supply nutrients and maintain joint function.

- SYNOVIAL (JOINT) MEMBRANE: A thin layer of tissue that filters blood and produces synovial fluid which when released into the joint provides nutrients and lubrication to the joint surface.

- SYNOVIAL FLUID: Fluid released by cells of the synovial membrane that helps cushion the joint. It also provides nutrients to the cartilage and lubrication that facilitates joint movement.

- CARTILAGE: A fibrous, white covering over the ends of the bones that makes up the actual gliding surface of the joint. The cartilage also has shock-absorbing properties that help distribute stresses placed on the joints during movement.

- SUBCHONDRAL BONE: The layer of bone directly below the cartilage that helps absorb shock, and carries nutrients and waste to and from the joint.

- PERIARTICULAR SUPPORT STRUCTURES: Tendons and ligaments surrounding the joint that help maintain stability. Most joints have a pair of collateral ligaments on the medial (inside) and lateral (outside) that provide support.

Tendons

Tendons provide the attachment of muscle to bone, and are structures that provide the pulley through which muscles have their effect. Basic tendon structure consists of a series of parallel fibers that come together in a bundle, similar to the small wires within an electrical cord.

Ligaments

Ligaments are connective tissue structures that attach bone to bone across joints to help provide stability and control movement. They can be situated within the joint capsule (intracapsular), can attach to the joint capsule (capsular), or can be completely outside of the joint capsule (extracapsular). Like tendons, ligaments consist of a series of parallel fibers that come together in a bundle. In general they are less elastic (stretchy) than tendons.

Muscles

The muscles are responsible for producing movement. They are composed of individual muscle fibers bundled together into larger units that make up the actual muscles. The structure of the individual muscle cells allows them to slide back and forth along one another. This action combines to produce a shortening (contraction) or lengthening of the muscle itself—thus producing movement through the tendinous attachment of the muscle to bone or connective tissues.

Regional Anatomy

Detailed below are the regions of the horse's body most critical for producing movement, with special emphasis on the structures most likely to be the source of problems associated with the musculoskeletal system.

The Foot   FIGURE 4.1

The foot consists of the hoof wall and associated hoof structures, as well as the internal bones, joints, and ligaments. The hoof itself is made up of a horny tissue that derives from the skin and grows down from the coronary band, which forms the junction between the skin and hoof. The wall is divided into three layers, the stratum externum, stratum medium, and

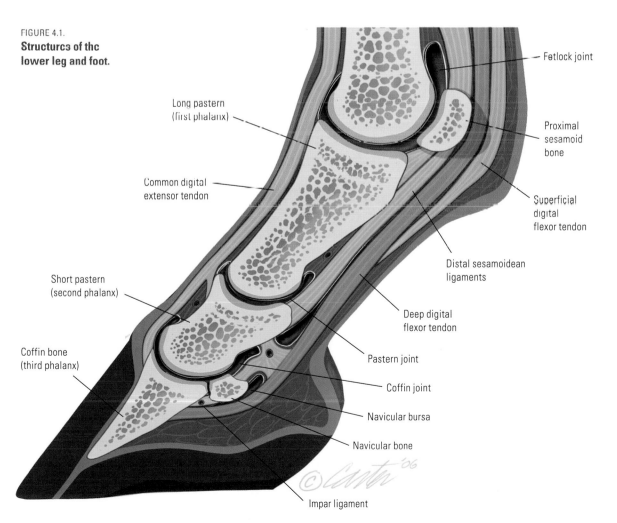

FIGURE 4.1.
Structures of the lower leg and foot.

Fetlock joint

Long pastern (first phalanx)

Proximal sesamoid bone

Common digital extensor tendon

Superficial digital flexor tendon

Distal sesamoidean ligaments

Short pastern (second phalanx)

Deep digital flexor tendon

Coffin bone (third phalanx)

Pastern joint

Coffin joint

Navicular bursa

Navicular bone

Impar ligament

stratum internum. At the inner layer, the hoof wall attaches to the coffin bone through a network of tiny fingers or "laminae." The laminae on the inside of the hoof wall are hard and insensitive, while those lining the coffin bone are soft and sensitive. Hence the terms sensitive and insensitive laminae used to describe the hoof's attachment.

At the sole of the foot is the V-shaped structure called the frog, which blends in with the heel bulbs at the back of the foot, and the sole at the toe and sides. Beneath the frog is a fatty, fibrous mass of tissue called the digital cushion, which helps provide shock absorption to the foot.

Bones of the foot include the hoof-shaped coffin bone (third phalanx), the end of the short pastern (second phalanx), and the small, wing-shaped navicular bone that rests just beneath the coffin bone. The coffin joint forms the junction between the coffin bone and the short pastern bone.

The navicular bone helps distribute stress and determine the angle of insertion of the deep digital flexor tendon. This tendon crosses beneath the navicular bone to its attachment at the bottom of the coffin bone. A fluid-filled sac called the navicular bursa rests between the navicular bone and the deep digital flexor tendon. It helps cushion and absorb stress.

Other soft-tissue structures within the foot include the impar ligament, a fibrous sheet that extends from the lower edge of the navicular bone to the bottom of the coffin bone, and a pair of small ligaments called the navicular suspensory ligaments that attach from each side of the navicular bone to the end of the long pastern bone (first phalanx) further up the leg. Both of these ligaments help stabilize the navicular bone.

The Lower Leg   FIGURES 4.2–4.3

The lower leg consists of the pastern, fetlock, cannon bone, and associated soft-tissue structures. The anatomy of the forelimb and the hind limb is comparable, so for this discussion, the details of the forelimb need only be described.

The pastern joint forms the connection between the long and short pastern bones (first and second phalanges), and is located in the middle of the pastern between the coronary band and the fetlock joint. This low-motion joint commonly develops osteoarthritis, referred to as high ringbone (see page 85). Just above the pastern joint is the high-motion fetlock joint that forms the connection between the cannon bone (third metacarpus), and the long pastern bone. This joint has a large joint space with a prominent pouch that extends up the back. At the back of the fetlock joint, two small bones, called the proximal sesamoids, sit side by side, where they help distribute stress from the important structures that run along the back of this area.

The Horse's Body: Health and Disease

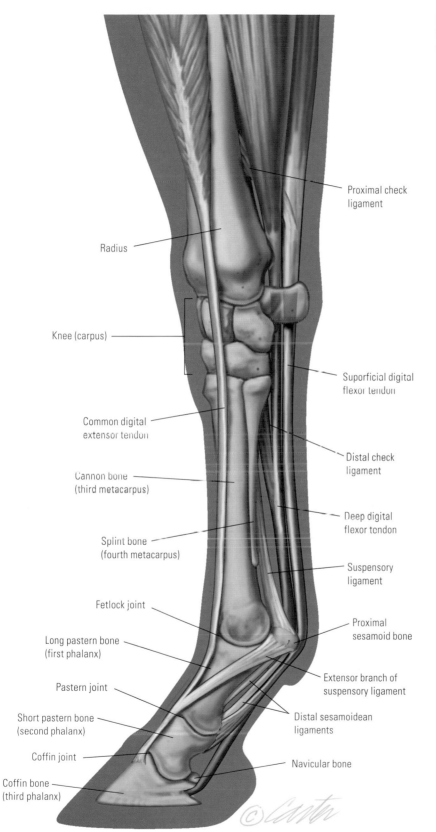

FIGURE 4. 2.
**Structures
of the forelimb.**

Proximal check
ligament

Radius

Knee (carpus)

Superficial digital
flexor tendon

Common digital
extensor tendon

Distal check
ligament

Cannon bone
(third metacarpus)

Deep digital
flexor tendon

Splint bone
(fourth metacarpus)

Suspensory
ligament

Fetlock joint

Proximal
sesamoid bone

Long pastern bone
(first phalanx)

Extensor branch of
suspensory ligament

Pastern joint

Distal sesamoidean
ligaments

Short pastern bone
(second phalanx)

Coffin joint

Navicular bone

Coffin bone
(third phalanx)

©Carta

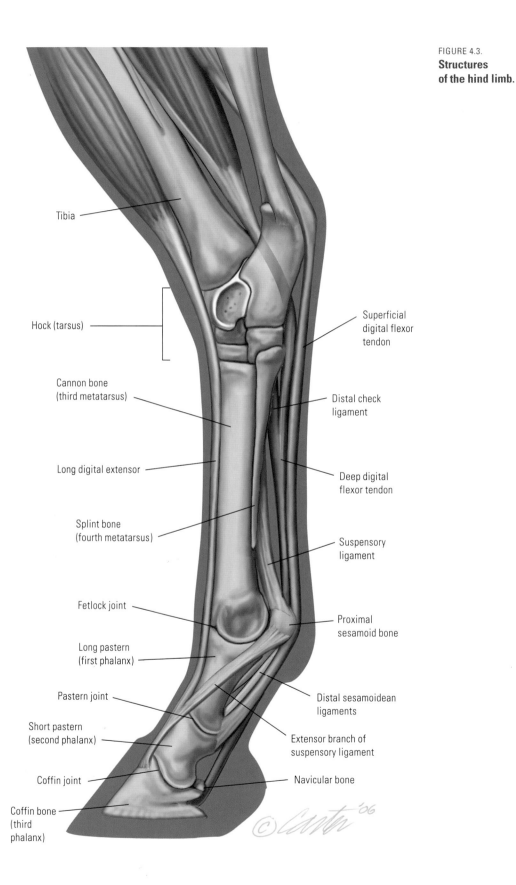

FIGURE 4.3.
**Structures
of the hind limb.**

Tibia

Hock (tarsus)

Cannon bone
(third metatarsus)

Long digital extensor

Splint bone
(fourth metatarsus)

Fetlock joint

Long pastern
(first phalanx)

Pastern joint

Short pastern
(second phalanx)

Coffin joint

Coffin bone
(third
phalanx)

Superficial
digital flexor
tendon

Distal check
ligament

Deep digital
flexor tendon

Suspensory
ligament

Proximal
sesamoid bone

Distal sesamoidean
ligaments

Extensor branch of
suspensory ligament

Navicular bone

A number of soft-tissue structures provide support for the lower leg, including:

- COMMON DIGITAL EXTENSOR TENDON: It runs down the front of the forelimb and forms the attachment of the group of muscles that extend (straighten) the knee, fetlock, pastern, and coffin joint. It attaches to the long and short pastern bones and the coffin bone. It can be palpated as a cord-like structure that runs down the front of the cannon bone.

- LATERAL DIGITAL EXTENSOR TENDON: It works with the common digital extensor tendon as an attachment for the extensor muscles. It originates from the extensor muscles on the outside of the forelimb and attaches to the long pastern bone. It can be palpated as a cord-like structure just to the outside of the common digital extensor.

- SUPERFICIAL DIGITAL FLEXOR TENDON (SDF): It arises from the muscles that flex (bend) the knee, fetlock, and pastern joints on the back of the leg. It has two attachments at the top of the long and short pastern bones and is the outermost tendon situated at the back of the horse's leg.

- DEEP DIGITAL FLEXOR TENDON (DDF): It arises from another muscle that flexes the fetlock, pastern, and coffin joints and runs just underneath the SDF. It has an important attachment point at the bottom of the coffin bone, after it runs across the back of the fetlock and across the navicular bone and bursa. This structure is a common site for injury.

- SUSPENSORY APPARATUS: This apparatus is a key supporter of the fetlock joint and the structures below it. It consists primarily of the suspensory ligament, which begins at the back of the cannon bone just below the knee, and runs along the length of the cannon bone until it splits into two branches that form a sling around the fetlock joint to incorporate the proximal sesamoid bones. The branches then wrap around to the front of the pastern area, where they finally attach at the top of the coffin bone.

Three additional ligaments contribute to the support of the suspensory apparatus: the distal sesamoidean ligaments (the superficial or straight, the middle or oblique, and the deep or cruciate ligaments). These small ligaments attach from the base of the proximal sesamoid bones to the long and short pastern bones to help support the fetlock.

- DISTAL CHECK LIGAMENT (DCL): It starts at the back of the cannon bone and joins with the DDF to provide additional support to this tendon.

- PROXIMAL CHECK LIGAMENT (PCL): Similar to the DCL, it starts at the back of the bone in the upper forelimb and joins with the SDF to provide additional support to this tendon.

- DIGITAL TENDON SHEATH (DTS): It is a structure that looks like a "sausage casing." It extends from the middle of the cannon bone, along the back of the fetlock, and through the pastern area. This fluid-filled sheath provides lubrication for the tendons to glide smoothly through as they work. The DTS is held in place by several flat ligaments (the annular ligaments) that run horizontally across the back of the fetlock and pastern.

The Forearm

The forearm (or upper front leg) consists of the knee (carpus), elbow, and shoulder joints. The knee is comparable to the human wrist and consists of two rows of small bones with three joint spaces between them that allow the knee to flex and extend. The elbow is a hinge-type joint with a single joint capsule that allows this joint to open and close. The shoulder has more of a ball-and-socket structure that gives it a wider range of movement on more than one plane (although soft-tissue structures surrounding this joint still restrict its primary movement to opening and closing on a single plane).

The carpal sheath, a fluid-filled structure similar to the DTS, encases the flexor tendons where they run across the knee and provides lubrication that allows them to glide smoothly. Another important fluid-filled structure in this area, the bicipital bursa, lies under the tendons that run across the shoulder joint to provide cushioning and support.

The Pelvis and Sacroiliac Connections   FIGURES 4.4–4.5

The pelvis consists of the ilium, the ischium, and the pubis, which come together to form a ring of bones. At the top and inside of this ring sits the sacrum, which is comprised of a set of fused vertebrae at the end of the spinal column. The sacrum attaches to the pelvis through the paired sacroiliac joints. These are flat, fibrous connections that hold it in place. Contributing to the stability of this connection is the dorsal sacroiliac ligament, a strong, cord-like soft-tissue structure that runs from the prominence at the top of the ilium (the tuber sacrale) and along the top of the sacrum. In addition, two smaller ligaments help hold things in place: the ventral sacroiliac ligament (between the bottom of the sacrum and the ilium) and the intraosseous ligament (a flat sheet of tissue on either side of the sacrum between the sacrum and the ilial wing).

Although they contribute little to the horse's actual movement, the sacroiliac joints provide support for the weight-bearing portion of the stride and help transmit the propulsive forces of the hind limbs through the vertebral column. With this function, the sacroiliac connections form

The Horse's Body: Health and Disease

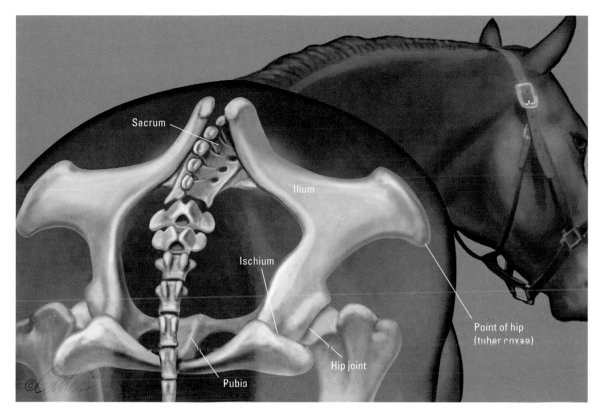

FIGURE 4.4. **Structures of the pelvis and sacroiliac area, hind view.**

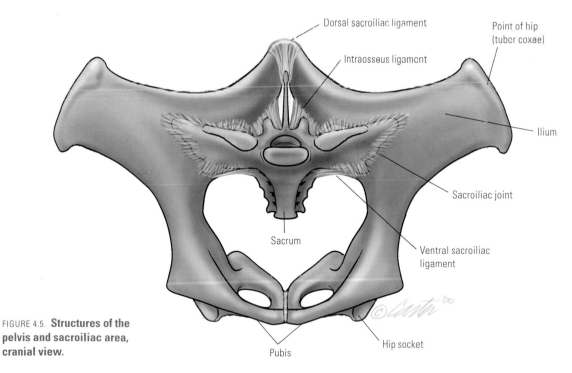

FIGURE 4.5. **Structures of the pelvis and sacroiliac area, cranial view.**

the all-important link between the horse's hindquarters and the rest of his body.

The hip (coxofemoral) joint is a ball-and-socket type joint that joins the top of the femur (the large upper leg bone) to the pelvis at a ring-like structure called the acetabulum. This is the socket formed by the ilium, ischium, and pubis. The head of the femur is secured into the acetabulum through two small ligaments. This large joint has a single joint space, and allows for a large range of movement that includes flexion, extension, and rotation.

Stifle   FIGURE 4.6

The stifle, one of the most complicated joints of the horse's body, is a very important structure that supports and controls hind limb movement. Three joint spaces (isolated joint capsules) make up the stifle joint: the femoropatellar joint (between the top of the femur and the patella, or kneecap), the medial femorotibial (on the inside of the leg, between the femur and the tibia), and the lateral femorotibial (on the outside of the leg, between the femur and the tibia).

The femoropatellar joint space has a large gliding surface on the top of the femur that allows the patella to slide up and down to perform its function of distributing stress from the large quadriceps muscle group that extends this joint. This joint space communicates with the medial femorotibial joint space in most horses. The paired femorotibial joint spaces contain the medial and lateral menisci, half-moon shaped cartilage pads that provide both cushioning and a smooth gliding surface for the joint.

Between the medial and lateral femorotibial joint spaces lie the paired cruciate ligaments. These two small ligaments help stabilize the joint, resist hyperextension, and control rotation. The medial and lateral collateral ligaments connect the femur and tibia on each side of the stifle joint to provide additional support.

Finally, three other very important ligaments act as a tendon of insertion for the quadriceps muscle on the top of the tibia: the medial, middle, and lateral patellar ligaments. These ligaments help distribute stress from the quadriceps muscles. In addition, they will lock the stifle into an extended position by forming a loop of the medial (inside) and middle ligaments over the large inner portion of the femur. This locking function is the foundation of the hind limb stay apparatus, the mechanism that allows the horse to "sleep on his feet."

Hock

The hock (tarsus) consists of four separate joint spaces: the tibiotarsal, proximal and distal intertarsals, and tarsometatarsal. The tibiotarsal joint is the uppermost space between the tibia and the small bones of the hock.

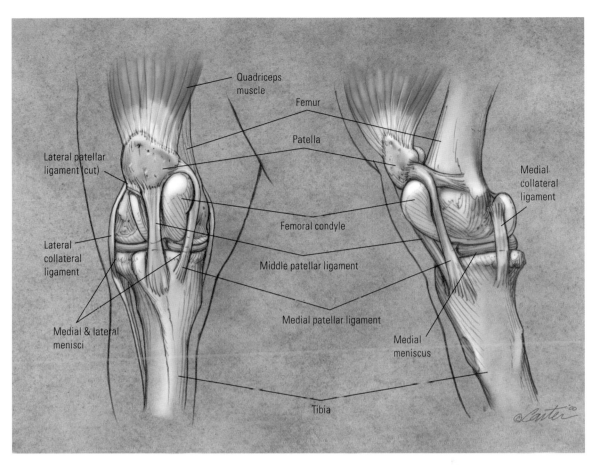

Quadriceps
muscle

Femur

Patella

Lateral patellar
ligament (cut)

Femoral condyle

Medial
collateral
ligament

Lateral
collateral
ligament

Middle patellar ligament

Medial & lateral
menisci

Medial patellar ligament

Tibia

Medial
meniscus

FIGURE 4.6.
**Structures of the
stifle joint.**

This joint has a large capsule, and is where most of the hock's movement comes from. Fluid accumulation (effusion) in this joint space can result in what is commonly called a bog spavin, a visible swelling that appears at the front of the hock joint. The proximal intertarsal is the space between the first two rows of small bones within the hock. It communicates with the tibiotarsal joint in most horses. The lower two joint spaces of the hock are the distal intertarsal (between the second and third rows of tarsal bones) and the tarsometatarsal (between the hock and the cannon bone). These are low-motion joints that together provide only 5 to 10 percent of the total movement of the hock. The most common location of degenerative joint disease of the hock (referred to as bone spavin) is in these two lower joints (see page 83).

A number of ligaments surrounding the hock, including two pairs of collateral ligaments, provide support on the inside and the outside of the joint. The plantar ligament runs along the back of this joint from the point of the hock (the protruding bone at the back) to the top of the cannon bone. Injury to this ligament is called a "curb" (see page 91).

How the Horse Moves

Movement in the horse can be summed up as the contraction (shortening) of muscles and how those muscles function through their tendinous attachments at bones and joints. With this in mind, an understanding of the function of individual joints depends on understanding the structures described above. To fully comprehend how the horse moves, one must understand basic gait patterns.

The four basic gaits of the horse are the walk, trot, canter, and gallop. (*Note: There are many different gait patterns that are variations of these basics, as is evident in different breeds of horses. An understanding of the basic four will help establish a foundation for an overall understanding of how the horse moves.*)

The Walk

The walk is a four-beat gait, meaning each of the horse's feet lands on the ground separately. There is no period of suspension (a time when the horse's body is off the ground).

The Trot

The trot is a two-beat gait, with diagonal pairs (left front/right hind; right front/left hind) hitting the ground together. There is a period of suspension in the trot, between the time when each pair of legs is on the ground. A variation of the trot is the pace, which is also a two-beat gait but with lateral pairs (legs on the same side) contacting the ground together, and a period of suspension between each step.

The Canter

The canter is a three-beat gait, with a single hind limb contacting the ground first, followed by the diagonal pair, followed by the final forelimb and then a period of suspension after pushing off before another stride begins (e.g., left hind, diagonal pair: right hind/left front, left front, and suspension). Because the canter is an asymmetrical gait, it has two possible variations, called leads. The right lead refers to the canter when the right front leg is the last to hit the ground, and the left lead refers to the canter when the left front leg is last to hit the ground.

The Gallop

The gallop is a four-beat gait that's similar to the canter, the difference being that the footfalls of the diagonal pair are split, with the hind leg striking the ground before the foreleg. Because is it asymmetrical, it also has left and right leads determined by the last front leg to hit the ground.

The Lameness Examination

Where does it hurt? If the horse is holding one leg up in the air and there's a large swelling visible from across the stall, it's not hard to tell where the lameness is coming from. In most cases, however, it's not so simple. Because the horse can't come into the vet's office and say, "It hurts right here," the vet must first localize the lameness to a specific area of the leg. Only after he determines where it hurts can he begin to take the necessary steps to find out exactly what's wrong. The following diagnostic steps may be taken to localize and define a musculoskeletal problem.

Hoof Testers

These large metal pinchers are used to apply pressure to areas of the horse's hooves. Sensitivity in a specific area can help pinpoint a bruise, sole abscess, or pain from structures like the navicular bone or coffin joint that lie deep within the horse's foot.

Palpation and Limb Manipulation

Swelling, heat, or sensitivity when pressure is applied to specific areas of the horse's legs or body can help the vet detect an injury. For example, an injury to a joint might result in visible accumulation of fluid within that joint. A tendon injury may cause swelling and sensitivity within the tendon.

Observation and Stress Testing

The veterinarian will watch the horse moving in order to determine which leg is affected. He may even be able to pinpoint the lameness to an area of the leg or a specific structure. He may observe the horse under the following conditions.

- Walking and trotting on a straight line in hand
- Walking small figure-8's on hard ground in hand
- Walking, trotting, and cantering on a lungeline on soft footing
- Walking and trotting on a lungeline on hard ground
- Working under saddle

He will also perform stress tests as a part of the observation process. Stress tests involve applying pressure to certain parts of the limb. The vet will hold a joint flexed for a period of time, then watch the horse trot away. If the horse's lameness becomes more pronounced when a certain structure is flexed, it's possible that's the area that has been injured.

Diagnostic Blocks

Perhaps the most important part of any lameness examination is the diagnostic block. To perform this test, a local anesthetic is injected into the nerves supplying a specific area of the horse's leg (nerve blocks), or directly into a specific structure such as a joint, bursa, or tendon sheath.

If the lameness disappears when a specific structure is "blocked," that's the most accurate means of pinpointing the source of the lameness. In general, the vet will begin at the bottom of the leg and work his way up when he performs peripheral nerve blocks. Joint blocks can be performed as isolated tests if a specific joint, bursa, or tendon sheath is suspected as the source of the lameness based on the clinical examination. Once a lameness has been specifically blocked, the vet is able to move on to the question of identifying exactly what's wrong.

Nuclear Scintigraphy

In cases where the lameness is very subtle, the vet is unable to block the lameness, it appears in multiple limbs, or there are other difficulties in pinpointing the source of the lameness, nuclear scintigraphy may help. This test involves injecting a radioactive substance into the horse's bloodstream. After a period of time, a gamma camera is used to detect areas of increased radioactivity in the horse's body, indicating increased blood flow. Because inflammation is generally associated with increased blood flow, the camera will detect an increased uptake of radioactivity in inflamed areas. This diagnostic technique primarily detects an area of bone inflammation or an inflammation at the attachment site of ligaments to bones. Soft-tissue injuries may not be identified.

Radiographs

Radiographs allow visualization of skeletal structures and are taken to evaluate bone-related problems, such as fractures, bone infections, or degenerative joint disease.

Ultrasound

Ultrasound allows visualization of soft-tissue structures and is performed to evaluate soft-tissue problems, such as a tendon or ligament tear.

Blood Work

Blood tests may be recommended for some types of lameness problems, particularly where muscle disorders are suspected, or where an underlying metabolic disease may play a role.

Muscle Biopsy

In cases where a muscular disorder is suspected, a sample of muscle may be taken and submitted to a lab for evaluation. Because a fairly large section of muscle is necessary, it is usually obtained from the hindquarters, just to the side of the tail head where scarring will be minimal.

Magnetic Resonance Imaging

This advanced diagnostic technique (MRI) is becoming more widely available for horses. It allows for visualization of both bones and soft-tissue structures and it can help pinpoint the site of an injury.

The following are the most common causes of lameness or muscular disorders.

Sole Bruise

WHAT IT IS. Bruising on the bottom of the foot.

DIAGNOSIS. The horse may be reluctant to put his foot on the ground and digital pulses will be increased in intensity. The vet may detect a specific area of sensitivity with the hoof testers, and visible discoloration may be present on the horse's sole.

TREATMENT. Anti-inflammatory medications will be administered, and warm foot soaks or poultices may be recommended to draw out accumulated fluid. Special shoeing or trimming might help to relieve pressure on the area and facilitate healing.

HOW SERIOUS IS IT? The horse should recover completely with no long-term complications, although full recovery may take as long as 6 to 8 weeks.

POTENTIAL COMPLICATIONS. In some cases, a sole bruise may develop into an abscess.

FIGURE 4.7.
A sole abscess involves a pocket of infection that builds up pressure within the foot, and can cause severe lameness.

Subsolar Abscess   FIGURE 4.7

WHAT IT IS. An infection that causes a pocket of pus to form under the sole of the foot.

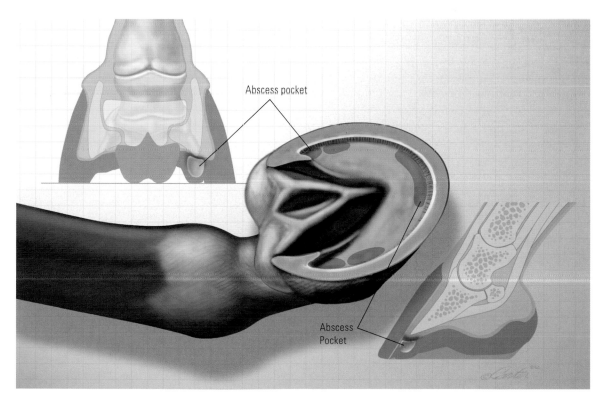

Abscess pocket

Abscess Pocket

DIAGNOSIS. Severe lameness may be present, and the horse may refuse to bear any weight on the foot if pressure buildup within the abscess pocket is extreme. A sensitive area may be detected with hoof testers.

TREATMENT. Warm-water soaks with a drawing agent such as Epsom salts may be recommended to try to draw out the infection and relieve pressure. Some abscesses will travel up under the hoof wall, and open for drainage at the top of the coronary band or heel area. If the abscess fails to open on its own or in response to soaking, the vet will attempt to open the pocket to allow drainage. The opening area will then be packed with an antibacterial agent and protected with a boot or bandage until the area has healed.

HOW SERIOUS IS IT? The horse should recover completely with no long-term complications.

POTENTIAL COMPLICATIONS. Very rarely, infection can extend to the coffin bone or other deep structures, causing long-term or even permanent lameness. A coffin bone fracture can easily be misdiagnosed as a sole abscess during an initial evaluation.

Quarter Crack   FIGURE 4.8

WHAT IT IS. A vertical crack that extends up the hoof, in the back quarter of the foot. A severe quarter crack will extend up through the coronary band.

DIAGNOSIS. A visible crack can be identified extending up the side of the hoof. If lameness is present, a nerve block performed on the side of the crack can confirm that the lameness is due to the quarter crack.

TREATMENT. In order for a quarter crack to resolve, it must be stabilized. Ideally, shoeing to provide support while eliminating pressure on the sole area behind the crack will prevent the crack from moving, and allow it to grow out and heal. Some veterinarians or farriers will recommend lacing or patching in an effort to stabilize the crack.

HOW SERIOUS IS IT? If a crack can be stabilized, it may grow out completely, returning the foot to its normal state. If the coronary band is damaged at the origin of the crack or it is very difficult to stabilize because of the horse's individual foot characteristics, it may never return to normal. In these cases, soundness can be maintained with good, balanced shoeing that prevents movement of the crack.

POTENTIAL COMPLICATIONS. A quarter crack can become infected, causing increased lameness and damage to underlying tissues.

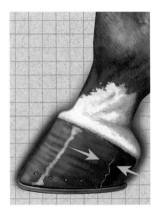

FIGURE 4.8: **A quarter crack can work its way up the hoof wall, causing inflammation and pain.**

Navicular Syndrome   FIGURES 4.9–4.12

WHAT IT IS. Pain originating from the horse's heel area and resulting in lameness. This syndrome can include numerous specific problems, including inflammation of the coffin joint, actual degeneration of the navicular bone, or injuries to the small ligaments that attach in the area. Symptoms most commonly appear between the ages of 7 and 9 years, and Quarter

Horses, Thoroughbreds, and warmbloods (specifically Dutch Warm-bloods) have a higher incidence than other breeds.

Most commonly navicular problems have an insidious onset that can begin with a subtle shortening of the stride or sensitivity on hard ground. An affected horse might shift his weight back and forth when standing, and may stand with one front foot pointed out in front of him. Stumbling is common due to the altered flight pattern of the foot during movement. Because both front feet are often affected, lameness may not be detected easily—especially during the early stages. As the problem progresses, the horse will become more uncomfortable, and actual lameness is likely to prompt a call to the veterinarian.

DIAGNOSIS. The veterinarian may suspect navicular issues in a horse that moves with short strides. Typically, the horse will draw the front feet back slightly before placing them on the ground in order to minimize stress to the heel area. The lameness most commonly appears when the horse is trotting in a circle on hard ground, with the most affected foot to the inside of the circle. Some horses will be sensitive to hoof testers applied across the heel area of an affected foot. The lameness will usually improve when the nerves that supply the heels are blocked, or when the anesthetic is placed directly into the coffin joint. Some practitioners will recommend blocking the navicular bursa (the small fluid-filled sac between the navic-ular bone and the deep digital flexor tendon) for a more specific diagnosis. Radiographs will usually be recommended, and may confirm a more spe-cific cause of the condition, such as degeneration of the navicular bone.

In a case where a soft-tissue injury is suspected, such as a tear in the impar ligament or injury to the deep digital flexor tendon deep within the foot, ultrasound examination may help identify a specific area of injury. With the increasing availability of MRI in lameness referral practices, this technique can also be used in some instances to help determine a specific diagnosis.

TREATMENT. Corrective shoeing can go a long way toward managing this condition, with the focus on providing heel support and easing breakover of the horse's foot. This is often accomplished through the use of egg-bar shoes with rocker or rolled toes, and as many as 50 percent of affected horses will improve with this type of shoeing. Sometimes heel wedges to raise the angle of the foot may be recommended to restore proper balance. NSAIDS (nonsteroidal anti-inflammatory drugs such as phenyl-butazone or flunixin meglumine) will be recommended. Isoxsuprine may be recommended to help improve circulation in the foot. The coffin joint or navicular bursa may be injected with an anti-inflammatory (cortisone) and joint lubricant (hyaluronic acid), especially if the lameness was specifically blocked in one of these two structures. Systemic medications designed to improve joint health, such as Adequan® and Legend®, may be recommended.

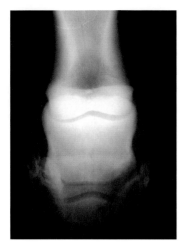

FIGURE 4.9. **A normal navicular bone can be seen in this radiograph.** (Author photo)

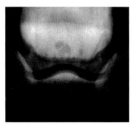

FIGURE 4.10. **In a severe case of navicular disease the small navicular bone within the foot would show signs of degeneration indicated by the irregular margins along the bottom edge of the bone.** (Photo courtesy of Jan Palmer, DVM, Diplomate ACVS)

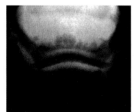

FIGURE 4.11. **This large cyst in the navicular bone would be the likely underlying cause of lameness originating from the heel area.** (Photo courtesy of Jan Palmer, DVM, Diplomate ACVS)

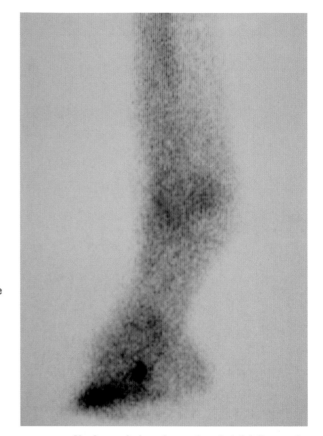

FIGURE 4.12. **Nuclear scintigraphy can be a helpful diagnostic technique for evaluation of foot problems. In this image, the navicular bone and toe of the coffin bone both show increased uptake of radioactivity, indicating active inflammation in these areas.** (Photo courtesy of Mark Revenaugh, DVM)

Some practitioners report success with extracorporeal shockwave therapy, treatment that is particularly useful for helping to stimulate healing for soft-tissue injuries. (See sidebar on p. 91)

For advanced cases, the nerves that supply the heels may be surgically cut (a procedure known as a neurectomy) to help manage chronic pain. It is important to recognize that this treatment can have a number of potential drawbacks. It is a temporary solution, as nerves will grow back after a period of 2 to 3 years. Complications from the surgery can include the development of a disorganized ball of nerve fibers (known as a neuroma) at the surgical site that can be extremely painful. Because the horse will have no sensation in the heel area, it is easy to overlook a problem stone bruise, an abscess or a foreign body, such as a nail in the foot, without vigilant monitoring. Finally, the deep digital flexor tendon can rupture fol-

The Horse's Body: Health and Disease

lowing surgery, and a horse with an injury to this structure should not be considered good a candidate for a neurectomy.

HOW SERIOUS IS IT? Problems tend to be chronic and often frustrating, although they can be managed quite successfully in many cases. Horses with chronic navicular problems can even be successful high-level performance horses with proper management.

POTENTIAL COMPLICATIONS. None.

Pedal Osteitis

WHAT IT IS. An inflammation of the coffin bone that may result in degeneration of the bone over time, although whether it really can be considered a specific abnormality is controversial. Some practitioners believe that this diagnosis actually incorporates a host of different problems that range from something as simple as thin soles that cause the horse to have front foot sensitivity, to mild or low-grade chronic laminitis. Lameness associated with these kinds of problems can be very subtle or pronounced, depending on severity.

DIAGNOSIS. There will be sensitivity to hoof testers around the sole of the foot. The lameness and sensitivity will disappear when the feet are blocked. Characteristic changes on radiographs, such as enlarged channels where blood vessels run or signs of degeneration around the edge of the coffin bone, may accompany these findings, although their significance is also controversial as similar things are commonly seen in normal horses.

TREATMENT. Good shoeing to protect the sole and minimize ongoing trauma to the coffin bone will help most horses. Anti-inflammatory medications and medications intended to improve circulation, such as isoxsuprine, will be recommended. In some cases, an injection of an anti-inflammatory medication (cortisone) into the coffin joint will help quiet inflammation affecting the coffin bone.

HOW SERIOUS IS IT? Conditions likely to be diagnosed as pedal osteitis are usually manageable, although many require long-term management. If the horse is diagnosed with pedal osteitis, he's likely to require treatment forever, including careful shoeing and medications.

POTENTIAL COMPLICATIONS. If diagnosed, pedal osteitis is related to low-grade laminitis, and an acute worsening of inflammation could lead to a more severe founder episode.

Coffin Bone Fracture   FIGURES 4.13–4.14

WHAT IT IS. A fracture (break) of the small hoof-shaped coffin bone within the foot. A coffin bone fracture will cause a horse to become suddenly very lame and will usually be accompanied by a strong digital pulse.

DIAGNOSIS. Most coffin bone fractures will be identified with a radiograph. Scintigraphy may identify a coffin bone fracture that is not seen on radiographs.

TREATMENT. Fractures that are nondisplaced (the bone on either side of the fracture line has not moved) will usually be stabilized with a bar shoe. The bar shoe in combination with the rigid nature of the horse's hoof acts like a cast to prevent movement of the fracture line. An extended period of rest of several months will be recommended. Healing may be monitored with sequential radiographs, although it's important to know that some coffin bone fractures heal with fibrous tissue instead of bone, meaning the radiographs will continue to appear abnormal even when the fracture has completely healed.

HOW SERIOUS IS IT? A nondisplaced coffin bone fracture that's identified immediately has a good chance for full recovery. If the fracture extends into the coffin joint, there may be risk of permanent unsoundness due to damage to the joint.

POTENTIAL COMPLICATIONS. A horse with a coffin bone fracture will have symptoms very similar to one with a sole abscess. Because of this, radiographs may not be recommended immediately, which can delay identification of the fracture and increase the risk of poor healing. In addition, a nondisplaced fracture line may not be visible on radiographs taken immediately after the injury. Over a period of several weeks, however, the bone begins to demineralize and the fracture may become visible. Because of this, the veterinarian may recommend repeating radiographs after 3 to 4 weeks if he suspects a coffin bone fracture but does not see one immediately. Finally, joint disruption from a fracture that extends into the joint can lead to arthritis and permanent lameness.

Laminitis (Founder) FIGURES 4.15–4.19

WHAT IT IS. Laminitis is an inflammatory condition that affects the sensitive laminae, the fingerlike projections that line the surface of the bones within the hoof. These sensitive laminae connect to horny insensitive laminae on the inner surface of the hoof wall and help stabilize the coffin bones inside the hooves. Laminitis results in a disruption of blood flow that can have wide-ranging consequences. Most important, if stresses on the laminae overcome the ability of these fingerlike projections to hold the coffin bone in position, the coffin bone can either rotate or drop down within the hoof capsule—a potentially life-threatening situation. At best, if rotation occurs initially but can

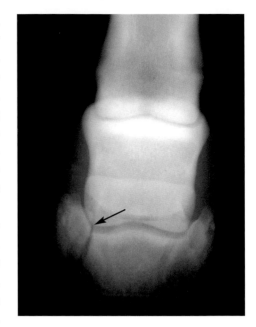

FIGURE 4.13. **A fracture of the coffin bone is easily seen on this radiograph.** (Author photo)

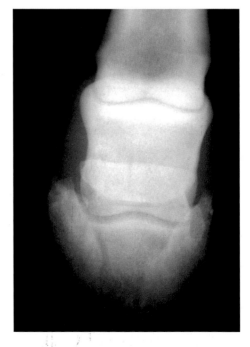

FIGURE 4.14. **After several months of confinement and stabilization with a bar shoe, the fracture is healing well.** (Author photo)

be stopped and stabilized, the horse becomes a chronic founder victim and will most likely require lifelong management.

A horse with laminitis will become suddenly lame in both front feet and may walk gingerly, as if he's "walking on eggshells." With each step he's likely to land on his foot heel first. The lameness will be more pronounced on hard surfaces, and the horse may exhibit the typical founder stance, with his front feet out in front of his body. The foot sensitivity will usually be accompanied by strong digital pulses in the affected feet. Laminitis commonly affects both front feet, although sometimes the hind feet can also be involved.

WHY DOES LAMINITIS OCCUR? It can be related to a variety of factors including obesity, ingestion of a large amount of carbohydrates (for example, if a horse breaks into the grain room and consumes large quantities of grain, or if he's turned out on a green-grass pasture for an extended period of time), direct trauma to the feet from work on hard surfaces, metabolic diseases such as endotoxemia, or endocrine imbalances such as Cushing's disease.

DIAGNOSIS. An uncomplicated case of laminitis will be identified based on the characteristic signs of foot sensitivity and an increased intensity of the digital pulses. Radiographs will be recommended to evaluate the position of the coffin bones within the hooves. Because laminitis is often related to some underlying cause (such as Cushing's disease, peripheral metabolic syndrome, or endotoxemia), diagnostic steps, such as blood work to identify the underlying cause, are often needed.

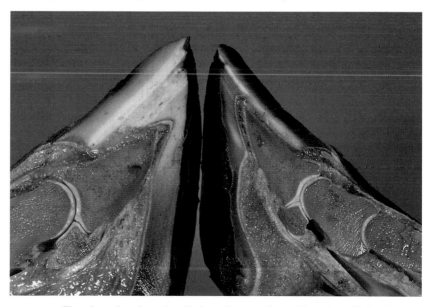

FIGURE 4.15. **The triangular-shaped coffin bone is normally positioned parallel to the hoof wall, as seen in the specimen on the right. When rotation of this bone occurs during a laminitis episode, it tips down, resulting in pressure on the sole.** (Photo courtesy of Jan Palmer, DVM, Diplomate ACVS)

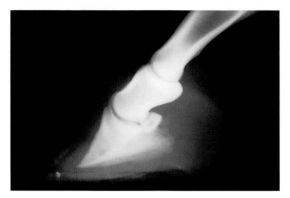

FIGURE 4.16. **Radiographs of the foundered horse's feet demonstrate the rotation of the coffin bone as seen here.** (Photo courtesy of Jan Palmer, DVM, Diplomate ACVS)

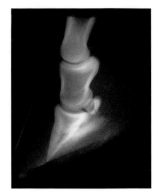

FIGURE 4.17. **In this severe case of founder, the coffin bone has rotated to the point of penetrating the sole of the foot—a situation that can easily be life threatening.** (Photo courtesy of Jan Palmer, DVM, Diplomate ACVS)

TREATMENT. If an underlying cause can be identified, treatment directed toward that cause may be critical for successful management. Recommendations for treating acute laminitis are varied, but will be directed toward reducing inflammation, improving blood flow by either dilating blood vessels or reducing clot formation, and providing physical support. Acute cases may be treated with intravenous DMSO to reduce inflammation as well as nonsteroidal anti-inflammatory medications, such as phenylbutazone or flunixin meglumine. Acepromazine injections can help improve blood flow to the feet during an acute episode. Oral isoxsuprine and topical nitroglycerine may also help resolve the disrupted blood flow. Immediate foot care may include squaring back the toes to reduce stress on the laminae at the front of the feet and taping foam pads to the feet to provide support. Rest and soft footing will be recommended.

Management of the horse with chronic laminitis is directed toward maintaining optimal foot balance to minimize stress to the laminae and help maintain stability of the coffin bone within the hoof. This includes careful shoeing to support the bone column, often with some type of bar shoe and supportive pad. Regular radiographic evaluation will be recommended to assess the position of the coffin bone and maintain optimal hoof balance.

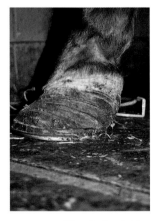

FIGURE 4.18. **Chronic laminitis leads to the abnormal shape and appearance of the hoof seen here.** (Photo courtesy of Jan Palmer, DVM, Diplomate ACVS)

In extremely severe cases, surgical options may be suggested as possible salvage procedures, including transection of (cutting) the deep digital flexor tendon to relieve stress on the coffin bone and slow rotation. For example, a mare in late-term pregnancy who founders severely might be a candidate for this procedure in order to save the foal. However, most of these procedures have a guarded prognosis for long-term success in a severely foundered horse.

HOW SERIOUS IS IT? A mild founder episode can be an isolated incident that resolves completely without long-term consequences if it's recognized early and treated appropriately. Severe founder is a very serious condition, however, that can often be life threatening.

POTENTIAL COMPLICATIONS. Abscesses that can progress to severe infections are common with serious founder cases, because of the pressure to the

The Horse's Body: Health and Disease

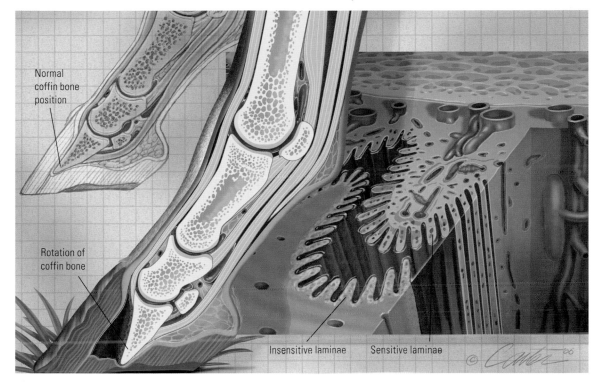

Normal
coffin bone
position

Rotation of
coffin bone

Insensitive laminae   Sensitive laminae

FIGURE 4.19. **With laminitis, weakening of the finger-like projections that hold the coffin bone in place within the hoof wall can lead to rotation of the coffin bone—a potentially life-threatening consequence.**

sole from the tip of the rotated coffin bone. If rotation is severe, it's possible for the toe of the coffin bone to penetrate the bottom of the sole, causing extreme pain and potentially irreversible damage to the bone.

Clubfoot   FIGURES 4.20–4.21

WHAT IT IS. A clubfoot is a defect in the alignment of the bones of the pastern and foot, resulting in a broken forward pastern/foot axis. Depending on the severity of the condition, the coffin bone will remodel or change its shape, due to abnormal stresses on the bone.

Clubfeet can be congenital or acquired. A congenital club foot may be hereditary, and is common in Arabians and Saddlebreds. An acquired clubfoot can develop secondary to another condition that is causing pain higher up the leg.

DIAGNOSIS. A clubfoot can be diagnosed based on its external appearance. It will have an elongated heel, upright position of the foot, and dished dorsal hoof wall. Radiographs will be recommended to evaluate the relationship of the pastern to the coffin bone, and the shape of the coffin bone.

TREATMENT. Treatment of the underlying condition is necessary to minimize development of an acquired clubfoot. A congenital clubfoot in a foal can be managed initially with regular trimming to lower the heels. The vet or farrier may recommend protection for the toe to prevent excessive wear, either with a steel toe shoe or acrylic material applied to the toe. Surgical cutting of the distal check ligament may be recommended to correct a severe clubfoot that is not responding to conservative treatment. Some veterinarians may recommend a single dose of the antibiotic oxytetracycline, which is believed to bind calcium and lead to relaxation of the tendons, to encourage the heel of the foot to drop. This treatment will be used in combination with support wraps or splints that allow relaxation and encourage stretching of the soft tissues. In a mature horse with an established clubfoot, a short shoeing interval and an experienced farrier will be necessary to maintain soundness.

HOW SERIOUS IS IT? Clubfeet result in asymmetries that can affect the horse's movement even in the absence of pain, causing actual lameness. The toe of the coffin bone often becomes traumatized, and abnormal stress to both the deep digital flexor tendon and the suspensory ligament can result in chronic lameness.

POTENTIAL COMPLICATIONS. Tendon and ligament injuries are likely in a horse with a clubfoot.

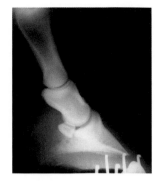

FIGURE 4.20. **This radiograph illustrates the normal shape and alignment of the coffin bone.** (Author photo)

Fractures   FIGURES 4.22–4.25

WHAT IT IS. A broken bone, which can include an unlimited number of specific injuries, depending on the bone involved and type of fracture. Usually, a fracture will appear as an acute, severe lameness, often following a known traumatic event. Fractures are classified in the following ways:

- COMPLETE. The fracture involves the whole bone.

- COMPOUND. The fracture fragments have penetrated the skin, often when a fracture is accompanied by a laceration.

- DISPLACED. The fragments are well separated.

- NONDISPLACED. There is a fracture line in the bone, but the pieces are still together in their normal orientation.

- CHIP. A small fragment of bone has broken away from a joint or section of bone.

- STRESS. A fracture line at the surface of the bone that has not completely penetrated.

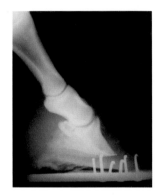

FIGURE 4.21. **With this clubfoot, the coffin bone is tipped down and remodeled into an abnormal shape.** (Author photo)

DIAGNOSIS. Most fractures will be identified on radiographs. Scintigraphy can be useful for nondisplaced fractures or stress fractures that do not show up on radiographs.

TREATMENT. Treatment for fractures varies widely. Complete, displaced fractures generally require surgery to repair with plates, screws, or other devices. Arthroscopic surgery will often be recommended for chip fractures involving joints. For stress fractures or nondisplaced fractures that appear stable, prolonged stall rest may be all that is necessary for successful healing.

HOW SERIOUS IS IT? A severe fracture can be life threatening, particularly if it involves one of the large upper bones of the upper leg that cannot be sur-

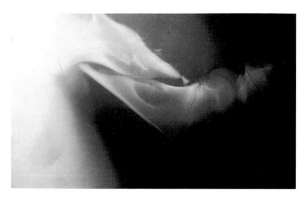

FIGURE 4.22. **This complete, displaced fracture would cause severe lameness and have a guarded prognosis for recovery.** (Photo courtesy of Jan Palmer, DVM, Diplomate ACVS)

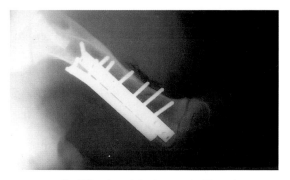

FIGURE 4.23. **Stabilization of the fracture with a plate may allow it to heal.** (Photo courtesy of Jan Palmer, DVM, Diplomate ACVS)

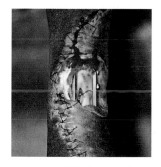

FIGURE 4.24. **This fracture is complicated by the fact that the bone has been exposed due to extensive damage to the skin.** (Photo courtesy of Jan Palmer, DVM, Diplomate ACVS)

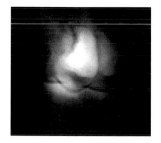

FIGURE 4.25. **This fractured sesamoid bone may be accompanied by damage to the attachment of the branch of the suspensory ligament in this area. A successful outcome is likely to require not only removal of the fracture fragment, but also treatment of the damaged ligament.** (Author photo)

gically repaired. Fractures involving joints generally have a poor prognosis compared with fractures where joints are not involved.

POTENTIAL COMPLICATIONS. Osteoarthritis is always a concern when a joint surface is disrupted by a fracture.

Splints   FIGURES 4.26–4.27

WHAT IT IS Inflammation of the interosseous ligament that lies between the small splint bone and the cannon bone. The periosteum, or lining of the splint bone, may also become inflamed, resulting in a visible bony bump. Splints can occur because of a direct trauma, such as a blow from the horse's opposite foot, or secondary to the stress of hard work. Most commonly they occur on the inside of the forelimbs, although they can be found on the inside or outside of all four legs. Splints are common in youngsters first beginning work.

DIAGNOSIS. Lameness may or may not be present. If the splint occurs on the inside of the forelimb, the horse is most likely to be lame when lunged with the affected leg on the outside of the circle. If the splint is not palpable or visible, diagnostic blocks of the affected area may help pinpoint the abnormality. A visible bump that's painful when pressure is applied may be enough to confirm a diagnosis. Radiographs may provide more complete information about the degree of bone response. Sometimes, the small splint bone may actually fracture, which would show on radiographs.

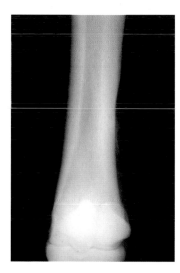

FIGURE 4.26. **This fracture at the end of the splint bone is surrounded by new bone as it attempts to heal itself. However, surgical removal of the fractured tip of the bone may still be recommended if the healing is unsuccessful.** (Author photo)

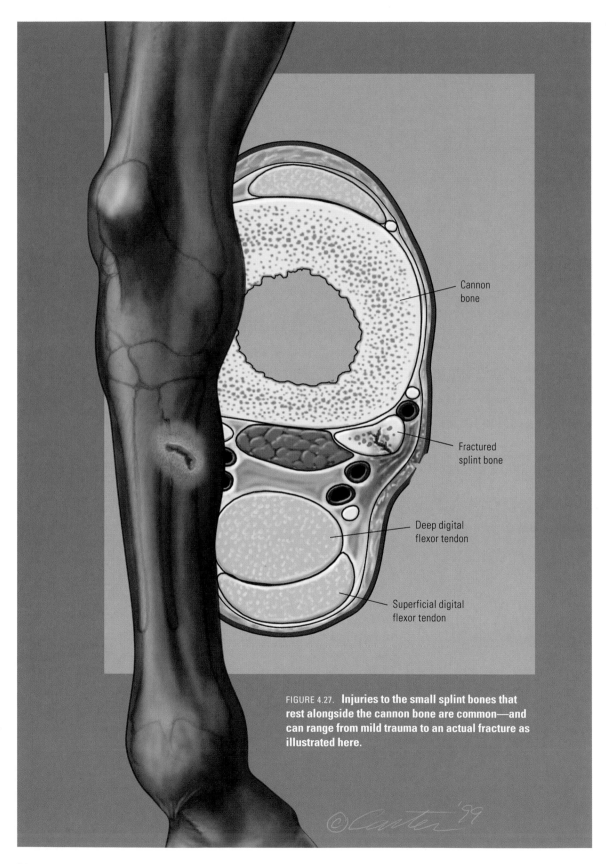

Cannon
bone

Fractured
splint bone

Deep digital
flexor tendon

Superficial digital
flexor tendon

FIGURE 4.27. **Injuries to the small splint bones that rest alongside the cannon bone are common—and can range from mild trauma to an actual fracture as illustrated here.**

The Horse's Body: Health and Disease

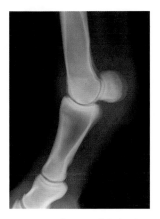

FIGURE 4.28. **A normal fetlock appears smooth along the margins of the joint space as seen on this radiograph.**

(Author photo)

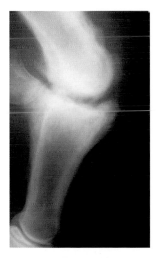

FIGURE 4.29. **The proliferation of bone at the margins of the fetlock joint seen on this radiograph is a sign of severe degenerative joint disease or arthritis.**

(Photo courtesy of Jan Palmer, DVM, Diplomate ACVS)

TREATMENT. If a splint is small, and the horse is not demonstrating any lameness, no treatment may be required. Rest and anti-inflammatories may be recommended if a splint is more severe. Topical treatment with an anti-inflammatory, such as DMSO, DMSO combined with a corticosteroid, or diclofenamic acid (Surpass®), can help quiet the area. In some cases, the area will be injected with an anti-inflammatory for more direct and effective treatment. Rarely, a fractured splint may require surgery to either remove the lower portion of the bone or stabilize and repair the fractured area.

HOW SERIOUS IS IT? Most splints will heal without complications, although it can take as long as 6 to 8 weeks for a lameness to completely resolve. A fractured splint that requires surgery to repair or remove will have a longer healing time, depending on the amount of damage and disruption.

POTENTIAL COMPLICATIONS. If the bony reaction of a splint is very large, it's possible for it to interfere with the suspensory ligament, resulting in damage to that structure (see page 88). A splint that's placed high can interfere with the knee joint and cause problems.

Degenerative Joint Disease (DJD) FIGURES 4.28–4.30

WHAT IT IS. A progressive deterioration of the joints leading to osteoarthritis, believed to be primarily due to mechanical stresses that result in damage to the cartilage at the joint surface. It has been proposed that underlying abnormalities of the cartilage structure predisposes the horse to degenerative joint disease and eventual development of arthritis.

DJD begins with stress to the periarticular structures, or the ligaments and other soft-tissue structures that provide support to the joint. The synovium becomes inflamed, resulting in the release of enzymes and other substances that can cause damage to the cartilage lining the joint. In response to this sequence of events, osteophytes (bone spurs) may form at the joint surface as the tissues attempt to stabilize the joint. At this point, the degenerative joint disease cycle has progressed to osteoarthritis.

Two specifically named diseases that are in this disease category are bone spavin (arthritis of the lower hock joints) and ringbone (arthritis of the pastern joint) (see pages 83 and 85).

DIAGNOSIS. Degenerative joint disease is characterized by lameness, a decrease in range of motion of the affected joint due to stiffening of the support structures in an attempt to stabilize the joint and reduce pain, and effusion (fluid) buildup within the joint. Stress tests of the affected joint will be positive. If these signs are observed, diagnostic blocks may be performed to confirm that the abnormal appearing joint is truly the source of the lameness.

Radiographs of the joint in question will be recommended in most cases, although they are not always a very sensitive diagnostic tool. Significant radiographic changes are usually only seen when the condition is fairly advanced. Subtle changes, such as a narrowing of the joint space, may be detected early in the course of the disease.

More advanced diagnostics, including scintigraphy and MRI, may provide better information during the early stages of joint disease. In recent years, techniques for evaluating the joint using ultrasound have proved useful for early signs of degenerative joint disease.

TREATMENT. NSAIDS will be recommended as a part of the basic management plan for most horses with degenerative joint disease. Joint injections with cortisone to reduce inflammation and with hyaluronic acid to improve nutrition and lubrication of the joint are likely to be recommended. Systemic treatments focused on improving joint health, including polysulfated glycosaminoglycans (Adequan®) and hyaluronic acid (Legend®) as well as oral joint supplements containing chondroitin sulfate, or glucosamine may be prescribed as well.

HOW SERIOUS IS IT? Degenerative joint disease is one of the most important, performance-limiting problems seen in athletic horses. It can progress to the point where chronic lameness prohibits the horse from continued use.

POTENTIAL COMPLICATIONS. Complications secondary to joint injections used for treatment are possible, including infection within the joint that can be life threatening.

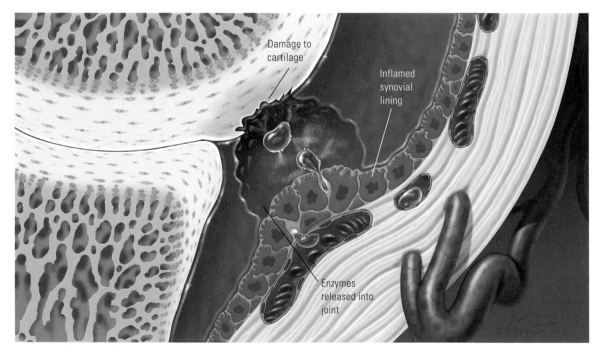

FIGURE 4.30. **Inflammation causes the release of enzymes into the joint and that can ultimately damage the cartilage lining and underlying bone, resulting in degenerative joint disease.**

The Horse's Body: Health and Disease

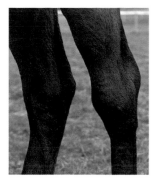

FIGURE 4.31. **The fluid accumulating in these hock joints, commonly called bog spavin, may be a sign of a more serious problem within the joint.**

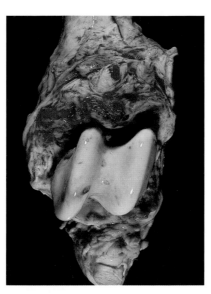

FIGURE 4.32. **Damage on the gliding surface of this hock, typical of degenerative joint disease, can easily be seen on this specimen.** (Author photo)

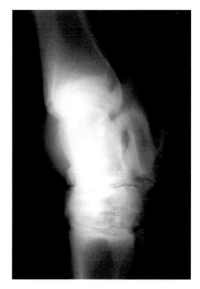

FIGURE 4.34. **In this severe case of bone spavin or hock arthritis there is an extensive amount of bone proliferation at the joint margins, as well as obvious collapse of the joint spaces.** (Author photo)

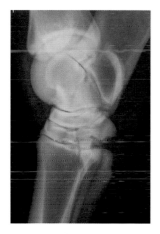

FIGURE 4.33. **A normal hock has four visible joint spaces and smooth edges surrounding the joint margins.** (Author photo)

Bone Spavin (Hock Osteoarthritis) FIGURES 4.31–4.35

WHAT IT IS. Arthritis of the hocks, usually involving the lower two (low motion) joint spaces. Many performance horses experience hock pain as a result of stresses to these joints, which can appear as an acute lameness, or simply as a decline in performance and noticeable stiffness or laziness of the hind limbs. A syndrome of juvenile-onset bone spavin has been described in young horses and is believed to be related to developmental orthopedic disease.

DIAGNOSIS. Hock pain may be suspected in a horse that becomes unwilling to work, drags his toes behind, or begins to have difficulty holding his canter leads behind (changes leads with the hind legs while cantering), or performing flying lead changes. He may have positive flexion tests observed during a lameness examination, although many horses with degenerative joint disease of the hocks continue to have a normal flexion response. Diagnostic blocks of the lower hock joints may help confirm a diagnosis of hock pain, and radiographs will show signs of osteoarthritis in advanced cases. Although it is rarely necessary to make a diagnosis, inflammation of the lower hock joints will be seen on nuclear scintigraphy images.

TREATMENT. Injections of the lower hock joints with cortisone, with or without hyaluronic acid, are likely to be recommended for a confirmed case of bone spavin. Joint treatments including Legend®, Adequan®, or oral chondroitin sulfate/glucosamine supplements may be beneficial. Non-steroidal anti-inflammatory medications will usually be recommended

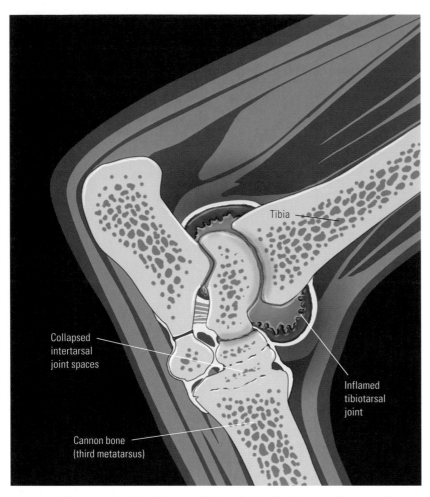

Tibia

Collapsed
intertarsal
joint spaces

Inflamed
tibiotarsal
joint

Cannon bone
(third metatarsus)

FIGURE 4.35. **Degenerative joint disease of the hock often includes cartilage erosion at the joint surface as well as proliferation of bone along the margins. As the condition progresses, the joint spaces may completely collapse and fuse together.**

to help manage the condition. A number of more aggressive treatments are occasionally recommended for cases that do not respond well to treatment. These include surgery to fuse the lower joints to prevent movement, thus minimizing discomfort, and extracorporeal shockwave therapy, which is theorized to reduce pain.

HOW SERIOUS IS IT? Most horses with degenerative joint disease of the hocks can be managed and continue as performance horses, even at the highest levels. However, it can be performance-limiting in some cases, due to chronic lameness.

POTENTIAL COMPLICATIONS. Some practitioners believe that degenerative joint disease of the hocks is a risk factor for injury to the proximal suspensory ligament of the hind limbs. Complications due to repeated corticosteroid injections are possible, including joint infection or weakening of the small bones within the joint, which can lead to fractures.

The Horse's Body: Health and Disease

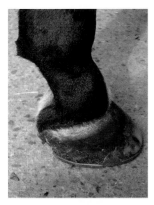

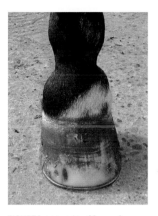

FIGURES 4.36–4.37. **The enlargement of this horse's pastern joint is easily visible from every angle.** (Author photos)

Ringbone (Pastern or Coffin Joint Osteoarthritis)   FIGURES 4.36–4.38

WHAT IT IS. Arthritis of the pastern joint (high ringbone) or coffin joint (low ringbone). A horse with ringbone will often be extremely lame as a result of osteoarthritis of one of these two lower joints. Classic ringbone involves the pastern joint, and often appears as a visible bony enlargement over the pastern area.

DIAGNOSIS. High ringbone can often be diagnosed based on the typical appearance of this condition. Response to nerve blocks will confirm the location of the lameness, and radiographs will confirm the presence of arthritis.

TREATMENT. Initial treatment will usually involve trimming or shoeing to shorten the toes and potentially raise the heels in an effort to relieve stress during breakover. This is done in combination with administering non-steroidal anti-inflammatory medications to relieve pain and minimize lameness. Joint treatments such as IV Legend) or (IM Adequan® may be recommended, as well as oral supplementation with chondroitin sulfate or glucosamine. In certain instances, joint injections with hyaluronic acid and corticosteroids can be extremely help-ful. Because the pastern is a low-motion joint, surgery to arthrodese (fuse) the joint may be suggested for advanced cases. This surgical procedure eliminates movement in the joint, thus eliminating pain.

HOW SERIOUS IS IT? Ringbone is usually performance limiting owing to some degree of lameness. Sometimes, a horse with this condition will be extremely lame.

POTENTIAL COMPLICATIONS. Complications due to repeated corticosteroid injections may be a consequence, including joint infection or weakening of the bones surrounding the joint.

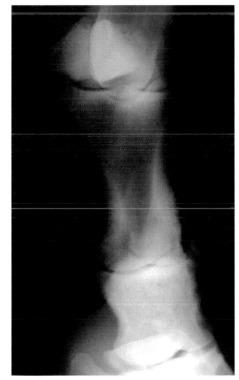

FIGURE 4.38. **On radiographs, the bony proliferation that creates the enlargement can be seen.** (Author photo)

Osteochondrosis FIGURE 4.39

WHAT IT IS. Osteochondrosis is an abnormality in joint development. It results in abnormal bone and cartilage either at the surface of the joints or in the form of bone cysts just below the surface of the joints. If an osteochondrosis lesion results in a loose flap of cartilage or cartilage and bone at the surface of the joint, it is referred to as an osteochondrosis dessicans. *(Note: All types of osteochondrosis are commonly called OCD by horsemen, an inaccurate term that should be reserved for cases where an actual fragment of bone or cartilage is present.)* Osteochondrosis most commonly occurs in the stifle, hock, fetlock, and shoulder joints, although it can appear in any joint of the body.

Causes for osteochondrosis are widely varied, and include heredity, nutrition and trauma. Studies show that certain factors are important to minimize the conditions. These include proper, balanced feeding of trace minerals including copper, zinc and manganese; calcium: phosphorous ratios of the diet; and appropriate amounts of energy (calories) to pregnant mares as well as foals during the first months of life . A recent study that examined a large number of young horses conclusively demonstrated that adequate exercise for youngsters was critical for lessening the risk of osteochondrosis.

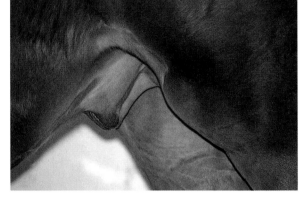

DIAGNOSIS. Osteochondrosis will be suspected with lameness in a young horse, especially if a fluid accumulation (called effusion) is detected in a joint at the same time. Lesions can be identified on radiographs. In many cases, osteochondrosis lesions are detected on radiographs taken of young horses during prepurchase examinations or other screening examinations before associated lameness is detected.

TREATMENT. Treatment for osteochondrosis will depend on the location and type of lesion. Surgical removal of bone fragments and unhealthy cartilage at the surface of the joints may be recommended, particularly for large defects on important, weight-bearing surfaces of the joints. In other cases, treatment will not be necessary.

Treatment with substances targeted to help promote joint health such as polysulfated glycosaminoglycan (Adequan®) or hyaluronic acid (Legend®) may be recommended.

HOW SERIOUS IS IT? Severity of osteochondrosis depends on the location and type of lesion. In some cases, severe performance-threatening lameness is likely. In others, long-term consequences are minimal.

POTENTIAL COMPLICATIONS. Degenerative joint disease may develop in a joint affected by osteochondrosis due to instability and uneven stresses across the joint surface.

FIGURE 4.39. **The fluid buildup, called effusion, in this horse's stifle joint, can be easily seen, and is a common finding with osteochondrosis.** (Photo courtesy of Jan Palmer, DVM, Diplomate ACVS)

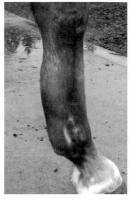

FIGURE 4.40. **This visible enlargement of the tendons at the back of the cannon bone is typical of a severe tendonitis or bowed tendon.** (Author photo)

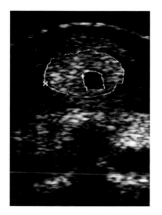

FIGURE 4.41. **The circular area that appears dark in the center of the deep digital flexor tendon, seen on this ultrasound image, represents a serious tendon injury.** (Author photo)

Tendonitis   FIGURES 4.40–4.42

WHAT IT IS. Injury or strain to one of the tendons of the lower leg, most commonly the superficial or deep flexor tendon. This condition is referred to as a "bowed tendon" in horsemen's terms.

DIAGNOSIS. A visible and/or palpable swelling is usually present, and the horse will be lame on the affected leg. If necessary, diagnostic blocks can be performed to confirm that the swollen tendon is actually the source of the lameness. Ultrasound examination will help pinpoint the actual structure involved and quantify the extent of the damage.

TREATMENT. Treatment varies according to the degree of injury, intended use of the horse, and veterinarian's preferences. In the acute stage, ice, rest, and anti-inflammatory medications, such as flunixin meglumine or phenylbutazone, will be recommended. To help stimulate good, strong healing a rehabilitation program will be suggested that involves gradually increasing the periods of controlled exercise. (See Table 4.1.) Movement is beneficial because the gentle stress applied along the tendon encourages fibers to heal in a normal, linear pattern. Extracorporeal shockwave therapy, which involves stimulation of the area with pressure waves, has proven to be beneficial for speeding up the healing process. Injection of

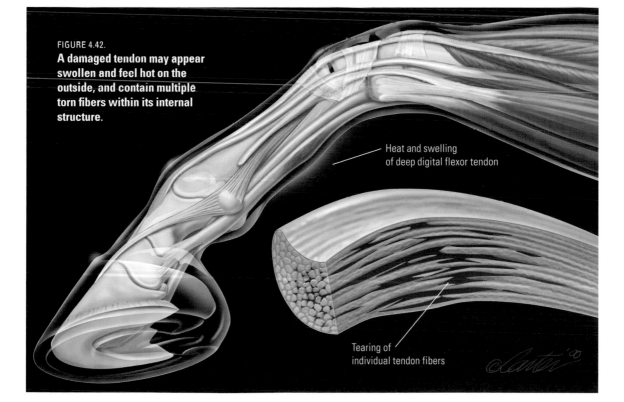

FIGURE 4.42.
A damaged tendon may appear swollen and feel hot on the outside, and contain multiple torn fibers within its internal structure.

Heat and swelling
of deep digital flexor tendon

Tearing of
individual tendon fibers

various substances into the damaged area may be advised if healing is not progressing favorably after a period of time.

HOW SERIOUS IS IT? The consequences of a tendon injury vary widely depending on the location and extent of injury. A simple tendon injury that heals well means the horse is likely to be sound and back at work within a period of several months. If he has a very demanding job, such as racing or jumping, however, his injured tendon may not hold up to his previous work demands. If a tendon is injured in a location where it runs underneath a tendon sheath, it may cause long-lasting pressure within the sheath and chronic lameness.

POTENTIAL COMPLICATIONS. Annular ligament constriction requiring surgical correction. Tenosynovitis. Chronic lameness.

Proximal Suspensory Desmitis (PSD) FIGURES 4.43–4.44

WHAT IT IS. Injury or strain to the suspensory ligament in the lower leg, at its point of attachment at the back of the cannon bone. A horse with this problem will exhibit a consistent lameness that appears most severe when the affected leg is on the outside of a circle. The problem can occur in both the front and hind limbs, and may have a slow, insidious onset. In other cases, the horse will suddenly become very lame. There is usually no detectable heat or swelling associated with this injury.

DIAGNOSIS. The veterinarian will perform a full lameness examination. Typically, a horse with a proximal suspensory injury will have a positive response to flexion of the fetlock and knee (front) or fetlock and hock (hind). The lameness will improve when the origin of the suspensory ligament is blocked, and an ultrasound examination will confirm the diagnosis and determine the extent of damage. Radiographs might be recommended to determine whether there has been damage to the top of the cannon bone at the point of attachment of the ligament. In some instances, small fragments of bone may be pulled away.

TREATMENT. Rest in a confined area and a very careful rehabilitation program are at the core of the recommended treatment. (See Table 4.1.) Extracorporeal shockwave therapy has proved very useful for this condition, and a series of three treatments might be recommended at 2 to 3-week intervals to help stimulate healing. Some practitioners might suggest injecting the area with anti-inflammatories such as cortisone or a combination of cortisone and hyaluronic acid. Although this can be very helpful for reducing initial inflammation, caution must be taken with this approach for a number of reasons. Immediate improvement may be seen with a resolution of lameness. However, if the horse is put back into work too soon, reinjury is likely. Complications such as calcification of the soft tissues or infection at the injection site are also possible.

HOW SERIOUS IS IT? A proximal suspensory injury can be a very serious, performance-limiting problem. The incidence of recurrence is high, and

Soft-Tissue Rehabilitation

Many soft-tissue injuries require a careful rehabilitation program to allow for proper healing. Low-stress, repetitive movement such as walking under saddle is ideal because the movement encourages tendons, ligaments, and even muscles to heal with proper alignment of individual fibers rather than with disorganized scar tissue. The following rules for basic rehabilitation apply:

- All walking and trotting should be performed in straight lines on solid, even footing. Lateral movements should be discouraged due to uneven stresses that can result.
- If necessary, sedation should be administered to the horse to keep him quiet in his stall and maintain control during exercise sessions.
- Evaluation of lameness and ultrasound examination should be performed at regular intervals to assess healing. These exams are generally best scheduled prior to increasing the workload, and increases in exercise intensity should only happen if healing is progressing well.
- Introduction of canter work, circles, or other sports-specific activities should occur gradually, only after the horse has been trotting for 25 to 30 minutes daily for at least 2 weeks, with no setbacks in the healing process.

---

severe damage may be extremely slow to heal. Expect a minimum of 3 to as many as 12 months of rest and rehabilitation following this diagnosis. POTENTIAL COMPLICATIONS Fragmentation of the bone at the site of the injury is a potential complication of this injury.

Degenerative Suspensory Ligament Desmitis (DSLD) FIGURE 4.45

WHAT IT IS. DSLD is a progressive degeneration of the suspensory ligaments, most commonly seen in both hind legs of older horses. An inherited form of this disease is seen in Peruvian Paso horses that affects all four legs, often appears at a younger age, and may involve other soft-tissue structures throughout the body in that breed.

Typically, a horse with DSLD will have enlarged, dropped hind fetlocks, with palpable enlargement of the branches of the suspensory ligaments. The hocks and stifles become very straight over time, resulting in a post-legged appearance, with the fetlocks having more angulation than normal. In severe cases, the fetlock joint might even come close to touching the ground. The horse will usually be very sore, and may shift his weight between the two hind legs. Flexion tests performed on the hind fetlocks will have a very strong positive result.

FIGURE 4.45. **The enlarged, dropped fetlock seen here is typical for degenerative suspensory ligament desmitis, a severe progressive condition.** (Photo courtesy of Scott Wenzel)

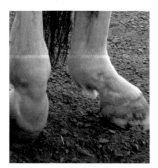

TABLE 4.1

Sample Program

This is a moderately aggressive rehabilitation program that might be recommended for the initial 10 weeks following a soft-tissue injury such as a superficial or deep digital flexor tendonitis. *(Note: Timing and medication for rehabilitation will vary with the location and severity of a particular injury. Consult with your vet before embarking on a specific program with your horse.)*

TIME FOLLOWING INJURY	EXERCISE	PHYSICAL THERAPY OPTIONS	MEDICATION	VETERINARY EVALUATION
Week 1	Stall rest.	Ice injury area.	NSAIDS.	Lameness examination and diagnosis. Ultrasound exam.
Week 2	Stall rest.	Ice injury area.	NSAIDS.	None.
Week 3	10–15 minute walk.	Ice injury area after work.	None.	None.
Week 4	20–30 minute walk.	Ice injury area after work.	None.	None.
Week 5	30 minute walk, 2 minute trot.	Ice injury area after work.	None.	Evaluation of lameness. Ultrasound exam.
Week 6	30 minute walk, 5 minute trot.	Ice injury area after work.	None.	None.
Week 7	30 minute walk, 10 minute trot.	Ice injury area after work.	None.	None.
Week 8	30 minute walk, 15 minute trot.	Ice injury area after work.	None.	None.
Week 9	30 minute walk, 20 minute trot.	Ice injury area after work.	None.	None.
Week 10	30 minute walk, 25 minute trot.	Ice injury area after work.	None.	Evaluation of lameness. Ultrasound exam.

DIAGNOSIS. Most cases of DSLD in older horses can be diagnosed simply based on the appearance of the legs, and a strong response to flexion. Abnormalities of the suspensory ligaments can be seen with ultrasound examination. Diagnosis of the condition in Peruvian Pasos can be more difficult in the early stages, as signs are subtle. Positive flexion tests and pain with palpation of the branches of the suspensory ligament are the most sensitive and consistent diagnostic tests for these horses.

TREATMENT. This is a progressive disease that does not respond well to treatment. Shoeing with heel extensions may help provide support for the fetlocks and may make the horse more comfortable. NSAIDS may also be administered for pain relief.

HOW SERIOUS IS IT? This disease is progressive, extremely painful, and often leads to euthanasia when the horse becomes too uncomfortable to manage.
POTENTIAL COMPLICATIONS. None.

Curb

WHAT IT IS. Injury to one of the structures that run along the back of the hock, including the plantar ligament, deep digital flexor tendon, or superficial digital flexor tendon. The horse may or may not be lame, depending on the specific structure injured and the degree of injury.

DIAGNOSIS. Ultrasound of the area will be recommended for a horse with an enlargement at the back of the hock typical of a curb. In some cases, radiographs might demonstrate an underlying bony abnormality.

TREATMENT. Treatment recommendations will vary depending on the specific injury. Nonsteroidal anti-inflammatory medications are likely to be recommended. Shockwave therapy might be suggested to encourage healing of a tendon or ligament.

HOW SERIOUS IS IT? If serious, injuries may be performance limiting due to marked lameness.

POTENTIAL COMPLICATIONS. None.

Extracorporeal Shockwave Therapy

Shockwave therapy is a treatment modality that's gained popularity in recent years for treating a wide variety of lameness problems. This therapy involves a device that allows the veterinarian to pass pressure waves through the tissues, and has been most successful for treating soft-tissue injuries such as proximal suspensory desmitis. The precise mechanisms within the tissues are still not completely understood, although tendon and ligament tears seem to heal faster, stronger, and with better alignment of the tissues (fewer scar tissues) when shockwave treatment is used. A typical treatment course would involve a series of three treatments at 2-week intervals for most soft-tissue injuries.

Shockwave therapy is also used for some bone and joint conditions, such as fractures that are slow to heal and even cases of osteoarthritis. Again, the mechanisms aren't completely clear, but treatment success has been reported by some practitioners.

It has been well established that shockwave therapy results in short-term pain relief for some conditions, primarily due to its impact on innervation of the tissues that are treated. For this reason, it must be used with extreme caution to prevent a horse from causing further damage when an injury first feels better following treatment. Because of these effects, the use of this treatment has been restricted prior to competition in some disciplines.

Upward Fixation of the Patella ("Locking" Stifles) FIGURE 4.46

WHAT IT IS. The medial and middle patellar ligaments hook over the medial trochlea of the femur (the enlarged portion at the inside of the bottom of the bone) causing the stifle joint to become locked into extension. Although this locking is a part of the normal functioning of the stifle under some circumstances, it becomes a problem when it happens inappropriately. In severe cases, the hind limb actually becomes "stuck" and the horse is unable to bend the stifle or hock joints to take a step. More mildly affected horses will experience intermittent locking or "catching" of this joint. This condition is most likely to occur in horses with straight hind limb conformation, and may have a hereditary component. It is prevalent in young horses or ponies, especially if they are lacking muscle development.

DIAGNOSIS. In severe cases, a locked stifle is easy to identify in a horse where the limb is stuck in extension. More subtle cases can be detected by a characteristic catching observed in the stifle area, often accompanied by a popping sound. In some situations, the horse will appear to trip

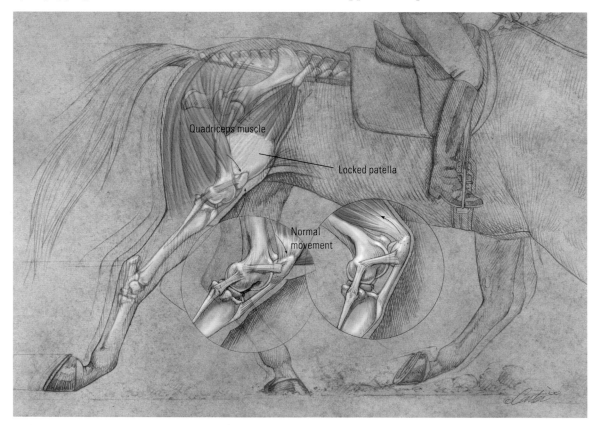

FIGURE 4.46. **Upward fixation of the patella or "locking" stifles occurs when the patella becomes trapped over the enlarged inner portion of the femur due to a loop that forms between the inner (medial) and middle patellar ligaments. The limb will lock into extension, which may prevent the horse from bending his leg and lead to a visible "catching," stumbling, or complete inability to move.**

behind by catching a toe, as the delayed flexion of the upper joints prevents him from bringing his foot underneath his body in time. The vet can often manipulate the stifle into a locked position in order to identify inappropriate laxity (looseness) of the joint.

If lameness is present in addition to the catching or locking, diagnostic blocks may be advised to determine whether the lameness is actually coming from the stifle. Radiographs of the stifle joint might also be suggested, as some horses with this problem have underlying abnormalities within the joint.

TREATMENT. If the horse is stuck in the locked position, he can usually be unlocked by asking him to step backwards. If this is unsuccessful, the vet can manually manipulate the patella while asking the horse to move in order to unlock it. For recurrent cases, the first stage of treatment usually involves exercises to strengthen the quadriceps muscle group, which may include sets of backing up, hill work, or work over cavalletti. Shoeing modifications might also be recommended. For example, wedges to raise the heels can help by closing up the angles of the hind legs.

If there has been no improvement within 60 to 90 days of careful conditioning, the vet might suggest injecting the medial and middle patellar ligaments with an irritant (usually some combination of iodine in oil). This treatment causes scarring, which ultimately shortens the ligaments to reduce the incidence of locking. Although it is very effective in many cases, it does result in permanent scar tissue. Most practitioners agree that it's best to correct the problem through strengthening before using this technique.

Finally, there are a number of surgical treatments that can be applied for severe cases that fail to respond to more conservative treatments. Traditionally, a medial patellar desmotomy (cutting the medial patellar ligament) has been the surgical treatment of choice. Although this procedure is successful for solving the problem, it has been associated with consequential long-term negative effects. These include fractures of the patella and instability of the joint that then leads to arthritis. Recently, newer surgical techniques, including the "splitting" of the medial patellar ligament (performing a series of small incisions into the ligament to encourage it to scar and shorten as it heals), have been suggested, with good results.

HOW SERIOUS IS IT? This condition can cause the horse a significant amount of discomfort and anxiety, and often limits performance. However, the majority of affected horses will respond well to conservative treatment and the condition is usually manageable.

POTENTIAL COMPLICATIONS. If the locking or catching is persistent, damage to the joint can occur, leading to more serious lameness.

Sacroiliac Desmitis or Osteoarthritis FIGURE 4.47

WHAT IT IS. Problems in the sacroiliac region are generally due to a ligament injury in the sacroiliac ligaments (desmitis) or arthritis of the flat, immobile sacroiliac joints themselves. These problems produce a wide range of symptoms that primarily result in poor performance, including low-grade hind limb lameness, dragging of one or both hind limbs, poor pushing power (propulsion) in the hind limbs during work, and general resistance. There may be a visible asymmetry of the hindquarters, and the horse may be painful to palpation over the sacroiliac area.

DIAGNOSIS. Specific diagnosis of these problems can be very challenging. Scintigraphy is the most useful diagnostic tool in the majority of cases. Diagnostic blocks of the area are possible, although they are difficult to perform and not always as specific as they need to be to pinpoint problems. Ultrasound examination can be helpful in enabling very experienced practitioners to identify ligament injuries.

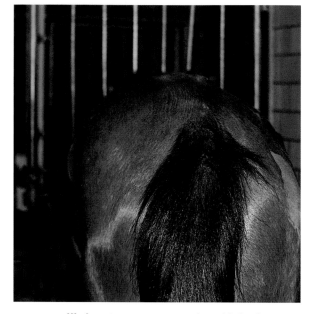

FIGURE 4.47. **Hindquarter asymmetry such as this is often seen with conditions involving the sacroiliac ligaments or joints.** (Photo courtesy of Jan Palmer, DVM, Diplomate ACVS)

TREATMENT. Treatment is almost as frustrating as diagnosis for sacroiliac problems. Many affected horses respond well to alternative therapies, including acupuncture and chiropractic manipulation. The sacroiliac joint can be injected with cortisone and/or long-acting blocking agents, and sometimes shockwave therapy can be helpful.

HOW SERIOUS IS IT? Sacroiliac problems tend to be chronic and frustrating, meaning they can have a serious impact on long-term performance.

POTENTIAL COMPLICATIONS. None.

Fibrotic or Ossifying Myopathy

WHAT IT IS. An injury to the hamstring muscles that heals with scarring or calcification of the muscle tissue. These injuries commonly occur with hyperextension of the hocks and stifles. This can happen, for example, during a sliding stop performed by a reining horse, when a horse slips in the pasture with his hind legs extended underneath his body, or when a horse pulls back when tied. A reaction to an intramuscular injection in this part of the body can also cause this problem. A horse with fibrotic myopathy will exhibit a typical gait pattern where the hind legs slap down to the ground after the forward phase of the stride, like a "goose step."

DIAGNOSIS. Fibrotic myopathy can usually be diagnosed based on the typical clinical appearance, along with palpation of scar tissue in the hamstring muscles.

The Horse's Body: Health and Disease

TREATMENT. Once present, this condition is difficult to treat. Surgical resection of the scarred area may be recommended, and can be beneficial in some cases. If an acute muscle injury occurs to this area, aggressive treatment to minimize inflammation, in combination with a careful physical therapy program, can help minimize the chances that scarring or calcification will occur.

HOW SERIOUS IS IT? Established fibrotic myopathy is usually a mechanical lameness, meaning the horse exhibits the gait abnormality because of the loss of range of motion of the affected muscle, although he does not experience pain. The condition can be performance-limiting in some cases but most horses will be able to maintain some level of work.

POTENTIAL COMPLICATIONS. None.

Exertional Rhabdomyolysis
(Tying-Up, Azoturia, or Monday Morning Disease)

WHAT IT IS. The muscles suddenly cramp and individual muscle cells break down at the onset of exercise. The horse will suddenly become stiff and reluctant to move. He may sweat and paw due to pain. A horse is most likely to tie up if he is asked to exercise after a period of rest—particularly if he has been fed full rations during the rest period.

DIAGNOSIS. An episode of exertional rhabdomyolysis is usually recognized due to typical symptoms, along with a palpable hardening of the muscles of the hindquarters—the most commonly affected area of the horse's body. Blood tests will show elevations of enzymes released during breakdown of muscles (AST and CPK), and will also be recommended to evaluate the horse's hydration status and kidney function following an episode.

TREATMENT. When a horse begins to tie up, exercise should be discontinued. For mild cases, a dose of acepromazine (a common tranquilizer) will be recommended to help relax the horse, relieve anxiety, and improve blood flow through the muscles by its effect of dilating blood vessels. In more severe cases, oral or intravenous fluids will be recommended to ensure that the horse is well hydrated and to help protect the kidneys. Myoglobin released during muscle breakdown can be extremely damaging to the kidneys, especially if the horse is dehydrated. The horse should be closely monitored for darkening of the urine, an indicator that myoglobin is present. Following an episode, care must be taken to avoid a recurrence when the horse is returning to work. In general, to minimize the risk of tying up, carefully return the horse to work after a period of rest.

HOW SERIOUS IS IT? This disease can range from a mild, isolated occurrence that has few long-term effects to a severe, recurrent condition that causes ongoing problems for the horse. If the horse has recurrent episodes, the veterinarian may recommend further diagnostic tests such as a muscle biopsy to determine whether there is an underlying muscle abnormality. Diet and management changes may be recommended. (See below.)

POTENTIAL COMPLICATIONS. Muscle breakdown products released during a serious bout of exertional rhabdomyolysis can damage the kidneys—even to the point of causing kidney failure. Although it is tempting to administer nonsteroidal anti-inflammatory medications (such as flunixin meglumine or phenylbutazone) to provide pain relief when a horse ties up, this should be discouraged due to the risk of further kidney damage with these medications.

Equine Polysaccharide Storage Myopathy (EPSM)

WHAT IT IS. Abnormal storage of sugars, including a form of stored energy called glycogen, in the muscles. This muscle abnormality can result in episodes of tying-up, weakness, muscle spasms, hind limb lameness, and exercise intolerance. An affected horse may even exhibit colic symptoms, and during a severe episode, the horse may go down and be unable to stand. The disease occurs at all ages and in all breeds of horses, although it is most common in draft horses, ponies, Quarter Horses, and some warmbloods.

DIAGNOSIS. Episodes of tying-up may be observed, and confirmed, with increased levels of the muscle enzymes (CPK and AST) in the blood. If suspected, the disease can be confirmed with a muscle biopsy, where abnormal amounts of polysaccharides are seen within muscle cells. The veterinarian may also recommend measurement of blood selenium levels, which can be low in affected horses.

TREATMENT. Treatment during an acute episode is similar to that described for exertional rhapdomyolysis. (See above.) Long-term treatment depends on diet changes that include the elimination of carbohydrates (grain) and the addition of fat. The goal is to provide approximately 20 to 25 percent of the total daily calories from fat. Either grass or alfalfa hay, or a combination of both, can still be fed. Fat can be added to the diet in a number of different ways. The least complicated way is the addition of corn oil to the horse's ration, poured over a low-carbohydrate pellet such as alfalfa pellets. As with all diet changes, oil should be added gradually. Begin with ¼ cup of oil daily, and increase to approximately 2 cups daily over a period of 2 to 3 weeks for the average 1000-pound horse. If the horse won't tolerate oil in the diet, a number of high-fat supplements such as rice bran can be used as an alternative. It takes 4 months for muscles to completely fat-adapt and for the full benefits of the diet to be observed, although many horses will demonstrate a noticeable improvement after as little as 1 to 2 weeks.

If blood selenium levels are low, selenium can also be supplemented. However, because of the narrow toxicity range of this mineral, levels should be rechecked following diet adjustments and reduced if needed.

In some horses, selenium levels will increase following diet changes, even without additional supplementation.

HOW SERIOUS IS IT? EPSM can be a serious condition that affects the horse's ability to move. Even mildly affected horses may experience compromised performance. The good news is that most affected horses respond well to diet changes, with significant improvement in performance.

POTENTIAL COMPLICATIONS. If EPSM is associated with severe tying-up, muscle-breakdown products can damage kidneys and lead to kidney failure.

Hyperkalemic Periodic Paralysis (HYPP)

WHAT IT IS. A genetic disease seen in Quarter Horses that traces back to the sire named Impressive. Horses with HYPP have an abnormality in the exchange of electrolytes (sodium and potassium) across muscle cells. This abnormality causes them to have periodic episodes of weakness, muscle fasiculations (twitching), sweating, and cramping. During severe episodes, the horse may stagger and even collapse. Typical episodes last between 15 and 60 minutes, and an affected horse will appear completely normal between episodes.

HYPP has autosomal dominant inheritance, meaning a horse will be affected if it has a single gene inherited from either the mother or the father, and that any affected horse has at least a 50 percent chance of passing the disease on to its offspring. A horse that inherits the gene from both parents will be more severely affected, and would pass the disease on to 100 percent of its offspring.

DIAGNOSIS. HYPP will be suspected in any horse with Impressive bloodlines that shows typical symptoms. Elevated potassium levels can be measured in the blood of an affected horse during an episode. Genetic testing can be performed to identify the gene, and to determine whether the horse is heterozygous (carries only one gene from either parent) or homozygous (carries two genes, one from each parent).

TREATMENT. Mild episodes may resolve without treatment. If treatment is necessary, it may involve administration of grain or corn syrup orally in order to stimulate the release of insulin that helps to move potassium back into the cells. For more severe episodes, intravenous calcium gluconate will be administered to quiet the excitable muscle cells, along with dextrose to stimulate the same insulin response and help rebalance potassium.

Long-term management of horses with HYPP involves avoidance of high-potassium feeds such as alfalfa hay and molasses grains. Regular exercise and frequent small meals can help minimize attacks. The diuretic medication acetazolamide may be recommended to help stabilize potassium and glucose levels in the blood.

HOW SERIOUS IS IT? HYPP has been a very serious condition for the Quarter Horse breed because affected horses should not be breed. The American

Quarter Horse Association (AQHA) has imposed registration restrictions on horses affected with this condition. The disease itself can usually be well managed in mild to moderately affected horses, allowing them to continue to perform normally with minimal difficulties.

POTENTIAL COMPLICATIONS. Severe episodes can be fatal in some situations.

TABLE 4.2

Things That Go Bump

You're examining your horse's leg and can't help wondering what those lumps and bumps are all about. "Was it there yesterday?" you ask yourself. "Should I worry?"

This table describes the most common, abnormal lumps and bumps you're likely to encounter on your horse's legs, and will help you decide how much to worry.

BUMP	CATEGORY	WHAT IS IT?	CAUSE	BLEMISH OR MENACE
Sidebone	Bony bump.	Calcification of the collateral cartilages that sit on either side of the coffin bone.	Poor conformation, leading to too much stress on the quarters of the foot; poor shoeing, leading to increased pressure on either quarter; trauma to area.	Usually a blemish, although sidebones can cause low-grade forelimb lameness.
Ringbone	Bony bump.	Excess bone formation at the surface of the pastern bone.	Stress due to conformation, hard work, poor conformation, or trauma that leads to development of osteoarthritis.	Menace. Often accompanied by chronic, serious lameness.
Windpuff FIGURE 4.48	Fluid bump.	Accumulation of fluid within the fetlock joint (articular windpuffs) or digital tendon sheath (tendinous windpuffs).	Stress to the area due to conformation, hard work, or a traumatic injury.	May be either. Some horses develop windpuffs with no accompanying lameness. A tendon sheath injury or underlying joint problem will also result in this type of swelling.
Splint	Bony bump.	Excess bone formation on the surface of the splint bone. Rarely may involve a fracture.	Direct trauma such as a blow from the opposite limb, or stress of hard work.	Short-term menace, then a blemish. Splints may cause lameness initially. Most heal leaving behind a bump but no residual problems.
Bowed tendon	Soft-tissue bump.	Injury to either the superficial or deep digital flexor tendons.	Stress from a traumatic injury, or accumulated over a period of hard work.	Menace when it first occurs, although with proper healing it can become a blemish with minimal impact on soundness or performance.

The Horse's Body: Health and Disease

BUMP	CATEGORY	WHAT IS IT?	CAUSE	BLEMISH OR MENACE
Carpal hygroma FIGURE 4.49	Fluid bump.	Fluid accumulation in a bursa (fluid-filled sac) over the knee.	Direct trauma.	Can be a menace if there's underlying damage to the joint. Usually a blemish if the bone is not damaged.
Bog spavin	Fluid bump.	Fluid accumulation within the upper hock joint (tibiotarsal space).	Stress or an underlying abnormality of the hock that leads to excessive fluid production.	Can be a menace when it first appears. If underlying bone abnormalities are ruled out, it becomes a blemish.
Capped hock FIGURE 4.50	Fluid bump.	Fluid accumulation in a bursa under the tendons that run over the point of the hock.	Direct trauma.	Blemish. Rarely causes problems.
Thoroughpin FIGURE 4.51	Fluid bump.	Fluid accumulation within the tendon sheaths on the side of the hock.	Stress from trauma or hard work. May appear with minimal cause.	Blemish. Rarely causes problems.
Bone spavin	Bony bump.	Bony proliferation on the lower hock joints due to osteoarthritis.	Conformation and accumulated stress of hard work.	Menace. Usually accompanied by chronic lameness.

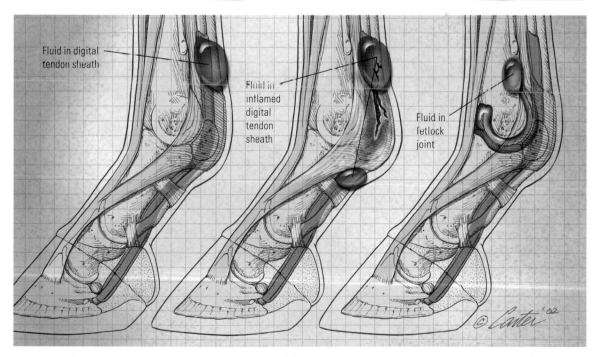

FIGURE 4.48. **Fluid accumulation in the digital tendon sheath is referred to as a tendinous windpuff, whereas fluid accumulation in the capsule of the fetlock joint is referred to as an articular windpuff. A windpuff may simply be cosmetic, or can be a sign of underlying inflammation due to injury.**

The Musculoskeletal System

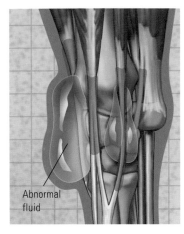

Abnormal
fluid

FIGURE 4.49. **Fluid accumulation within a bursa over the knee joint is called a carpal hygroma. In most instances it is a cosmetic problem, although it can appear with more severe underlying damage.**

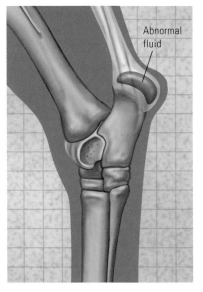

Abnormal
fluid

FIGURE 4.50. **A fluid-filled pouch at the point of the hock is called a capped hock and is a common blemish seen in horses who have experienced trauma to that area—often due to kicking.**

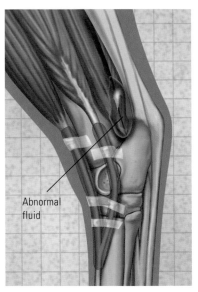

Abnormal
fluid

Abnormal
fluid

FIGURE 4.51. **Fluid accumulation within a tendon sheath running alongside the hock is called a thoroughpin.**

CHAPTER 5

The Gastrointestinal Tract

THE HORSE'S DIGESTIVE TRACT consists of the organs he needs to eat and process his food. We can trace his digestive organs beginning with his sensitive lips, which he uses to carefully select potential food items, through his stomach and intestines where that food is digested and absorbed into his system to keep his body going. The following structures make up the horse's gastrointestinal system: FIGURES 5.1–5.2

Oral Cavity

The horse's lips, tongue, jaws, and teeth form the portal for food entering his digestive tract. He uses his lips to carefully sort through the food items he wants to take into his mouth. His front teeth or incisors are also important for this function as he uses them to tear forage grasses from the pasture. Once food enters his mouth, his strong tongue helps position it for grinding by his back teeth or molars, through the crushing action of his muscular jaws. Food that's taken in and processed in his mouth is then swallowed and passed into the next portion of the tract. (See chapter 14 for a complete description of the horse's dental anatomy.)

Esophagus

This muscular tube connects the horse's mouth to his stomach. It is approximately 125 to 150 centimeters long and is divided into three sections, the cervical (neck) portion, the thoracic (chest) portion, and the abdominal (belly) portion. It runs along the neck, on the left side of the trachea or breathing tube. Muscular contractions of the esophagus help push food along from the mouth, and through the cardia, the opening into the stomach.

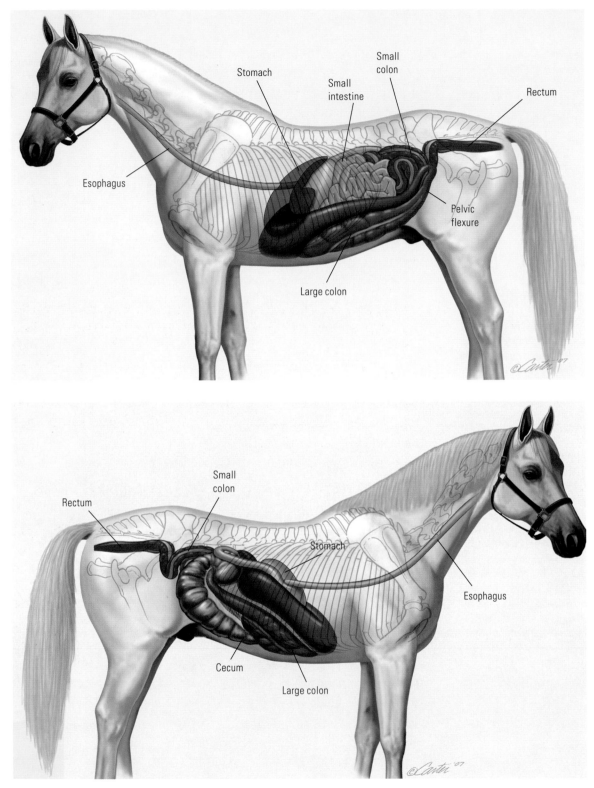

Stomach

Small intestine

Small colon

Rectum

Esophagus

Pelvic flexure

Large colon

Rectum

Small colon

Stomach

Esophagus

Cecum

Large colon

FIGURES 5.1–5.2. **The gastrointestinal tract.**

The Horse's Body: Health and Disease

Stomach

The horse's stomach is a curved muscular sac with a capacity of approximately 8 to 15 liters. It consists of glandular and nonglandular portions, divided by a distinct line called the margo plicatus. After ingested feed is processed in the stomach, it passes through a valve called the pylorus, into the small intestines for further digestion.

Small Intestines

The small intestines consist of three sections, the duodenum, jejunum, and ileum. The small intestine is a coiled tube approximately 5 to 7 centimeters in diameter, with a total length between 19 and 30 meters. The final portion of the small intestine, the ileum, empties ingested matter into the large, blind sac called the cecum, which represents the first part of the large intestine.

Large Intestines

The cecum is a sac approximately 1 meter long, with an average capacity of 33 liters. It rests on the right side of the horse's abdominal cavity, where it acts as a fermentation vat for fiber. The cecum opens into the remainder of the large intestine or colon through the cecocolic valve. The colon is a very large diameter (25 to 30 centimeters) tube that is approximately 6 to 9 meters long and is divided into right and left, upper, and lower portions. After time in the colon, processed food passes into the rectum where it is eventually passed as feces.

Liver

The liver is considered a part of the digestive system of the horse because of its role in the digestive process. It is the second largest organ in the body (second to the skin) and makes up approximately 1 percent of the total body weight of the adult horse. It is a brownish red structure that consists of a right and left section or lobe. The liver rests under the ribs between the heart and the intestinal tract, with most of its bulk situated on the right side of the horse's body. The horse is one of the few species that does not have a gall bladder, meaning that bile (the substance released from the liver to aid digestion) empties from the liver directly into the duodenum through the bile duct. The liver is also responsible for processing and detoxifying many of the substances taken into the horse's body.

How the Horse Digests His Food

Digestion begins in the horse's mouth, where the teeth physically grind ingested food and mix it with saliva-containing enzymes that begin breaking the food down. Once the chewed food passes through the esophagus to the stomach, it is mixed with gastric juices, including the enzymes pepsin and rennin, as well as hydrochloric acid (HCl), that aid chemical breakdown. Muscular contractions of the stomach help mix ingested feed with gastric juices, and gradually move it into the duodenum, or the first portion of small intestine.

The small intestine is the area where most enzymatic digestion occurs. Bile released from the liver assists with breakdown and processing. The majority of sugars are absorbed from the small intestine, resulting in an increase in blood glucose (sugar) levels approximately 30 minutes following a high-carbohydrate (grain) meal. The small intestine absorbs most of the vitamins and minerals as well.

The large intestine is the site of microbial fermentation of material that was not digested in the small intestine. This process produces substances called volatile fatty acids (VFAs), which are critical for energy. The large intestine also plays an important role in water balance as the site for resorption of the large volumes of fluid that were emptied into the small intestine during the digestive process. Finally, the bulk of proteins are processed and absorbed in the large intestine.

Gastrointestinal Evaluation

Auscultation

Examination of the horse's gastrointestinal tract usually begins with auscultation (or listening for GI sounds) by using a stethoscope at his flanks. The vet listens in four different locations, high and low on each side. A normal horse will have 2 to 4 small sounds (bubbles and gurgles) every minute, and 1 large sound (a rumble) every 2 to 3 minutes.

Rectal Examination

This exam requires the veterinarian to pass his or her hand into the horse's rectum, in order to palpate or feel various structures of the back portion of the GI tract. Typically palpable structures include portions of the large and small colon as well as non-GI organs such as the bladder, uterus, and ovaries of the mare, and the tip of the spleen.

Nasogastric (NG) Intubation   FIGURE 5.3

A long, flexible tube passed through the nose and into the stomach might also be included in a thorough examination of the GI system. An NG tube will help identify an obstruction in the esophagus (choke). Once passed into the stomach, it might also help detect a buildup of fluid in the

The Horse's Body: Health and Disease

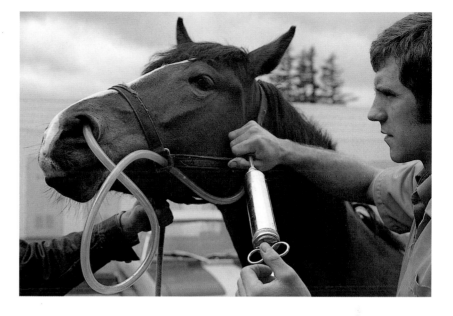

stomach that could accompany a problem with the stomach or small intestines. In this situation, stomach fluids might flow out of the tube, a condition known as gastric reflux.

Abdominocentesis (Belly Tap)

The veterinarian inserts a metal teat cannula or a needle into the abdominal cavity in an attempt to obtain fluid. The fluid can then be analyzed for red or white blood cells, high protein levels, or other abnormalities that could indicate inflammation or infection.

Ultrasound

In some cases, an ultrasound examination will be used to evaluate the horse's GI system. An ultrasound allows the veterinarian to visualize soft-tissue structures and can help detect gas buildup in sections of the intestine, thickening of intestinal walls, displaced segments of intestines, or other abnormalities of organs within the abdomen.

Radiographs

Rarely, a radiograph of the abdomen will be recommended—most commonly if the veterinarian suspects an enterolith, or intestinal stone. In most situations, radiographs of the abdomen have limited usefulness because the large size of the horse makes penetration with X rays difficult.

Endoscopy

If a problem with the esophagus or stomach is suspected, an endoscopic examination may be performed. This involves passing an instrument through the same route as the nasogastric tube in order to permit direct visualization of these structures by means of either fiberoptic or video technology.

Blood Tests

A variety of different blood tests may be recommended, especially if weight loss or neurologic symptoms accompany the GI problems. Blood tests can help pinpoint liver diseases, as well as identify anemia or other disruptions in basic body functioning that may be associated with gastrointestinal disorders.

WHEN THINGS GO WRONG

Choke   FIGURE 5.4

WHAT IT IS. A blockage in the horse's esophagus, caused by a mass of dry forage or grain, a solid object such as a large piece of carrot or apple, or any other obstruction.

DIAGNOSIS. A choked horse will cough repeatedly, often with his neck extended. He may appear distressed, and is likely to have a discharge, at both his mouth and nostrils, that includes copious amounts of foamy saliva combined with food material. He may take food or treats if offered, but will be unable to swallow them. His attempts to eat will stimulate a coughing episode. In some cases, a hard mass can be palpated on the left side of his neck in the jugular groove, where the esophagus runs alongside the jugular vein. A diagnosis is generally made based on clinical signs. It will be confirmed if the vet attempts to pass a nasogastric tube into the horse's stomach but is prevented from doing so by the obstruction.

TREATMENT. Many cases of choke resolve on their own within a fairly short period of time. Gentle massage of the esophagus using a thumb stroke along the length of the jugular groove on the left side of the horse's neck can help to break up an obstruction. If a choke hasn't resolved within an hour, the vet will usually sedate the horse and pass a nasogastric tube in an attempt to push the obstruction down the esophagus and into the stomach. In more severe cases, water will be used to help break up the obstruction, along with multiple manipulations of the tube.

FIGURE 5.4. **This mass of feed material resulted in a prolonged choking episode that severely damaged the esophagus.** (Author photo)

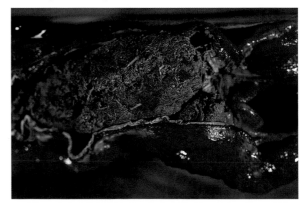

HOW SERIOUS IS IT? Although it's distressing to watch, choke is generally not a life-threatening situation for the horse (unlike the human version of "choke," which involves an obstruction of the airway). Most cases of choke can be easily resolved without complications. In rare cases, choke will persist for extended periods of time, causing damage to the esophagus that can have severe consequences.

The Horse's Body: Health and Disease

POTENTIAL COMPLICATIONS. If a choke persists for an hour or longer and the veterinarian has to pass the nasogastric tube numerous times or use large amounts of water to break up the obstruction, there's the risk that fluids and feed material may be aspirated or sucked into the lungs. Antibiotics and anti-inflammatories may be recommended following a choke episode to protect the horse against aspiration pneumonia. Multiple passages of the tube past sensitive tissues can also cause a nosebleed that is frightening to watch but generally has no long-term ill effects. Damage to the esophagus that results in stretching or a stricture (a permanent narrowing) may have serious consequences, including chronic choke episodes that can't be controlled.

Equine Gastric Ulcer Syndrome (EGUS)

WHAT IT IS. Gastric or stomach ulcers are erosions in the surface of the stomach lining. Veterinary researchers have estimated that ulcers are present in as many as 60 to 90 percent of mature horses in training for athletic disciplines. Foals are also at high risk.

DIAGNOSIS. In many cases, gastric ulcers cause no symptoms or the symptoms are extremely subtle. Horses with ulcers may exhibit a wide range of symptoms including chronic, recurrent colic, weight loss and poor body condition, a change in attitude, and poor performance. Ulcers have even been associated with back pain and subtle hind limb lameness. If ulcers are suspected, they can be easily diagnosed through gastroscopy, or examination of the stomach using a flexible endoscope that allows direct visualization of the stomach lining. For this diagnostic test, the horse must be held off food for a minimum of 24 hours prior to the examination in order to ensure the stomach is empty and can be visualized.

TREATMENT. There are a number of different medications available for treatment of stomach ulcers, the most effective being omeprazole paste (GastroGard® by Merial). Omeprazole works by blocking the acid pump in the stomach, thus preventing acid secretion. This blocking effect lasts up to 27 hours following administration, allowing the medication to be effective when given once a day. Treatment at a dose of 4mg/kg for up to 4 weeks is recommended to completely heal gastric ulcers. A follow-up endoscopic examination may be warranted to assess treatment before discontinuing the medication. Once existing ulcers are healed, a half dose (2 mg/kg) administered daily may prevent recurrence. Because this medication is extremely expensive, long-term daily administration is not always practical. It may be suggested to administer half doses during periods of high stress, such as competition or transport, to help prevent ulcers in horses at risk.

Other medications for treating ulcers are available at a fraction of the cost of omeprazole. These include cimetidine (Tagamet) and ranitidine (Zantac®) which act by blocking receptors in the stomach that are involved with acid secretion, sucralfate (Carafate) which adheres to the ulcerated areas of the stomach to act as a protectant, and antacids such as aluminum/magnesium hydroxide (Maalox®) which help neutralize stomach acids. However, although these medications may help minimize symptoms or reduce severity of ulcers, they are not effective treatments when compared with omeprazole.

If a horse is diagnosed with ulcers, changes in management to help minimize recurrence are critical. Increased grazing time is one of the most important recommended management changes, and can be accomplished either by turnout on grass or more frequent small feedings throughout the day for stall-kept horses. Other efforts to minimize stress should also be taken, such as modified training schedules and care during transport.

HOW SERIOUS IS IT? Ulcers may have a significant impact on performance, making them a serious problem for an athletic horse, particularly given the fact that they have a tendency to recur. The good news is that, once identified, most cases of ulcers can be effectively treated and controlled through the use of omeprazole, along with management changes to decrease stress.

POTENTIAL COMPLICATIONS. In severe cases, a gastric ulcer may perforate or penetrate the stomach, resulting in leakage of stomach contents out into the horse's abdominal cavity. In rare cases, ulcers may also result in reflux of gastric contents into the esophagus where it enters the stomach, resulting in spasms and narrowing of the esophagus.

Colic   FIGURES 5.5–5.9

WHAT IT IS. Colic is defined as "abdominal pain." This can be attributed to a number of different underlying causes that include not only pain related to the gastrointestinal tract, but also pain from non-GI conditions such as kidney failure. Most commonly, however, colic is used to describe a disorder of the intestines in horses, ranging from gas pains, to impactions or blockages, to twisted, displaced, or strangulated loops of intestine. (See Table 5.1.)

DIAGNOSIS. Diagnosis of colic begins with a suspicion based on clinical signs. A horse experiencing abdominal pain from colic may sweat, paw, and turn his head to look at his flank area. His heart rate and respiratory rate will elevate and he may attempt to go down and roll. He will refuse food, and may have a decrease in manure output. (See Table 5.2 for more information about how to interpret your horse's colic signs.)

If colic is suspected, the vet will perform a thorough examination, including many of the tests described under GI evaluation above. He'll begin by assessing the horse's pain level by observing his behavior. An elevated heart and respiratory rate is also an indication of pain. Next, he'll listen to GI sounds. A horse with gas or spasmodic colic may have increased GI sounds, while a horse with an impaction, displacement, or

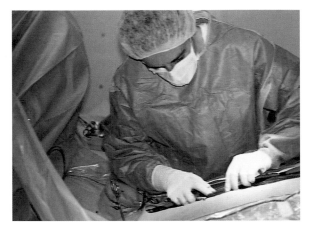

FIGURE 5.5. **When a horse requires surgery to correct a colic, the horse is typically placed on his back to allow the surgeon to enter the abdomen through a ventral midline incision.** (Photo courtesy of Jan Palmer, DVM, Diplomate ACVS)

FIGURE 5.6. **The intestines are then exposed and carefully evaluated to identify any potential abnormalities.** (Photo courtesy of Jan Palmer, DVM, Diplomate ACVS)

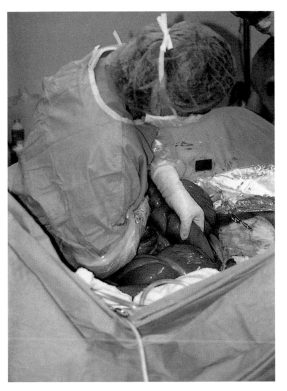

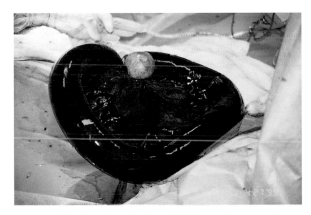

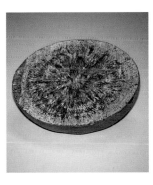

FIGURE 5.8. **This intestinal stone, or enterolith, has been removed from a section of the intestine. It may have caused chronic, intermittent colic symptoms for many years before it was discovered.** (Photo courtesy of Jan Palmer, DVM, Diplomate ACVS)

FIGURE 5.7. **The blackened color of this intestine means it has been severely compromised, in this case due to a lipoma or fatty tumor that has tightly wrapped around the intestine to cut off its blood supply. This severe condition, called a strangulating lipoma, is very common in older horses.** (Photo courtesy of Jan Palmer, DVM, Diplomate ACVS)

FIGURE 5.9. **This intestine is distended with gas, a situation that often accompanies an obstruction or displacement of a section of the GI tract.** (Photo courtesy of Jan Palmer, DVM, Diplomate ACVS)

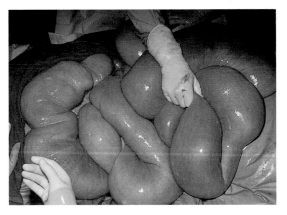

twist is likely to have decreased GI sounds. In general, decreased or absent GI sounds are a more concerning sign.

A rectal examination is one of the most important parts of the veterinarian's evaluation of colic. A rectal exam may reveal an impaction, build-up of gas in specific portions of the intestines, or even a displacement or torsion. It's important to recognize, however, that a rectal examination can't be 100 percent accurate, and may change as a colic episode progresses.

The vet will also often pass an NG tube to determine whether the horse has gastric reflux or an excess accumulation of fluid in the upper portion of the GI tract (the stomach and small intestines). If the vet obtains fluid through the tube, it means the source of the colic is likely to be the small intestines, and is considered a more serious sign. A belly tap may be performed to determine whether the intestines are becoming compromised—perhaps with a more serious condition such as a twist or strangulation.

TREATMENT. Treatment for colic will vary depending on the severity of the symptoms and the underlying cause. A simple spasmodic or gas colic may require nothing more than light exercise to relieve gas pains, and will often be self-limiting within 20 to 30 minutes.

A colic that involves an impaction or blockage of a section of the intestines may require administration of a laxative substance via an NG tube. If this fails to relieve the impaction after a period of time, intravenous fluids to "hyperhydrate" the horse may help loosen the impaction and enable it to pass.

In most cases, pain during colic will be controlled with a variety of different medications. The most commonly used medication is the anti-inflammatory flunixin meglumine (Banamine®), a potent pain reliever that may exert its effects for as long as 8 hours. Other medications that help relieve colic pain include the sedatives xylazine and detomidine, as well as the narcotic butorphanol. Finally, the antispasmodic medication butylscopolammonium bromide (Buscopan®) may be administered to a spasmodic or gas colic to help relieve painful spasms.

In colic cases where laxatives and intravenous fluids fail to relieve an impaction, when a loop of intestines is displaced or twisted, or when another factor has caused a section of intestine to die, surgery to correct the problem may be required. Colic surgery involves opening the horse's abdominal cavity under general anesthesia in order to identify and correct the underlying abnormality. This surgery may simply involve rearranging healthy intestines that have been displaced. It becomes more complex if the intestines must be opened to relieve an impaction or if sections of intestines that have been compromised must be completely removed.

In general, colic can be divided into two categories: surgical and medical. A surgical colic will not be resolved with medical treatment, and

The Horse's Body: Health and Disease

prompt surgical intervention is critical for success when surgery becomes necessary. This makes the decision to recommend surgery an extremely important one. The vet will recommend surgery based on the horse's overall condition, degree of pain and response to pain medications, and results of tests such as the rectal examination or belly tap.

HOW SERIOUS IS IT? The severity of colic ranges from a minor, self-limiting bellyache to a life-threatening condition requiring major surgical intervention for survival. Full recovery from colic surgery will take as long as 3 to 6 months, even in uncomplicated cases.

POTENTIAL COMPLICATIONS. Most medical colics will resolve without problems. However, a more serious colic requiring surgery can have a number of serious complications. Endotoxins resulting from the death of normal bacteria within the intestinal tract are common with severe colic, causing shock-like symptoms and a wide range of problems that affect the body's basic functioning. Laminitis is a potential serious condition resulting from endotoxemia.

Following surgery, adhesions may form between loops of intestine that have been opened, or between sites of intestinal repair and the body wall. These adhesions can lead to disruptions in motility (movement) of the intestines, gas buildups, and future colic episodes. Incisional hernias due to a breakdown of the incision in the belly wall can also occur.   FIGURE 5.10

Administration of pain medications without a thorough evaluation of the horse's condition can result in very serious complications. Potent pain relievers such as flunixin meglumine will mask symptoms of colic that are an important signpost for the veterinarian to evaluate the need for surgery. Their use can cause a delay in surgical intervention that compromises the horse's prognosis. It is even possible for them to mask pain to the point of rupture of the intestine, a fatal consequence. For this reason it's best to avoid administering any pain-relieving medications in a horse showing signs of colic without first consulting with the veterinarian.

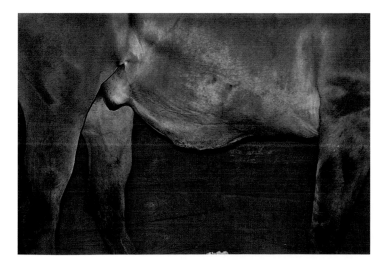

FIGURE 5.10. **This incisional hernia is a potential complication following colic surgery. The incision in the belly wall breaks down.** (Photo courtesy of Jan Palmer, DVM, Diplomate ACVS)

TABLE 5.1

Colic: What's Wrong?

TYPE OF COLIC	WHAT IT IS	SIGNPOSTS	TREATMENT	PROGNOSIS	COMMENTS
Spasmodic	Spasms or cramping of segments of the intestines.	Acute pain, often severe. Louder than normal GI sounds.	Often self-limiting. Pain management.	Good.	None.
Gas	Gas buildup within the intestinal loops.	Acute pain, often severe. Louder than normal GI sounds.	Often self-limiting. Pain management.	Good.	May progress to a displacement if gas accumulation persists.
Feed impaction	A blockage due to a ball of feed material that clogs the intestines.	Mild, intermittent pain that gradually progresses. Lowered fecal output. GI sounds quiet but present.	Pain management and laxative via NG tube. May require IV fluid therapy. Rare cases require surgery.	Good if uncomplicated. May worsen if impaction can't be easily resolved.	Rare cases can build up pressure and rupture the intestine, resulting in a life-threatening situation.
Enterolith	A stone that forms in the intestines, causing a blockage.	May be acutely painful. Often intermittent if stone moves in position from one location to another. May be identified with radiographs of the abdomen.	Mild episodes may resolve with pain management. Eventual surgical removal of stone will be necessary.	Will require surgery, but prognosis is good if stone is identified and removed without complications.	Common cause of chronic colic in some geographic areas, including Florida and California. May be associated with alfalfa hay.
Displacement	A loop of intestine moves into an abnormal position.	May be intermittent, mild colic symptoms. Can progress to an acute, severe episode. GI sounds generally decreased. May continue to pass feces in small amounts.	Pain management. Rolling techniques have been used to successfully resolve displacements. Surgery is often necessary.	Good if displacement is identified and resolved while horse is still in good condition. Usually does not require opening or removing sections of intestines.	A displacement can persist for days or even weeks. Eventually the displaced loop becomes trapped to the point where symptoms become more severe and surgery is often necessary.

TYPE OF COLIC	WHAT IT IS	SIGNPOSTS	TREATMENT	PROGNOSIS	COMMENTS
Torsion	A section of intestine twists around itself resulting in blockage and damage to the intestine involved.	Often acute, uncontrollable pain. Signs of toxicity such as a very high heart rate or dark, muddy mucous membranes. Lack of GI sounds.	Surgery is necessary.	Guarded. Many torsions occur rapidly, making time to surgery critical. If large portions of the intestinal tract are involved and intestinal health is compromised, prognosis can be poor.	Torsions can cause such pain and damage that it's not possible to get the horse to surgery in time. Complications with toxicity are possible if much intestinal death occurs.
Strangulation	A section of intestine is constricted by becoming trapped in between two structures, or by something wrapping around it. This leads to a blockage, gas buildup, and eventual death of the involved intestine.	Often acute, uncontrollable pain. Signs of toxicity such as a very high heart rate or dark, muddy mucous membranes. Lack of GI sounds.	Surgery is necessary.	Guarded. Best if surgery is performed quickly to minimize release of toxins resulting from intestinal death. May do well if a small section of intestine is involved, and condition is recognized early.	Most common cause is a lipoma or fatty tumor wrapping around a loop of intestine, an occurrence often seen in older horses.

TABLE 5.2

Colic: When to Call the Vet

This table describes symptoms you're likely to see during a typical colic episode. As a rule of thumb, if you observe two or more symptoms of moderate or severe colic, or your horse's symptoms continue for longer than 30 minutes, call your veterinarian. (Refer to "Taking Vital Signs" on pages 39–42 for instructions about how to assess your horse's condition.)

COLIC SYMPTOM	MILD	MODERATE	SEVERE
Heart rate	40–60 bpm.	60–80 bpm.	Over 80 bpm.
Respiratory rate	20–30 bpm.	30–40 bpm.	Over 40 bpm.
Temperature	99–100.5 degrees F.	99–100.5 degrees F.	Under 99/over 102.5.
Gum color	Pale pink.	Pale to dark pink.	Dark red or purplish.
Capillary refill time	1–2 seconds.	2–4 seconds.	Over 4 seconds.
Gut sounds	Normal or increased.	Decreased but present.	Absent.
Feces	Yes.	No.	No.
Passing gas	Yes.	No.	No.
Pain level	Sweating, intermittent pawing, looking at belly, lifting hind leg, stretching.	Same as mild but continuous. May try to go down and roll.	All other signs. Uncontrollable, continuous attempts to roll or thrash about.

After Colic Strikes

If your horse experiences a colic episode, you're likely to be a little nervous in the days that follow. The following is a guide to aftercare for your horse if he has a simple colic that resolves without surgery, such as an impaction or simple gas buildup. *(Note: For surgical aftercare instructions follow your surgeons advice to the letter, because the individual situation will determine the recommended post-surgery care.)*

Feeding

WHY IT MATTERS. It's important that your horse be given easily digestible feed in small amounts. You want to avoid feed that overworks his sensitive digestive tract and might cause more gas buildup. It's more important to give your horse small amounts of feed if your horse has experienced an impaction; feeding him large meals all at once could add to the blockage if it hasn't been completely resolved.

WHAT TO DO. Avoid grain for at least 24 hours following the colic episode, and feed only soaked hay, bran mashes, or equine senior feeds. Hand grazing on fresh grass is also acceptable. Begin with the equivalent of a one-pound coffee can of mash or senior feed every 2 to 3 hours. Gradually

The Horse's Body: Health and Disease

add hay by the handful, giving your horse a handful every hour or so. If all goes well, you can usually feed a normal meal of soaked hay 24 hours after the colic symptoms are completely resolved. *(Note: If your vet advises withholding hay longer because of a resolving impaction or other concern, follow his or her advice.)*

Water

WHY IT MATTERS. It's crucial that your horse take in adequate amounts of water to ensure he stays well hydrated. Lack of water consumption can be a component of his colic episode in the first place, especially during a cold winter. WHAT TO DO. Provide warm water during cold weather. When you begin feeding, make sure that he takes in water by soaking hay or feeding wet mashes. Monitor his water intake carefully—if you have automatic waterers, turn them off and provide buckets instead. *(Note: Some newer automatic watering systems offer a monitoring device to help you keep track of your horse's consumption.)*

Be aware that your horse may drink less during the first 24 hours of a colic episode if your veterinarian has administered water or oil via a nasogastric tube, or if your horse has been on IV fluids. By day 2, however, he should be drinking normal amounts.

Monitor Fecal Output

WHY IT MATTERS. Maintaining normal fecal output is critical, especially if you are concerned about an impaction or other blockage. If your horse is passing normal amounts of manure that are normal in size and consistency, chances are his GI tract is functioning properly. However, his output may be decreased slightly on day 2 following a colic episode due to his decreased feed consumption during the day following the episode. If he had a large impaction, he may pass huge amounts of manure once it has broken loose. WHAT TO DO. Notice and record you horse's fecal output—frequency, size, and consistency. If he's not back to normal after 48 hours, notify your veterinarian. If your veterinarian has administered oil, keep an eye out for it passing in your horse's feces. You'll detect the oil as a thin film on his rectum, or you may see oil in his tail or glistening in his manure. Although seeing oil isn't a guarantee that a blockage is completely resolved (oil can make its way around an impaction or displacement), it's clearly a good sign, and in most cases indicates your horse is on the mend.

Exercise

WHY IT MATTERS. Your horse is likely to be tired following a colic episode, even a mild one that resolves without veterinary intervention. In addition, exercise is important to ensure his GI tract keeps moving and functioning properly. WHAT TO DO. Hand walk, turn out, or provide other light exercise for the first 48 hours following a colic episode. Avoid hard, stressful rides, however, until your horse is feeling better.

Tips to Prevent Colic

- **MAINTAIN A REGULAR DEWORMING PROGRAM.** Intestinal parasites can damage your horse's intestines and/or the blood vessels that supply them, leading to life-threatening colic.

- **MAINTAIN A REGULAR FEEDING SCHEDULE.** Irregular feeding can produce changes in your horse's intestines and motility (movement). This can result in painful gas buildups, and even in intestinal twists or displacements.

- **FEED SEVERAL SMALL MEALS A DAY.** Frequent small feedings will help your horse's intestinal tract, which is designed for a grazing lifestyle, function normally. Occasional large meals are a recipe for disaster.

- **FEED NOTHING BUT THE BEST.** Feed your horse the best-quality feed available. Poor-quality, hard-to-digest feed can lead to an accumulation of gas.

- **GRADUALLY INCREASE PASTURE TIME.** Although grazing is natural, if your horse's digestive system isn't used to fresh green grass, unlimited grazing can result in gas colic—especially when the first lush grass of spring appears. Gradually introduce your horse to grass, beginning with 30 minutes for the first week, then adding an hour every 3 to 5 days, to give his system time to adjust.

- **PROVIDE DAILY EXERCISE.** Your horse's body is designed for the constant movement required by grazing and traveling to water. If a stall-kept horse doesn't get out of his stall at least an hour a day, his GI tract won't function normally.

- **PROVIDE ACCESS TO FRESH WATER AT ALL TIMES.** Without an adequate water supply to lubricate your horse's GI tract, he may become dehydrated and develop an impaction colic.

- **SCHEDULE REGULAR, ROUTINE DENTAL WORK.** Sharp edges or imbalances in your horse's mouth can make chewing difficult. Poorly chewed food can mark the beginning of a digestive disturbance.

Proximal Enteritis (Duodenitis-Proximal Jejunitis)

WHAT IT IS. Inflammation of the upper portion of the small intestine that results in large amounts of fluid being secreted by the small intestine and leads to gastric reflux. Horses with this condition will be in extreme pain and are likely to have a small-intestine obstruction. The underlying cause of this problem is not known, although it is believed that a bacterial organism may be involved.

DIAGNOSIS. The diagnosis of proximal enteritis depends on clinical signs of abdominal pain, large amounts of gastric reflux obtained through a nasogastric tube, and a distended small intestine identified during a rectal exam or an ultrasound. In some cases, the horse will be taken to surgery for a suspected small-intestinal obstruction and enteritis will be identified at that time.

TREATMENT. Treatment is primarily supportive, and consists of intravenous fluid therapy to replace fluids lost through gastric reflux, decompression of the stomach by removing fluids through the nasogastric tube at regular intervals, and nonsteroidal anti-inflammatory medications such as flunixin meglumine to control pain and minimize the toxic effects of substances released from the damaged intestine (endotoxemia). It's recommended that the horse be held off feed, and nutrition may be provided intravenously in cases that do not resolve within a period of days.

HOW SERIOUS IS IT? Proximal enteritis is a very serious disease that can be life threatening.

POTENTIAL COMPLICATIONS. Because it is difficult to distinguish proximal enteritis from a small-intestine obstruction, many horses with this disease are taken to surgery. Unfortunately, the prognosis for recovery following surgery is poor (as low as 17 percent) compared with those treated medically (as high as 94 percent). In addition, many horses with this disease will develop adhesions (loops of intestine "stick together") following recovery that can increase risk of future colic episodes. Finally, laminitis is a possible complication of this disease due to endotoxemia.

Colitis

WHAT IT IS. Colitis is a condition of the large intestine that results from inflammation and a disruption in the microbial balance within the intestines, and leads to severe diarrhea as its primary sign. There are a number of different underlying causes of colitis, including infectious organisms, drug reactions, or even grain overload. (See Table 5.3.)

DIAGNOSIS. A diagnosis of colitis is based on signs of abdominal pain (colic symptoms) and diarrhea. If an infectious agent is involved, the horse may have a fever. Signs of toxicity may also occur: depression, elevated heart and respiratory rates, and disruptions of the circulatory system that lead to darkened mucous membranes. Blood tests will often reveal dehydration due to fluid losses in diarrhea, as well as nonspecific findings such as a low white blood cell count. If a particular infectious organism is suspected, specific blood tests or fecal tests may help identify the culprit.

TREATMENT. In general, treatment for colitis depends on fluid therapy to help keep up with fluid losses through diarrhea, and medications such as flunixin meglumine, which helps counteract endotoxemia. Specific causes of colitis may require treatment with specific antimicrobial agents (See Table 5.3.)

HOW SERIOUS IS IT? Severe colitis can have a number of serious consequences, including laminitis due to endotoxemia that can accompany the

TABLE 5.3

Common Causes of Colitis

COLITIS CAUSE	SPECIFIC SIGNS	IDENTIFIED HOW	SPECIFIC TREATMENT	COMMENTS
Salmonellosis	Fever and sudden onset of diarrhea with a low white blood cell count.	Tests on fecal samples to identify the organism. Multiple samples are required for accurate results.	Treatment with antibiotics targeted against the salmonella organism is controversial.	The salmonella organism may be carried by horses that show no signs of disease. A salmonella outbreak can have extremely serious consequences in a barn environment, and strict isolation is recommended if salmonellosis is suspected.
Colitis X *(Clostridium perfringens* type A*)*	Extremely severe, acute diarrhea that may lead to death within 24 hours.	Identification of clostridial (bacterial) organisms in feces may be possible. Otherwise specific diagnosis is difficult.	Aggressive measures to maintain hydration and counteract toxicity may be necessary, including shock doses of corticosteroids in severe cases.	Many cases are fatal.
Potomac Horse Fever *(Ehrlichia risticii)*	Fever followed by diarrhea, similar to salmonellosis.	Antibody levels in blood specific to the organism can help pinpoint the diagnosis.	Oxytetracycline (6.6 mg/kg one time daily).	Vaccination is available and may help reduce chances of becoming ill, or severity of clinical signs.

condition. In addition, some bacterial causes of colitis such as salmonella or Potomac Horse Fever can spread throughout a barn. Strict isolation is likely to be recommended if a horse is found to have a high fever, low white blood cell count, and sudden onset of severe diarrhea.

POTENTIAL COMPLICATIONS. The most frightening complication of colitis is laminitis, which can be life threatening. Other consequences can also be significant, including severe shock and circulatory collapse.

GI Neoplasia

WHAT IT IS. Cancer involving either the stomach or the intestines. A number of different types of cancers can occur, the most common being squamous cell carcinoma of the stomach or lymphosarcoma of the stomach or intestines.

COLITIS CAUSE	SPECIFIC SIGNS	IDENTIFIED HOW	SPECIFIC TREATMENT	COMMENTS
Nonsteroidal anti-inflammatory drugs	Diarrhea following NSAID administration. Most common with higher than recommended doses.	History of NSAID use.	Discontinue use of NSAIDS.	NSAID toxicity can damage colon lining, even at recommended dosages, resulting in colitis.
Antibiotics	Diarrhea following antibiotic administration. Most common antibiotic culprits include penicillin, trimethoprim-sulfa, erythromycin, tetracycline, and ceftiofur.	History of antibiotic administration.	Discontinue use of antibiotics.	Antibiotics can disrupt normal GI balance, resulting in colitis.
Grain overload	Diarrhea following overeating of carbohydrates, typically grains such as corn or barley.	History of consuming large amounts of carbohydrates. Horse "breaks into the feed room."	Remove carbohydrate source. If overeating is discovered, immediate administration of mineral oil to speed passage or activated charcoal to absorb toxins via NG tube may help prevent problems.	Sudden large amount of carbohydrates introduced to large intestine disrupts natural balance.

DIAGNOSIS. Cancer of the stomach or intestines may be suspected in older horses with a history of weight loss, anemia, or intermittent colic. A specific diagnosis is often difficult to pinpoint. Stomach cancers may be seen during endoscopic examination, whereas intestinal cancers often won't be identified as such unless the horse undergoes surgery for colic. Blood tests may show lowered protein levels if protein is leaking out of damaged intestines, and high calcium levels can be suggestive of a neoplastic process.

TREATMENT. Most GI cancers in horses are untreatable except in rare instances where an isolated tumor is identified and can be removed.

HOW SERIOUS IS IT? In the majority of cases, GI cancer is a fatal condition.

POTENTIAL COMPLICATIONS. Tumors that cause obstruction could lead to a serious colic episode.

Liver Disease

WHAT IT IS. Liver disease refers to any abnormality affecting the liver which may or may not progress to liver failure. In general, liver failure fits into two categories, acute and chronic. Acute liver failure occurs quickly and is often accompanied by a sudden onset of severe signs, whereas chronic liver failure is likely to have a more slow and insidious onset. Because the liver has so many important functions, failure of this organ results in a wide variety of symptoms including depression, weight loss, and jaundice (yellowing of the skin and mucous membranes). In severe cases, neuro-logic symptoms can occur (referred to as hepatic encephalopathy) such as circling, head pressing, or even seizures due to a buildup of toxins.

DIAGNOSIS. Liver disease may be suspected based on clinical symptoms, but further tests will be necessary to make a determination, beginning with blood tests that measure enzymes released during liver cell death. The most reliable and specific of these enzymes is gamma-glutamyl trans-ferase (GGT). Other enzymes that may indicate liver disease are aspartate aminotransferase (AST), sorbitol dehydrogenase (SDH), and alkaline phosphatase (AP). Bilirubin (a substance found in bile) is also elevated in the blood during liver failure, which is an indicator of liver function rather than actual cell damage. However, it's important to know that bilirubin may also be elevated simply because a horse is not eating.

If liver disease is diagnosed based on blood tests, ultrasound examina-tion may help determine a specific cause. Abscesses, tumors, or other abnormalities of the liver's structure, such as scarring, may all be seen with ultrasound. Finally, a liver biopsy, or sample of tissue examined under a microscope, provides further information. Potential underlying causes of liver disease are outlined in Table 5.4.

TREATMENT. In general, a horse with a compromised liver should be main-tained on a high-carbohydrate, low-protein diet to minimize ammonia production that contributes to hepatic encephalopathy. Frequent small meals will also help reduce demands on the liver during the digestive process. During an acute liver failure crisis, supportive treatments with intravenous fluids and medications such as lactulose or the antibiotic metronidazole that minimize absorption of ammonia will be recommended to help control hepatic encephalopathy. If a specific underlying cause of liver failure is identified, other treatments may be warranted.

HOW SERIOUS IS IT? Both acute and chronic liver failure have a poor prog-nosis, and often lead to death. However, because the liver has a large reserve capacity, it may be possible to manage a horse with liver damage and some degree of chronic liver failure for many years.

POTENTIAL COMPLICATIONS. The most serious complication in a horse with chronic liver disease is progression to acute liver failure, which may be impossible to control. Hepatic encephalopathy that leads to seizures or collapse can result in trauma.

The Horse's Body: Health and Disease

TABLE 5.4

Common Causes of Liver Disease

CAUSE	SPECIFIC SIGNS	IDENTIFIED HOW	SPECIFIC TREATMENT	COMMENTS
Theiler's disease (Serum hepatitis)	Acute severe hepatic encephalopathy, jaundice, and dark urine.	Liver biopsy shows characteristic tissue death. May be associated with administration of tetanus antitoxin (4–10 weeks prior to signs occurring).	No specific treatment available. Supportive measures to contol acute crisis.	Cause not completely determined, but may be associated with tetanus antitoxin. Prognosis depends on ability to manage acute crisis.
Cholangiohepatitis (Infection of the bile duct which may or may not be associated with choledcholithiasis or a bile stone)	Fever, loss of appetite and weight loss. Colic symptoms may occur.	Ultrasound will show liver enlargement and a distended bile duct. Stones may be observed. Biopsy will confirm the diagnosis, and may help identify a specific microorganism.	Antibiotic treatment may be curative if a specific organism is identified. Stones causing obstruction may require surgical removal.	Prognosis is good if stones are not present and damage to the liver is minimal. In long-standing cases, chronic liver damage may result.
Hyperlipemia (Accumulation of fat in the bloodstream)	Sudden onset of depression, loss of appetite. May have edema (fluid accumulation in tissues) under the belly.	Suspected in obese horses and most common in miniature horses and donkeys. May occur with Cushing's disease. High levels of fat measured in blood samples.	Primary disease such as Cushing's should be treated. Other treatment is supportive, and includes maintaining nutrition ideally with small amounts of high-carbohydrate feeds.	Prognosis is poor if horse refuses to eat.
Tyzzer's disease (*Bacillus piliformis* Infection)	Affects foals 8–42 days old. Foal is usually found dead. If alive, down, convulsing, and severely depressed.	Suspected based on signs and blood tests consistent with liver disease. Diagnosis often made postmortem during microscopic evaluation of the liver.	Supportive treatment and high levels of antibiotics, including penicillin and amikacin or chloramphenicol.	Treatment is either not possible or unsuccessful.
Pyrrolizidine alkaloid toxicosis (A condition resulting from ingesting plants containing this toxin—see Table 5.5)	Weight loss, jaundice, behavior changes consistent with hepatic encephalopathy.	Exposure to pyrrolizidine alkaloid–containing plant. Confirmed with liver biopsy.	Removing offending plant from the environment to prevent ongoing toxicity. Supportive treatment depending on degree of chronic liver damage.	Most horses will not eat toxic plants due to their bitter taste, but if adequate feed is unavailable, they will. The best strategy to prevent toxicity is to remove toxic plants from the horse's environment.

TABLE 5.5

Pyrrolizidine Alkaloid–Containing Plants Found in the U.S.

BOTANICAL NAME	COMMON NAME
Senecio vulgaris	Common groundsel
Senecio jacobaea	Tansy ragwort
Senecio douglasii	Threadleaf groundsel
Senecio trianularis	Tar weed
Amsinckia intermedia	Fiddleneck
Crotalaria sp.	Rattlebox
Echium plantagineum	Salvation Jane/purple viper's bugloss
Heliotropium europeaum	Common heliotrope
Symphytum officinale	Comfrey
Cynoglossum officinale	Hound's tongue

CHAPTER 6

The Cardiovascular System

THE HORSE'S CARDIOVASCULAR SYSTEM, which consists of the heart, blood vessels, lymph nodes, and lymphatic vessels, is responsible for regulating blood-flow delivery of oxygen and nutrients throughout the body, as well as collecting and draining waste materials that form in body tissues. In general, the flow of blood can be divided into two categories: pulmonary (blood circulates through the lungs to collect oxygen) and systemic (blood circulates throughout the body to deliver oxygen). The lymphatic portion of the circulatory system is composed of the spleen and lymph nodes as well as a network of channels that filter, carry, and help eliminate waste products.   FIGURE 6.1

The following structures make up the horse's cardiovascular system.

The Heart   FIGURE 6.2

The horse's heart is located in the middle of his ribcage. It is divided into four chambers, the right and left ventricles and the right and left atria, which serve to circulate blood throughout the body through a sequence of coordinated pumping actions. The ventricles are the actual pumping chambers and are larger than the atria, which receive blood being returned to the heart by large blood vessels.

Valves help control blood movement between and out of the different chambers, and include the bicuspid (mitral) valve between the left atrium and ventricle, the tricuspid valve between the right atrium and ventricle, and the pulmonary and aortic valves between the ventricles and vessels that carry blood out into the organs.

The heart consists of three layers of muscle and connective tissue, including the endocardium (inner lining layer), myocardium (thick muscular layer), and pericardium (outer sac that separates the heart from other internal organs).

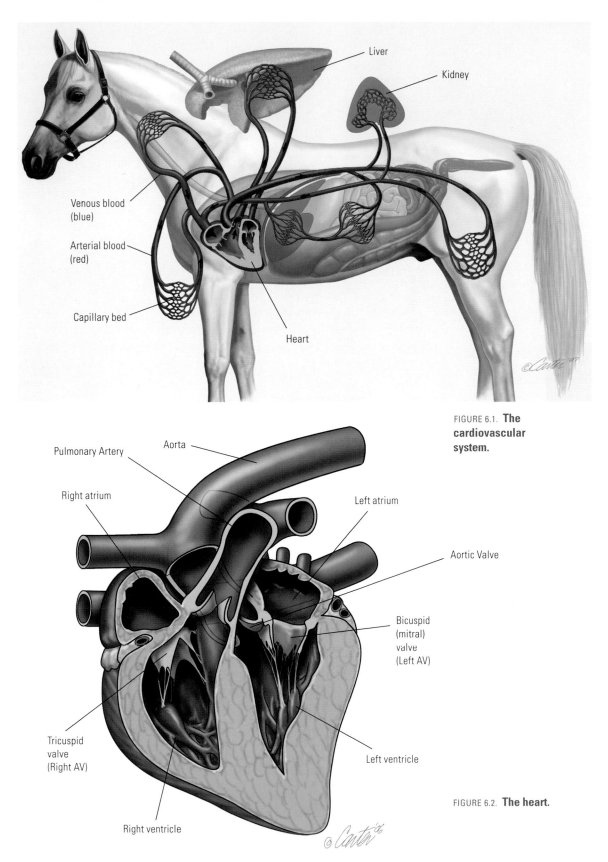

Liver

Kidney

Venous blood
(blue)

Arterial blood
(red)

Capillary bed

Heart

FIGURE 6.1. **The cardiovascular system.**

Pulmonary Artery

Aorta

Right atrium

Left atrium

Aortic Valve

Bicuspid
(mitral)
valve
(Left AV)

Tricuspid
valve
(Right AV)

Left ventricle

Right ventricle

FIGURE 6.2. **The heart.**

Arteries

The arteries are tubes constructed of layers of elastic tissues and muscles that help maintain the pumping action of the heart to propel blood to the other organs of the body. The expansion and constriction of the arteries with each heartbeat is what creates the "pulse" that can be felt in arteries near the surface of the body.

Veins

Veins are blood vessels that return blood to the heart from some part of the body. They are larger in diameter than corresponding arteries, have thinner walls, and lie closer to the body surface.

Capillaries

Capillaries, tiny vessels with very thin walls, form the connection between the arteries and veins in the tissues of the body. They provide the network where blood is transferred between the arterial and venous system.

Spleen

The spleen, a large glandular organ, is located on the left side of the body, between the stomach and the intestines. It helps to regulate the circulatory system by acting as a storage area for red blood cells and destroying damaged or worn-out red blood cells.

Lymph Nodes

Lymph nodes are masses of lymphocytes (a type of white blood cell) that are distributed throughout the body. They are usually encapsulated to create isolated structures, and function as filters to recognize and remove toxic substances that have accumulated within the body. Lymph nodes are also considered part of the immune system.

Lymphatic Ducts

Lymphatic ducts are a series of tubes that back up the veins in returning fluid and other substances to the heart. Fluids that enter the lymphatic ducts are filtered through the various lymph nodes situated along the way.

How the Cardiovascular System Functions

The flow of blood begins with a pump of the heart. Blood from the body and the lungs fills the right and left atria respectively. The filling of these two chambers stimulates them to contract, which then causes blood to be pushed through the AV valves and into the ventricles. After the ventricles are filled, they contract to actively pump blood out into the body and lungs. The pressure from the contracting ventricles then closes off the AV valves, allowing them to fill again to complete another cycle. The filling phase of the heart cycle is called diastole; the contracting phase is called systole.

The blood itself is made up of fluid (called plasma) as well as red (erythrycytes) and white (leukocytes) blood cells. The red blood cells contain a compound called hemoglobin, which is responsible for the oxygen-carrying capacity of the blood. The white blood cells are primarily responsible for fighting off infection and include five different types of cell: neutrophils, eosinophils, basophils, monocytes, and lymphocytes. A more detailed discussion of these different cells can be found in chapter 15, "The Immune System."

Function of the cardiovascular system depends on the heart. Blood pumped by the heart carries nutrients, oxygen, and essential components to the organs, where exchange takes place in the capillary beds. The blood then returns to the heart to be cleaned up, recharged, and pumped again.

The horse's amazing capacity as an athlete is partly due to his efficient cardiovascular system. At rest, the heart beats approximately 30 to 40 beats per minute. This heart rate elevates dramatically with exercise (70 to 120 bpm at the trot, 120 to 150 bpm at the canter, and as high as 240 bpm at maximum velocities) in order to meet oxygen demands.

Examination

The following diagnostic steps will be taken to fully evaluate a problem related to the horse's cardiovascular system.

Auscultation

The first step in examining the horse's cardiovascular system involves auscultation, or listening to the heart using a stethoscope. The vet will listen at several different locations on both sides of the chest in order to evaluate both the rhythm of the beats and the quality of the heart sounds.

The normal heart rhythm includes four sounds that correspond to the contraction of the ventricles (first heart sound or S1), contraction of the right and left atria (second heart sound or S2), rapid filling of the ventricles (third heart sound or S3) and contraction of the atria (fourth heart sound or S4). The typical "lub-dub" thought of as a heartbeat actually represents S1 and S2. Because of the large size of the horse's heart, however, all four sounds can often be heard (lub-ub—dub-ub). A normal heart rhythm consists of a regular sequence of beats, typically at a rate of 30 to 40 beats per minute.

The large size of the horse's heart also means that an occasional beat may be "dropped" and therefore not heard. This condition, called a second-degree AV block, occurs when a signal from the atria is not completely transmitted to the ventricle, resulting in a failure of the ventricle to contract. As long as the pattern of the dropped beats is regular, and the block resolves with exercise (the heart rhythm is regular when the horse is working), this fairly common irregularity in the heart rhythm should not be cause for concern. It has actually been reported to occur in as many as 44 percent of normal horses.

Murmurs, or abnormal sounds associated with blood flow through the heart, will also be detected during auscultation. If a heart murmur is detected, it will be classified according to one of the following categories:

- GRADE 1: Soft murmur heard only at a specific location on the chest.
- GRADE 2: Soft murmur easily heard over a larger area of the chest.
- GRADE 3: A moderately loud murmur heard over a wide area of the chest.
- GRADE 4: A loud murmur heard over a wide area of the chest and accompanied by a faint "thrill," or detectable vibration.
- GRADE 5: A loud murmur heard over a wide area of the chest with an obvious thrill.
- GRADE 6: A loud murmur that can be heard even when the stethoscope is no longer in contact with the chest.

Although murmurs often point to leaky heart valves or structural abnormalities within the heart, it is also possible to hear heart murmurs in horses that do not indicate an underlying abnormality. Again, because of the size of the horse's heart, blood bounding around in the heart's chambers can cause a whooshing sound. Called "physiologic murmurs," these sounds generally disappear during periods of exercise. However, it can be difficult to determine whether a murmur is simply normal for that horse, or if it indicates a problem. In some cases, further diagnostic tests may be recommended to determine the significance of a heart murmur.

Ultrasound

Echocardiography, or ultrasound examination of the heart, is one of the most useful diagnostic tools available. Sound waves passed through the tissues produce an image that allows for an evaluation of the size and wall thickness of the heart chambers, valve structure and function, and even structure of blood vessels. Blood flow can also be evaluated through a variety of techniques.

Electrocardiography (ECG)

Electrocardiography (ECG) measures the electrical activity of the heart that corresponds to nerve impulses involved with the heart cycle, and can help define variations in heart rhythm. To perform this test, electrodes are placed at various locations on the horse's skin where they detect electrical impulses. An ECG may even be performed remotely through radio-signal transmission on a horse during exercise. (*Note: Because of differences in the electrical functioning of the horse's heart compared with that of humans or small animals, ECG is of little value for determining anything about heart size in horses.*)

Exercise/Stress Testing

Because the cardiovascular system is crucial to oxygen delivery to the tissues, cardiovascular diseases that disrupt this delivery often result in exercise intolerance. Stress tests involving exercise and measurement of oxygen supplies in the blood can provide the veterinarian with information about the functioning of the heart and blood vessels.

WHEN THINGS GO WRONG

The following are the most common conditions likely to affect the cardiovascular system.

Atrial Fibrillation

WHAT IT IS. Atrial fibrillation is the most common rhythm disruption (arrhythmia) in the horse and occurs when the atrium vibrates ineffectively, therefore disrupting the normal pattern of electrical signals that stimulate a regular heartbeat rhythm. The ventricles contract on their own in an irregular pattern. In many cases, atrial fibrillation may occur secondary to some other heart disease, although it is possible for this arrhythmia to arise as an isolated primary condition.

DIAGNOSIS. The vet will hear an irregular heart rhythm during auscultation that has no detectable pattern. In addition, no fourth heart sound will be heard. A confirmation of atrial fibrillation would be based on an ECG. If fibrillation is accompanied by other signs of heart disease such as audible heart murmurs, exercise intolerance, or an elevated heart rate (greater than 60 bpm), ultrasound examination would be recommended to determine the extent and nature of the underlying heart condition.

TREATMENT. In horses with a recent onset of atrial fibrillation where no other signs of concurrent heart disease are seen, it is possible to convert the heart rhythm back to normal using a medication called quinidine. Recurrence is likely only in about 15 percent of these horses. In horses where atrial fibrillation has been established for 4 months or longer, conversion of the heart rhythm is still possible. It may be more difficult to do so, however, and the condition may reoccur in up to 60 percent of horses. Instances of atrial fibrillation can occur secondarily to another problem, including conditions unrelated to the heart itself, such as colic. Treatment in these cases depends on treating the underlying condition. In cases where atrial fibrillation is secondary to heart disease or heart failure, treatment to convert the atrial fibrillation is not recommended. Treatment in those cases should be aimed toward supporting the heart failure.

HOW SERIOUS IS IT? The seriousness of atrial fibrillation depends on how long it has been established, as well as whether it is associated with a more serious underlying condition. Uncomplicated atrial fibrillation that is recognized early is often easily converted back to a normal rhythm with no

further complications. Many horses with well-established atrial fibrillation can live healthy lives and even perform successfully in athletic disciplines. Where there is another underlying condition, prognosis will vary.
POTENTIAL COMPLICATIONS. These will vary with other underlying conditions.

Heart Failure

WHAT IT IS. The heart is unable to pump enough blood to meet the needs of the body. Heart failure can occur secondarily to other conditions that overstress the heart such as congenital abnormalities in heart structure (see below) or valvular disorders (see Table 6.1). It can also occur simply because the myocardium (muscle of the heart) becomes diseased and is no longer able to function properly.

DIAGNOSIS. Signs of heart failure include exercise intolerance, breathing difficulty, and pooling of fluid in the lower legs or belly area. If heart failure is suspected, ultrasound examination can help evaluate its severity and identify potential underlying causes.

TREATMENT. Medications such as digoxin are available to help improve the heart's ability to contract and function effectively, and diuretics such as furosemide, to help mobilize fluids that are accumulating in the body due to the heart's poor functioning, may help alleviate symptoms. However, long-term treatment for heart failure is usually impractical and frustrating.

HOW SERIOUS IS IT? Heart failure is often progressive and life threatening.
POTENTIAL COMPLICATIONS. None.

Congenital Heart Disease

WHAT IT IS. A congenital heart disease is an abnormality in the structure of the heart that is present at birth. Common congenital heart diseases seen in horses include the following:

- VENTRICULAR SEPTAL DEFECT: A hole in the wall between the two ventricles. When the heart pumps, blood is pushed from the left ventricle to the right ventricle, increasing blood flow to the lungs and decreasing blood flow to the internal organs. This is the most common congenital heart abnormality.

- PATENT DUCTUS ARTERIOSIS: A small duct (the ductus arteriosis) that is part of the fetal circulation fails to close. As a consequence, some of the blood pumped by the heart flows from the aorta to the pulmonary artery, resulting in increased blood flow to the lungs and decreased blood flow to the internal organs. This duct remains open for up to 7 days following birth in normal foals, but should close after that time.

- ATRIAL SEPTAL DEFECT: A hole in the wall between the two atria. Blood may flow back and forth through this hole between the two atria. This defect, although uncommon, can cause enlargement of the atria and may lead to atrial fibrillation.

- TRICUSPID ATRESIA: The right AV valve fails to develop normally, and is accompanied by a number of abnormalities in the structure of the heart that result in communication between both the two atria and the two ventricles. This leads to a severe disruption in blood flow, and affected foals usually will not survive beyond 6 months of age.
- TETRALOGY OF FALLOT: An abnormality that involves a number of different alterations in the heart structure, including a blockage of blood flowing out of the right ventricle, an abnormal aorta that allows outflow from both the right and left ventricles, and a ventricular septal defect. The amount of blood flowing into the lungs is restricted, resulting in a lack of oxygen.

DIAGNOSIS. Congenital heart diseases may be recognized because a murmur is heard at birth. If this is not the case, they may cause stunted growth that is noticeable within the first few months of life. If the abnormality does not cause significant alterations in blood flow, it may not be discovered until the young horse is started in work and exhibits exercise intolerance. In very mild cases, congenital heart defects may be identified only as incidental findings because a murmur is heard during a routine examination. Specific identification of the abnormality will be made through ultrasound examination of the heart.

TREATMENT. Treatment is generally not available. Rarely, surgery might be attempted to repair a defect.

HOW SERIOUS IS IT? The severity of a congenital heart disease is highly variable, depending on the degree to which blood flow is altered. It may be life threatening in severe cases, and lead to death at a very young age. At the other extreme, adult horses with mild abnormalities may perform normally, with no noticeable negative effects.

POTENTIAL COMPLICATIONS: None.

Valvular Disease

WHAT IT IS. A heart valve disorder involves a problem with one of the major valves that help to control blood flow in and out, resulting in blood leaking back through the valve. The left and right AV valves, pulmonary valve, and aortic valve may all be affected. (See Table 6.1 for details about individual valve problems.)

DIAGNOSIS. Most valve disorders are first identified by the presence of a murmur during auscultation. Ultrasound examination of the heart will allow the vet to determine which valve is affected and whether there are other heart abnormalities accompanying the leaky valve.

TREATMENT. If heart failure is not present, most valve disorders will not require treatment. However, a horse with a known "leaky valve" should be examined with ultrasound if a sign such as exercise intolerance, decline in performance, or difficulty breathing occurs.

The Horse's Body: Health and Disease

TABLE 6.1

Valve Disorders

VALVE AFFECTED	CAUSE	MURMUR	SYMPTOMS	PROGNOSIS
Left AV Valve (Mitral valve)	Degeneration of the valve; most commonly seen in older horses. May also be the result of inflammation.	Grade 3 or louder; heard loudest on the left side. Occurs during systole.	No symptoms in some horses. Exercise intolerance, poor performance, and breathing difficulties can occur.	If mild and non-progressive, continued performance may be possible. Can lead to heart failure if severe.
Right AV Valve (Tricuspid valve)	Uncommon; due to degeneration of valve. May occur with atrial fibrillation.	Grade 2 or louder; heard loudest on the right side. Occurs during systole.	Most have no symptoms. Edema in the belly, problems breathing due to fluid in the lungs, and distention of the jugular vein can occur if severe.	If mild and non-progressive, continued performance may be possible. Can lead to heart failure if severe.
Aortic Valve	Degeneration and thickening seen in older horses. Rarely can be congenital.	Grade 2 or louder; heard loudest on the left side. May sound "musical." Occurs during diastole.	Most have no symptoms.	If secondary to heart failure, symptoms consistent with failure will be present.
Pulmonary Valve	Very rare, due to degeneration of the valve. Occurs with heart failure.	Grade 2 or louder; heard loudest on the left side. May sound "musical." Occurs during diastole.	Good. Most affected horses have no associated problems.	May accompany heart failure.

HOW SERIOUS IS IT? Valve insufficiencies cause only mild disruptions in blood flow and should not be cause for concern. In some circumstances, though, they can be associated with heart failure.

POTENTIAL COMPLICATIONS. Valve insufficiency may lead to heart failure.

Bacterial Endocarditis

WHAT IT IS. Bacteria invade the heart and colonize tissues, most commonly the valves. Endocarditis may be secondary to another bacterial infection within the body, such as an abscess or pneumonia, and is more likely to occur if the horse has an existing heart disease such as a leaky valve.

DIAGNOSIS. Endocarditis may be suspected if the horse exhibits weight loss, depression, and an unexplained fever along with signs of cardiac disease such as a loud murmur or rhythm abnormality. Blood work will often have a very elevated white blood cell count, indicative of a bacterial infection, as well as a high fibrinogen level, which is an indicator of inflammation. Bacteria cultured or grown from a blood sample can confirm the diagnosis, and an ultrasound examination will often do so as well.

TREATMENT. Treatment depends on aggressive antibiotic therapy that is given intravenously for a period of as long as 8 weeks. Ideally, an appropriate antibiotic will be selected based on bacteria grown from a blood sample. This may not always be possible, so a broad-spectrum antibiotic must be chosen that's likely to affect most organisms.

HOW SERIOUS IS IT? Although the horse may respond well to initial treatment, the long-term outlook for survival is poor. It is difficult to completely clear the infection, and damage to valves or tissues in the heart can occur, meaning that symptoms will often reappear after therapy has stopped.

POTENTIAL COMPLICATIONS. Damage to the heart as a result of this infection can lead to progressive heart disease, failure, or even sudden death due to the rupture of structures within the heart.

Thrombophlebitis FIGURE 6.3

WHAT IT IS. Venous clotting and inflammation that may or may not be accompanied by infection. Most commonly, thrombophlebitis occurs in the jugular vein secondary to repeated intravenous injections or the presence of an intravenous catheter.

DIAGNOSIS. The affected vein will enlarge and become hot and painful. Edema, or the accumulation of fluids, may occur in the tissues surrounding the clot as blood flow is disrupted. If infection is present, the horse may also have a fever. Ultrasound examination of the clotted area can help evaluate the extent of the thrombus. If infection is suspected, a sample may be taken from the clot and submitted to a laboratory for culture and identification of an appropriate antibiotic to be used for treatment.

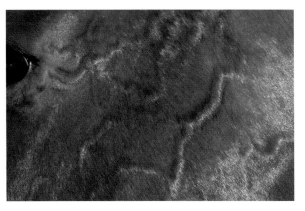

FIGURE 6.3. **The prominent blood vessels on the side of this horse's face will appear if the jugular vein has been damaged due to thrombophlebitis. These blood vessels provide alternative pathways for blood flow.**
(Photo courtesy of Scott Wenzel)

TREATMENT. Initial treatment would involve hot packs and topical anti-inflammatory applications. Systemic anti-inflammatories such as phenylbutazone or flunixin meglumine would also be recommended. When infection is suspected, broad-spectrum antibiotics will be administered. Ideally, the appropriate antibiotic can be chosen based on culture results. In cases that do not respond to treatment, surgical excision might be advised.

HOW SERIOUS IS IT? Uncomplicated thrombophlebitis will resolve without problems. In severe cases, however, a thrombophlebitis can result in permanent blockage of the involved vein. If this occurs, alternative routes for blood flow will develop and be apparent on the surface of the skin. For example, a horse with a permanently thrombosed jugular vein will have a visible network of abnormally large blood vessels that can easily be seen on that side of the horse's face. An extremely serious thrombophlebitis is one with bacterial involvement, which can lead to severe, even life threatening consequences.

POTENTIAL COMPLICATIONS. The most significant complication of a thrombophlebitis would occur with a bacterial infection that could enter the bloodstream to affect other organs. Specifically, bacterial endocarditis is a potential severe complication.

Anemia

WHAT IT IS. A decrease in the amount of red blood cells circulating in the bloodstream. Anemic horses may be lethargic, weak, and have poor tolerance for exercise. Their heart and respiratory rates will also be elevated, and mucous membranes may appear either pale or jaundiced (yellowed), depending on whether red blood cells are simply decreased in number or being destroyed within the bloodstream.

A number of different factors can lead to anemia, including blood loss due to either internal or external bleeding, inadequate production of red blood cells because of chronic diseases, or the destruction of red blood cells secondary to a virus or other infectious disease.

It is interesting that iron deficiency anemia is extremely rare in horses and is usually due to some kind of chronic blood loss, such as gastric ulcer disease or intestinal parasites. Rarely does dietary supplementation with iron help, although it is a common step taken by horse owners. A more effective approach is to identify and treat the underlying cause.

DIAGNOSIS. Anemia is diagnosed based on blood tests showing a decreased number of red blood cells. The specific cause of anemia may be more difficult to identify. If anemia of chronic disease is suspected, the vet will attempt to identify another problem. Cushing's disease, heaves, or chronic kidney failure could be the underlying cause of the anemia. Specific blood tests may be recommended.

TREATMENT. Treatment for anemia depends on identifying and treating the underlying cause.

HOW SERIOUS IS IT? The severity of anemia depends on the severity of the underlying cause. Anemia can lead to exercise intolerance and poor performance simply due to lack of adequate delivery of oxygen and nutrients to the tissues.

POTENTIAL COMPLICATIONS. None.

Vasculitis

WHAT IT IS. An inflammation of blood vessel walls that can be secondary to a number of other conditions, including respiratory infections, other viruses, or trauma. When blood vessels become inflamed, they enlarge and "leak," causing fluid to accumulate within the tissues. A horse with vasculitis will have swollen legs, fluid accumulation in his belly, and may have swelling around his face. In more severe cases, serum will leak from the skin, small hemorrhages may occur, and skin may blister or ulcerate.

DIAGNOSIS. A history of a viral condition, trauma, or a disease in conjunction with typical signs of fluid accumulation and limb swelling is usually enough to identify vasculitis. A diagnosis can be confirmed with a skin biopsy. If an underlying cause is not known, the vet will attempt to identify an existing problem that might require specific treatment.

TREATMENT. Initial treatment for vasculitis includes taking steps to control inflammation and reduce swelling. Icing or cold-hosing the legs, along with light work to dispel accumulated fluid, can be helpful in the early stages. Support bandages to limit the degree of swelling might also be recommended. Anti-inflammatories such as phenylbutazone or flunixin meglumine may be enough to control inflammation in mild cases, although more potent medications such as dexamethasone might be required in more severe cases. If limb edema becomes well established, sweat bandages may help draw out fluid to reduce the degree of swelling. If an underlying cause has been identified, treatment to manage that condition will be necessary.

HOW SERIOUS IS IT? The severity of a vasculitis often depends on the underlying cause. Severe vasculitis can have very serious consequences, including sloughing of skin and tissues if it does not respond to treatment.

POTENTIAL COMPLICATIONS. Although vasculitis commonly affects the skin, other organs may also be involved, leading to organ failure and potential death. If the skin is severely affected and sloughing occurs, bacterial infections can complicate healing.

Equine Infectious Anemia (EIA): A Regulatory Question

Equine infectious anemia, or "swamp fever," is a viral disease that leads to anemia. If a horse is exposed to this virus, he may develop clinical signs of fever and depression 30 days following exposure. The virus is transmitted by bloodsucking insects. The most troubling aspect of this disease is that once infected a horse can become a carrier for life. With the virus in his blood, he is a threat to other horses.

Although this disease is extremely uncommon, every horse owner is aware of its consequences. A simple blood test, the Coggins test, is available to detect a virus in the bloodstream. Government regulations do not permit a horse to be transported across state lines within the United States, or in or out of the country, if a positive Coggins test identifies him as a carrier of the EIA virus. In fact, a horse that tests positive is required to be maintained in strict isolation for life. Many infected horses are humanely destroyed.

As a general rule, Coggins testing is required any time a horse is to be transported, and is recommended as a screening prior to purchase and prior to the introduction of a new horse onto a farm. For horses participating in competitions, proof of a negative Coggins is often required.

CHAPTER 7

The Respiratory Tract

THEN AND NOW

A painting that hangs in the Louvre by Antonio Pisanello entitled Cavallo depicts a horse with surgically slit nostrils. This technique, popular in the 1500s, involved an incision several inches long made on the side of each nostril, and was used to increase airflow and aid endurance in the exercising horse.

Today, disruptions of airflow may be surgically corrected using a variety of different techniques, depending on the underlying cause. Nasal strips, designed to hold open the nostrils to improve airflow during exercise, offer a nonsurgical option. Their effect is not so different from what surgically slit nostrils of long ago achieved—but in a kinder, gentler way.

THE RESPIRATORY TRACT IS THE MEANS by which air is drawn into the horse's body so that oxygen can be extracted and delivered to the tissues. The respiratory tract, which is divided into the upper and lower portions, consists of the following structures: FIGURES 7.1–7.2

Nasal Passages

The nasal passages provide a conduit for air to travel from the nostrils to the pharynx (the chamber at the back of the horse's throat). These passages are composed of cartilage and bone with a moist soft-tissue covering (mucous membrane) that has fingerlike projections (called cilia) on its surface. As the air is drawn into the respiratory tract, it is both warmed by blood vessels in the lining of the nasal passages and filtered for dust particles and potential infectious organisms by the cilia, in preparation for passage into the airways. At the end of the nasal passages is a structure called the ethmoid turbinate, a mucous membrane–coated filter that helps prevent dust and particles from entering the horse's airways. The ethmoid is also a detector involved with the horse's sense of smell. The nostrils themselves are constructed with cartilage rings at their openings, and they can be expanded by small muscles to allow more airflow during exercise or at other times when extra oxygen is needed.

Guttural Pouches

The guttural pouches are a pair of blind sacs that arise from the tubes of the middle ear. Large blood vessels run through the center of these pouches that are located at the end of the nasal passages—at the beginning of the pharynx.

Sinuses

The horse has six pairs of sinuses that have openings into the nasal passages: the maxillary, frontal, sphenopalatine, and three sequential pairs of conchal sinuses. In the young horse (under 5 years of age), roots of the first three molar teeth fill up the maxillary sinus cavity. This opens into the

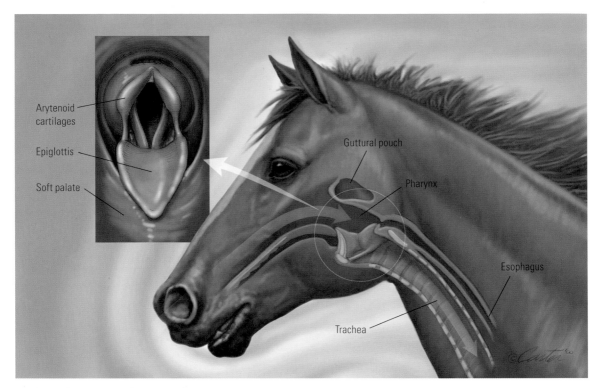

FIGURE 7.1. **Structures of the upper airway.**

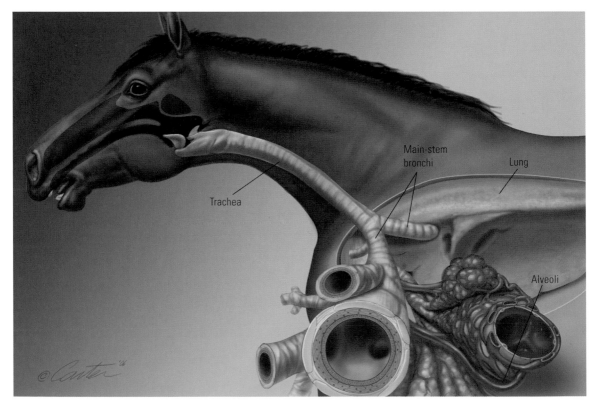

FIGURE 7.2. **Structures of the lower airway and lungs.**

The Horse's Body: Health and Disease

frontal sinuses. In part due to this communication, the frontal and maxillary sinuses are most commonly diseased.

Pharynx

This chamber at the back of the horse's throat helps to funnel air into the larynx and on into the lungs from the nasal passages. It also funnels food into the esophagus from the mouth.

Larynx

This membrane-covered cartilage structure controls the flow of air into the lungs. At the front of the larynx is a V-shaped flap of cartilage called the epiglottis, which helps separate the trachea from the esophagus. When air is drawn in, the epiglottis lays flat to close the communication between the two openings, allowing air to flow freely into the trachea. When the horse is eating and needs to swallow, the epiglottis is drawn over the opening of the larynx to prevent food from entering the trachea and lungs. This mechanism makes it very difficult for the horse to breathe through his mouth.

The arytenoid cartilages are also a part of the larynx. These paired cartilages are located at either side of the opening into the trachea and help control airflow. When air is taken in, they are pulled open to allow it to flow freely. Between breaths, they move back into a resting position.

Trachea

The trachea is the large tube that carries air from the larynx into the lungs, and marks the transition between the upper and lower respiratory tracts. Like the nasal passages, the trachea is covered by a mucous membrane with cilia that help filter and prepare air before it enters the lungs.

Bronchi

After entering the chest cavity, the trachea branches into two smaller tubes called the main-stem bronchi, which carry air into the right and left lungs. These bronchi then branch into smaller and smaller tubes until they reach the part of the lungs where they will exchange oxygen—similar to a tree's branches as they reach the leaves. The smallest branches at the end of the bronchial tree are called bronchioles.

Lungs

The lungs are divided into the right and left segments called lobes, which are further divided into the cranial (front) and caudal (back) lobes on the left side and the cranial, intermediate, and caudal lobes on the right side. Unlike in other species, the lobes of the horse aren't clearly divided from one another within their internal structures, making diseases of the horse's lung more likely to involve the entire lung rather than isolated areas. It's interesting that the right main-stem bronchus is oriented more horizontally than the left, which may make the right side of the lungs more susceptible to disease than the left side. Air passed through the bronchioles enters small sacs called alveoli within the lung tissue, which is where the actual transfer of oxygen takes place.

Diaphragm Muscle

The diaphragm is a dome-shaped muscle that separates the horse's thorax (chest) from his abdomen (belly). It controls expansion and relaxation of the chest cavity, which helps move air in and out of the lungs.

How the Horse Breathes

When the horse takes a breath, the diaphragm muscle and muscles of the chest wall contract to create negative pressure that draws air into the nasal passages. The air is warmed and filtered by the lining of the nasal passages until it passes through the pharynx into the laryngeal area. The epiglottis at the opening between the larynx and the trachea closes off the opening to the esophagus as the arytenoid cartilages are pulled open, allowing air to pass through the trachea, bronchi, and bronchioles on into the alveoli. It is there that oxygen carried in the air is transferred to the blood circulating through the lungs. At exhalation, the organs within the abdomen (including the stomach, liver, and intestines) push against the diaphragm to expel air, which is then passed back out through the trachea, larynx, and nasal passages.

At rest, the horse takes approximately 12 breaths per minute and each breath moves between 6 and 7 liters of air. When the horse is exercising, his respiratory rate increases in order to meet the increased need for oxygen by working muscles. When oxygen demands are very high, the muscles of the abdomen assist the diaphragm muscle, resulting in an obvious abdominal movement during breathing. A pattern of "abdominal breathing" is also a significant factor in respiratory disease.

An interesting pairing occurs when the horse breathes while cantering and galloping. As the horse moves during a canter or gallop stride, his chest and diaphragm are mechanically stretched and compressed. This action affects the passage of air in and out of the lungs, resulting in a coupling of breaths with each stride of the gallop.

Evaluation

Examination of the horse's respiratory system involves the following steps:

History

Information provided about the duration of the illness, progression of symptoms, exposure to possible infectious organisms, vaccinations, stabling conditions, and seasonality of symptoms can help the veterinarian determine whether a respiratory condition is more likely to be due to an infectious organism or an allergy. An accurate evaluation of the horse's living conditions will also help the veterinarian develop a practical treatment plan for many respiratory problems, as environmental control is a critical part of management in many cases.

Physical Examination

The physical examination will include observation of the breathing pattern of the horse at rest, measurement of respiratory rate, and careful auscultation, or use of a stethoscope to listen to the lungs during breathing. The veterinarian will listen to the horse in a quiet location, and for best results, may place a bag over the nostrils to encourage deep breathing. He'll also take note of any nasal discharge if one is present, and will look for enlargement of lymph nodes under the jaw that might indicate the horse is fighting an infection.

Endoscopy

An endoscopic examination is commonly used to diagnose respiratory disorders, especially those involving the larynx. With the endoscope, structures can be visualized, which is all that is needed to make a definitive diagnosis in many upper respiratory conditions. In addition, this instrument can be passed through the larynx and into the trachea to allow observation of discharge originating from the lower respiratory tract. A discharge can even be sampled for laboratory analysis using a tube passed through the endoscope. In some performance centers, high-speed treadmills make it possible to examine the horse with the endoscope during exercise.

Cytologic and Microscopic Analysis

Samples taken from the trachea or lower airways can provide information about the underlying cause of lower respiratory diseases. To obtain these samples, one of the following methods may be employed:

- TRANSTRACHEAL ASPIRATION: This method involves passing a type of needle through the skin into the trachea to collect fluid from it. Once a common sampling method, it is not used as much now because of the widespread availability of endoscopic equipment for obtaining samples. Unlike endoscopy, it has the limitation of not allowing for the direct visualization of the airways. Furthermore, it is invasive since a large needle must be passed through the tissue, and that can lead to inflammation or infection at the point of entry.

- ENDOSCOPIC COLLECTION OF TRACHEAL FLUID. A tube can be passed through an opening in the endoscope to allow fluid to be collected at the same time the airways are being directly visualized. This is a noninvasive, safe technique for sampling fluid and can provide good information about inflammation and infectious organisms, such as bacteria, involved with many lung diseases. However, it may not provide as accurate a sample of changes in the lungs as bronchoalveolar lavage, where samples are taken from deeper within the lungs. (See below.)

- BRONCHOALVEOLAR LAVAGE (BAL): Bronchoalveolar lavage provides the best information about chronic lung conditions. The procedure involves passing a tube down into the main-stem bronchi. The tube is then sealed off so that fluid can be pushed into the lungs and then collected in a syringe. Inflammatory cells that have accumulated in the lungs can then be evaluated.

Radiographs

Radiographs may be used to examine various parts of the horse's respiratory tract. Skull radiographs are useful for evaluating disorders of the sinuses or guttural pouches, as fluid lines within these normally gas-filled structures can be easily seen. Radiographs can also be used to examine the lungs, particularly in cases where abscesses or fluid filling is suspected. Unfortunately, the large size of the horse makes it difficult to obtain good-quality radiographs without specialized equipment, which limits the use of radiographs in many instances. Radiographs of the lungs are easily obtained in foals, however, and can be extremely helpful for evaluating foal pneumonia.

Ultrasound

Ultrasound is used to diagnose lung problems, particularly when abscesses are suspected with specific types of pneumonia.

WHEN THINGS GO WRONG

The respiratory tract is one of the most common sites of disease in the horse, and is second only to musculoskeletal disorders as a factor limiting performance in athletic disciplines. Problems in the respiratory system can involve either the upper or lower respiratory tract, and may have a number of potential underlying causes. The following are the most common respiratory system disorders.

Sinusitis FIGURE 7.3

WHAT IT IS. Just like humans, horses can develop infections in their sinus cavities—often due to dental problems or secondary to viral and bacterial infections of the upper respiratory tract. The sinuses can also be affected by cysts, hematomas (accumulation of blood), or cancer. A horse with a sinus problem will usually have a nasal discharge coming from only one nostril, on the same side as the affected sinus. If sinuses on both sides are involved, the nasal discharge will also be on both sides. The discharge

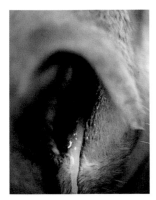

FIGURE 7.3. **A discharge from one of the horse's nostrils often means a problem in the nasal passages, guttural pouch, or sinuses. A two-sided nasal discharge is more likely to indicate a problem lower down the respiratory tract, such as pneumonia.** (Photo courtesy of Lisa Metcalf, DVM, Diplomate ACVT)

may be creamy white and foul smelling, especially if tooth roots are involved or the bone is infected.

DIAGNOSIS. The vet may suspect a sinus problem if there is a one-sided nasal discharge. Percussion or tapping on the sinuses may help him to detect fluid within the cavity and in some advanced cases a noticeable deformity of the face may be observed under the affected sinus. Radiographs of the horse's skull will usually confirm a diagnosis and may help identify an underlying problem with a tooth root. If dental problems are suspected, a thorough oral examination will be performed to identify loose, broken, or rotting teeth. Sometimes an examination of the sinus with endoscopic equipment (sinuscopy) may help pinpoint an underlying cause. Finally, samples of cells or tissue taken from the sinuses can identify bacterial organisms, cancer, or other specific causes of a sinus problem.

TREATMENT. If a dental abnormality has been identified as an underlying cause of sinusitis, the affected teeth will be removed. Extraction in combination with a thorough flushing of the sinus may be curative. With the horse sedated but still standing, flushing can be performed through a hole created in the sinus cavity using an instrument called a trephine. In more severe cases or cases involving cysts, cancer, or other abnormal tissues, the horse may need to be put under general anesthesia so that the sinus can be entered and tissues cleaned out through a large bone flap made over the sinus cavity. Following this type of surgery the sinuses will require regular flushing and the horse will be maintained on antibiotics and anti-inflammatory medications until healing is complete.

HOW SERIOUS IS IT? At best, sinus problems are a significant health problem that can be difficult and expensive to treat. At worst, they can be life threatening.

POTENTIAL COMPLICATIONS. If sinus problems go untreated, they can progress to the point where pressure buildup can cause pressure on the brain and neurologic symptoms.

Ethmoid Hematoma

WHAT IT IS. This hematoma, which tends to develop in older horses, is a blood-filled mass that forms on the surface of the ethmoid turbinates at the back of the nasal passages. It may be on one or both sides. A horse with an ethmoid hematoma will have a nasal discharge that is either blood or blood mixed with other fluid. Abnormal noises may be heard during breathing due to the obstruction of airflow caused by the mass.

DIAGNOSIS. If suspected based on the symptoms, an ethmoid hematoma can be identified on radiographs, and will also be seen during endoscopic examination of the upper airway.

TREATMENT. Surgical removal of the hematoma is required

HOW SERIOUS IS IT? If hematomas are causing serious symptoms, they do require treatment, which can be expensive and complicated.

POTENTIAL COMPLICATIONS. There is a high risk of hemorrhage during surgery and blood transfusions may be necessary if bleeding cannot be controlled. In addition, as many as 50 percent of ethmoid hematomas will recur following removal.

Guttural Pouch Infection   FIGURE 7.4

WHAT IT IS. An infection caused by a bacterial (guttural pouch empyema) or fungal (guttural pouch mycosis) organism. The most common clinical sign is a nasal discharge from the same side as the affected guttural pouch. Bacterial infections can occur secondary to other bacterial infections—for example, guttural pouch involvement is a common complication of strangles. (See page 150.)

DIAGNOSIS. This infection is high on the list of possibilities any time a horse has a one-sided nasal discharge. Radiographs of the skull and endoscopic examination of the pouch can confirm the diagnosis.

TREATMENT. A bacterial infection will require flushing with large volumes of saline solution and antibiotics in addition to treatment with an appropriate systemic antibiotic. In severe cases where flushing is not successful, surgery may be performed to clear the pouch.

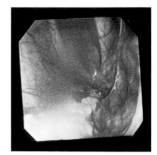

FIGURE 7.4. **This pus within the guttural pouch seen during endoscopic examination indicates infection.** (Photo courtesy of Jan Palmer, DVM, Diplomate ACVS)

Fungal infections can be very difficult to treat, as fungal accumulations (called plaques) can cause damage to the carotid artery (a major artery that passes through the pouch), putting the horse at risk for a fatal hemorrhage. For this reason, surgery to tie off this artery may be necessary before the fungus can be treated. In fact, it may not even be recommended to attempt to confirm a diagnosis of a fungal infection if blood is seen at the opening of the pouch. This is because of the risk of a fatal hemorrhage if an affected guttural pouch is entered with the endoscope.

HOW SERIOUS IS IT? Guttural pouch empyema can be difficult and expensive to treat, but it can be successfully resolved. Guttural pouch mycosis is often untreatable and may have fatal consequences.

POTENTIAL COMPLICATIONS. If a bacterial infection is present for a long period of time, material within the pouch can form stones called chondroids that are more difficult to treat. Fatal hemorrhage can occur due to rupture of the carotid artery with a fungal infection.

FIGURE 7.5. **The swelling in this foal's throat area is typical for guttural pouch tympany, a condition where air accumulates within the guttural pouches.** (Photo courtesy of Jan Palmer, DVM, Diplomate ACVS)

Guttural Pouch Tympany   FIGURES 7.5–7.6

WHAT IT IS. Accumulation of air within the guttural pouch, most commonly seen in foals. An affected youngster will have visible enlargement of the throat area and may have difficulty swallowing or breathing. The exact cause of this disorder is not clear, but is related to a disruption of normal airflow through the pharyngeal area.

DIAGNOSIS. Radiographs will show excessive air accumulation within the guttural pouches.

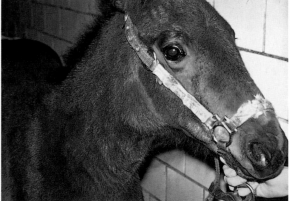

The Horse's Body: Health and Disease

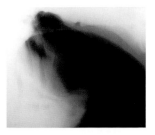

FIGURE 7.6. **This radiograph of the foal in Figure 7.5 confirms the presence of excessive air within the pouches.** (Photo courtesy of Jan Palmer, DVM, Diplomate ACVS)

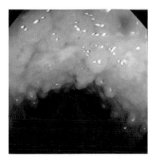

FIGURE 7.7. **These raised nodules on the lining of the pharynx, seen with endoscopic examination, are typical of pharyngitis.** (Author photo)

TREATMENT. If only one pouch is involved, surgery to create an opening between the two pouches will correct the problem. If both pouches are involved, surgery is more difficult and involves a more complicated procedure to equalize pressure within the pouches.

HOW SERIOUS IS IT? The prognosis for resolution of tympany of one guttural pouch is very good following surgery. If both sides are involved, it may be more difficult to correct.

POTENTIAL COMPLICATIONS. Pneumonia can occur secondarily to difficulties in breathing and chewing.

Pharyngitis (Lymphoid Hyperplasia) FIGURE 7.7

WHAT IT IS. Chronic inflammation of the pharynx, commonly seen in young horses between 2 and 3 years of age. It may have a number of underlying causes, including a previous viral respiratory infection and exposure to large amounts of respiratory irritants. An affected horse will have a nasal discharge that reoccurs even after antibiotic treatment, an intermittent cough that seems to originate from the upper airway or throat, and possibly enlargement of the lymph nodes between the lower jaw bones.

DIAGNOSIS. A diagnosis will be suspected based on the typical symptoms and confirmed with an endoscopic examination of the pharyngeal area. The vet will see small raised bumps or nodules on the pharynx where lymph tissue is activated. Severity of lymphoid hyperplasia may be graded according to the following guidelines:

GRADE I: A small number of tiny white nodules at the top of the pharynx. These are likely to be a normal finding in many young horses.

GRADE II: A larger number of tiny white nodules spread over the top and sides of the pharynx, accompanied by several larger, pinkish nodules scattered over the same area.

GRADE III: Many large pink and shrunken white nodules spread over the entire surface of the pharynx.

GRADE IV: Closely packed pink nodules covering the pharynx, epiglottis, and lining of the guttural pouches.

In many cases, a horse may have been administered an antibiotic in an effort to control bacteria that may be contributing to the nasal discharge with some success initially, only to have the discharge recur once the antibiotic is discontinued. This happens because bacteria involved with the nasal discharge are secondary to the existing pharyngitis, meaning the nasal discharge cannot be successfully eliminated unless the inflammation of the pharynx is controlled.

TREATMENT. Treatment is often unnecessary as youngsters tend to outgrow this condition over time. Topical treatment with anti-inflammatory solutions such as DMSO or systemic treatment with corticosteroids may be recommended in a young horse if the chronic nasal discharge and cough are affecting performance.

HOW SERIOUS IS IT? Most of the time lymphoid hyperplasia is more of a nuisance than a significant health threat. In the majority of cases it is self-limiting.

POTENTIAL COMPLICATIONS. None.

Laryngeal Hemiplegia (Roaring) FIGURE 7.8

WHAT IT IS. Damage or disease of a nerve called the recurrent laryngeal nerve that supplies the muscles that control movement of the arytenoid cartilages when the horse breathes. This results in partial or complete paralysis of one of the arytenoid cartilages, leading to an obstruction of airflow when the horse takes a breath. It usually affects the left side. The exact cause of this condition is unknown, although larger horses appear to be more at risk.

DIAGNOSIS. Laryngeal hemiplegia is suspected if the horse makes a loud noise during inspiration (referred to as "roaring"), and a diagnosis can be confirmed with an endoscopic examination of the horse's upper airway.

TREATMENT. Often treatment is unnecessary. Even with complete paralysis of one arytenoid cartilage, horses can continue to perform in many disciplines without compromise. However, for a horse that races or competes in other high-intensity sports such as barrel racing or 3-day eventing, laryngeal hemiplegia can cause a decline in performance because the restricted airflow limits the intake of oxygen. The noise can also be extremely distracting, and may become more pronounced in sports, such as dressage, where neck flexion is required. In all of these situations, surgical correction of the problem may be recommended. Surgery for laryngeal hemiplegia involves placement of large sutures to hold the cartilages open (called a tie-back). Sometimes this procedure will be combined with a second procedure called a ventriculectomy, which involves removing the small sac of tissue that sits next to the cartilage, which then scars down and helps hold the arytenoid cartilages out of the airway. In severe cases, an arytenoidectomy, or the removal of the affected cartilage, may be recommended.

HOW SERIOUS IS IT? This condition can be very mild and nothing more than an annoyance because of the noise heard during breathing. Depending on the degree of paralysis and the athletic demands on the horse, it can be performance limiting. Although surgery is usually successful at resolving the problem, it is a major procedure that can be expensive and risky. Furthermore, the surgical correction may fail after a period of time, and have to be repeated.

POTENTIAL COMPLICATIONS. Laryngeal hemiplegia may increase the risk for EIPH (see page 148) secondary to alterations in pressure balance in the lungs during breathing.

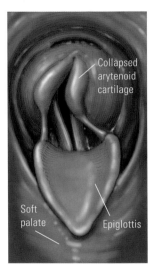

FIGURE 7.8. **Paralysis of the arytenoid cartilages of the pharynx is known as laryngeal hemiplegia, and causes the airway to become obstructed when the horse takes a breath.**

Collapsed arytenoid cartilage

Soft palate

Epiglottis

The Horse's Body: Health and Disease

Dorsal Displacement of the Soft Palate (DDSP)   FIGURE 7.9

WHAT IT IS. The soft palate (tissues that divide the pharyngeal area between the nasal passages and mouth) is displaced dorsally (up) over the top of the epiglottis, affecting its function of controlling breathing and swallowing. This can happen intermittently in normal horses, but if the palate remains displaced during high-intensity exercise the horse will have trouble breathing. Should this be the case, the horse will exhibit exercise intolerance and make abnormal breathing noises.

DIAGNOSIS. A diagnosis may be confirmed with an endoscopic examination. The vet must be careful not to overinterpret a finding that the soft palate is displaced, given that this can occur intermittently in normal horses. Endoscopy at exercise on a high-speed treadmill can confirm a diagnosis.

TREATMENT. Trainers may manage this condition by tying the tongue into a position that prevents displacement from occurring. If there is underlying inflammation of the pharyngeal area, treatment with anti-inflammatory washes may be recommended. A number of different surgical procedures may be suggested to correct the condition when it is a consistent problem. These include cutting some of the muscles that control movement of the larynx (sternothyrohyoideus myectomy), cutting away a part of the soft palate (staphylectomy), or enlarging the epiglottis with injection of Teflon.

HOW SERIOUS IS IT? This condition may cause no problems at rest, or for a horse that is not required to perform high-intensity exercise. It may have a negative impact on performance for horses involved in sports such as racing and can be difficult to eliminate even when surgery is performed.

POTENTIAL COMPLICATIONS. Permanent displacement of the soft palate can lead to pneumonia due to particles of feed being breathed into the lungs when eating. The epiglottis is prevented from performing its important function of closing off the airways when the horse is swallowing.

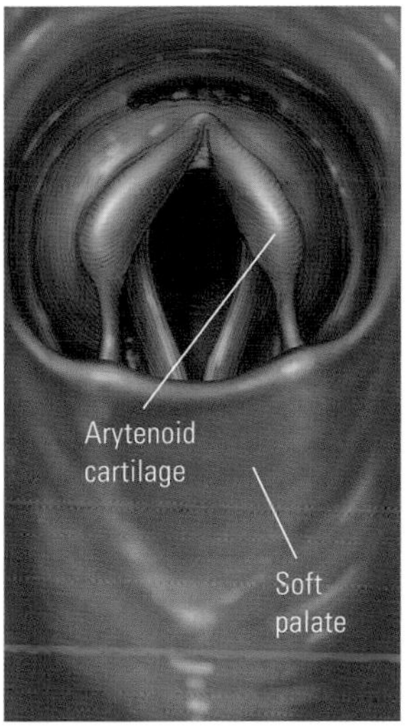

FIGURE 7.9. **The soft palate becomes positioned over the top of the epiglottis with the condition known as dorsal displacement of the soft palate.**

Epiglottic Entrapment

WHAT IT IS. The epiglottis becomes trapped in the tissues of the pharynx, preventing it from functioning properly to control breathing and swallowing. This may be due to a deformity or abnormally small-sized epiglottis. A horse experiencing problems due to epiglottic entrapment will have exercise intolerance, make abnormal sounds during breathing, and cough occasionally, especially during mealtime.

DIAGNOSIS. This condition is diagnosed through an endoscopic exam.

TREATMENT. Surgery is necessary to incise the tissues trapping the epiglottis and it can be performed with the horse sedated but still standing, or under general anesthesia. The surgery not only frees the epiglottis, but also prevents recurrence of the condition.

HOW SERIOUS IS IT? It is easily corrected, and horses can return to training as soon as 2 weeks after a standing surgical procedure is performed.

POTENTIAL COMPLICATIONS. Surgery can deform the larynx and affect breathing.

Arytenoid Chondritis

WHAT IT IS. An inflammation that results in the distortion and enlargement of the arytenoid cartilages, causing them to lose their mobility and begin to obstruct airflow through the larynx. A horse with this problem will begin to show exercise intolerance, and a noise may be heard with every breath while he is exercising. In severe cases, a horse may even have difficulty breathing at rest.

DIAGNOSIS. The abnormality of the arytenoid cartilages will be seen during an endoscopic examination. Radiographs of the larynx might also show mineralization of the cartilages.

TREATMENT. In most cases the arytenoids, or at minimum, the diseased area of the cartilages, must be surgically removed.

HOW SERIOUS IS IT? Even with a successful surgery, as many as 50 percent of affected horses will still have compromised breathing which will limit their ability to perform.

POTENTIAL COMPLICATIONS. None.

Inflammatory Airway Disease

WHAT IT IS. Inflammation of the respiratory tract caused by exposure to irritants such as dust or mold, or secondary to infectious diseases such as influenza. Mucous and inflammatory cells will be released, and small muscles may spasm to close the airways (bronchospasm). Signs of exercise intolerance, intermittent nasal discharge, and cough are seen most commonly in younger horses.

DIAGNOSIS. If this disease is suspected due to a decline in performance, nasal discharge, or intermittent cough, an endoscopic examination will be recommended. Samples obtained from the trachea or through BAL will contain mucous along with different types of inflammatory cells.

TREATMENT. In many cases, the most important component of treatment is to minimize exposure to respiratory irritants. This means careful environmental management to reduce airway inflammation. (See page 155.) Once the condition is established, treatment with bronchodilators such as clenbuteral to relieve bronchospasms and with corticosteroids such as dexamethasone or prednisolone to reduce inflammation is likely to be recommended. Medications administered through an inhaler may be appropriate prior to competition for young performance horses with chronic problems to help control the progression of damage by minimizing inflammation.

HOW SERIOUS IS IT? Inflammatory airway disease can cause a significant decline in the horse's performance, especially in sports such as racing or barrel racing where oxygen demands are high. However, if it is recognized early and treated appropriately, it should be a manageable condition.

POTENTIAL COMPLICATIONS. Inflammatory airway disease can progress to COPD if it is not managed and controlled. (See page 147.)

Chronic Obstructive Pulmonary Disease
(COPD, Heaves, or Reactive Airway Disease)

WHAT IT IS. Heaves is the most common lung disease seen in horses. It is due to inflammation of the airways, resulting in a thickening of airway walls, spasms of the small muscles that control the airways (bronchospasms), and a discharge of mucous and inflammatory cells. These changes within the lungs make it difficult for the horse to push air out, leading to an increased expiratory effort during breathing.

The underlying cause of heaves likely involves some degree of allergy, along with chronic inflammation due to exposure to dust, molds, and other airway irritants. Horses with a history of viral respiratory infections as youngsters may be more prone to heaves as they age, and horses kept in a stable are at higher risk than horses kept outside. A young horse with inflammatory airway disease may eventually develop COPD.

Depending on the severity of the disease, the signs of COPD range from mild exercise intolerance to labored breathing, a chronic cough, and a persistent nasal discharge. Symptoms may be seasonal, especially when allergy is an important underlying factor. A horse with dust sensitivity may show more severe signs during dry summer months, while a horse with mold sensitivity may have more severe symptoms during the winter. A horse seriously affected by heaves will exhibit a pattern of extremely labored breathing with a large amount of abdominal movement associated with each breath. In long-standing cases, the muscles running along either side of the horse's belly will become enlarged, forming a visible line known as a "heaves line."

DIAGNOSIS. A suspicion of heaves will be based on typical clinical signs. The vet will often hear wheezing during auscultation of the lungs. To confirm a diagnosis, an endoscopic examination may be recommended, and a sampling of discharge through the endoscope or with BAL will provide useful information.

In circumstances where allergies play a significant role, allergy testing will be suggested. (See chapter 15, "The Immune System.")

TREATMENT. What the vet recommends will depend on the severity of the signs as well as on how a horse responds to different treatments. In all cases, environmental management and reduction of exposure to all respiratory irritants will be recommended. As in treatment for inflammatory airway disease, bronchodilators and corticosteroids are likely to be a part of the management of this disease. Expectorants such as potassium iodide may also be recommended to help loosen mucous within the airways and enhance clearance.

Medications administered through an inhaler may be the most effective way for treating heaves with minimal side effects. Generally this involves administration of a bronchodilator first to open airways, followed by administration of a corticosteroid to help control inflammation. The purpose of the bronchodilator in this situation is to ensure that the corticosteroids reach deeper into the lungs in order to achieve the best results.

In cases where allergy is involved, hyposensitization with allergy shots can help minimize the allergic response and lessen the symptoms. (See chapter 15, "The Immune System.")

HOW SERIOUS IS IT? COPD is often a debilitating disease that can progress to the point where it is difficult or impossible to control, even with aggressive treatment. The best course is to take management steps to minimize risk of this disease.

COMPLICATIONS. Horses with heaves are more prone to infections and may be at risk for developing pneumonia or pleuropneumonia.

Exercise-Induced Pulmonary Hemorrhage (EIPH)

WHAT IT IS. The horse bleeds from his lungs into the airways following hard exercise. Horses involved in racing, barrel racing, or jumping tend to develop EIPH, and they are referred to as bleeders. The exact mechanisms behind bleeding are unknown, but it may be related to increased pressure within the small blood vessels in the lungs, secondary to demands on the heart during heavy exercise. Blood may be seen in the nostrils after exercise, although this occurs only in approximately 5 percent of affected horses.

DIAGNOSIS. A diagnosis of EIPH is usually made by an endoscopic examination. Blood is seen within the airways for up to several hours following exercise. If endoscopy cannot be performed right after exercise, a sample of discharge taken from the airways in the days following a bleeding episode may still show broken-down red blood cells within the "cleanup crew" of white blood cells.

TREATMENT. Treating EIPH usually involves giving the horse between 250 and 500 milligrams of the diuretic medication called furosemide one to four hours prior to exercise. Although not completely effective, this treatment appears to reduce bleeding in 50 percent of affected horses. Its use in performance horses is controversial, because of the belief that it may have performance-enhancing effects unrelated to EIPH. Racehorse trainers may also restrict a bleeder's intake of food and water on the day of a race, thus of reducing the mass within the intestines. In theory this would take pressure off of the diaphragm muscle and minimize the stresses that may encourage bleeding.

HOW SERIOUS IS IT? The actual effect of EIPH on performance is controversial, yet studies have supported the widespread belief that bleeding can cause a decline in performance. Many horses continue to compete at an acceptable level even though they bleed. Although the condition may be manageable it generally cannot be cured, and once a horse is identified as a bleeder he is likely to continue to bleed with high-intensity exercise.

POTENTIAL COMPLICATIONS. A horse with EIPH may be more prone to infections or airway irritation at the site of bleeding within the lungs. This could predispose him to pneumonia or inflammatory airway disease.

Pneumonia

WHAT IT IS. A bacterial infection that attacks the lungs. The most common bacterial organism to cause pneumonia in adult horses is *Streptococcus zooepidemicus*, a bacterium that normally lives within the respiratory tract but may overgrow and produce disease in lungs that are compromised by another condition, such as a viral infection, stress during transport, or chronic heaves. Other bacteria may be isolated in cases of pneumonia, including *Streptococcus equi* (see Strangles, page 150), *Staphylococcus aureus,* or *Streptococcus pneumoniae*. A horse with pneumonia will become anorexic and have a fever, abnormal respiration (fast or labored), nasal discharge, and cough.

DIAGNOSIS. Pneumonia will be suspected based on the symptoms. Abnormal lung sounds will be heard during auscultation, and blood work may have a high white blood cell count consistent with infection, as well as a high fibrinogen—a substance released into the blood during inflammation. Samples obtained from the trachea will have increased numbers of white blood cells along with bacterial organisms. Culture of these samples will help identify the specific cause of the pneumonia in order to determine an appropriate treatment. In serious cases, radiographs of the lungs might be recommended to help determine the extent of lung involvement.

TREATMENT. An appropriate antibiotic will be recommended. Ideally, the choice of antibiotic will be based on culture of the specific bacteria from tracheal samples. If this is not possible, the vet will choose a broad-spectrum antibiotic most likely to be effective against the organisms that commonly cause pneumonia.

HOW SERIOUS IS IT? If pneumonia is identified early and treated aggressively with the appropriate antibiotic, success is likely. However, if the pneumonia is not recognized and is allowed to become chronic, serious complications can result.

POTENTIAL COMPLICATIONS. Bacteria can form pockets or abscesses in the lungs that can be very difficult to treat. It's also possible for the pneumonia to spread from the lungs to the pleura, or lining of the chest cavity, causing pleuropneumonia, which can be life threatening.

Pleuropneumonia (Pleuritis)

WHAT IT IS. An infection that affects the pleura, or space surrounding the lungs. Most commonly it will be a complication of pneumonia. Pleuropneumonia is a potential risk of transport, as well as a possible complication of surgical procedures performed on the upper respiratory tract. A horse with pleuropneumonia will have a fever, refuse to eat, have a nasal discharge, cough, and labored breathing.

DIAGNOSIS. The vet may be able to detect fluid accumulating within the chest when he listens to the horse's breathing with a stethoscope. Blood work may show a high white blood cell count and high fibrinogen, typical of infections, and marked inflammation. A needle can be passed into the chest (a process called thoracocentesis) to obtain fluid, so that an analysis of bacteria and cell types can confirm a diagnosis. Radiographs and ultrasound may also be useful diagnostic tools.

TREATMENT. Antibiotics will be administered, and long-term treatment may be required (up to 8 weeks) to completely clear the infection. In severe cases, fluid may need to be drained from the chest.

HOW SERIOUS IS IT? Pleuropneumonia is a very serious disease that may not respond well to treatment, and can have life-threatening complications. Only about 50 percent of severely affected horses will survive, and of those, only 50 percent are likely to return to high-level competition.

POTENTIAL COMPLICATIONS. Laminitis.

Strangles

WHAT IT IS. A bacterial disease of the horse's upper respiratory tract caused by the organism *Streptococcus equi*. The disease is easily spread from horse to horse, either through direct contact or indirectly via handlers, shared equipment, or even flies transmitting the organism. Strangles begins with a fever as high as 103 to 106 degrees F, usually occurring 2 to 14 days after exposure to the organism. The horse will have a clear nasal discharge that becomes purulent (thick and creamy) and may be accompanied by a cough. Lymph nodes begin to enlarge, and often abscess open and drain approximately 2 weeks following the fever stage of the disease. Many horses will show minimal signs of illness beyond the abscessed lymph nodes, whereas others will be depressed and refuse food.

The vet is likely to suspect strangles if the horse shows characteristic signs of a fever and abscessed lymph nodes. A diagnosis can be confirmed by a culture of abscess material if draining lymph node abscesses are present. Or, it can be confirmed from a pharyngeal wash sample, which the vet will obtain by flushing a saline solution through a long catheter that is passed up the horse's nose and into the pharyngeal area (his throat) to collect a fluid sample. In some cases, the organism can be cultured from a nasal discharge, but this method for making a diagnosis is less reliable.

TREATMENT. Recommendations vary widely and can be highly controversial. Most practitioners agree that farm owners should monitor temperatures daily in barns where known exposure has occurred or during an actual outbreak, and immediately initiate treatment with an appropriate antibiotic if the horse develops a fever. By treating immediately, the organism is controlled before infection can become well established and involve lymph nodes or other organs.

If a fever stage is not identified and lymph nodes begin to swell, they should be encouraged to ripen and drain using hot packs or poultices. As abscesses mature they may open on their own, or the vet will lance and drain them when they have developed to the appropriate point. Following

The Horse's Body: Health and Disease

drainage, the abscesses are flushed with a dilute betadine solution, and may be infused with an antibiotic ointment. If the horse is bright, alert, and eating well at this point, systemic antibiotics may not be needed. In the majority of cases, strangles is self-limiting and clinical signs should resolve on their own within 2 to 3 weeks. When abscesses mature and drain and antibiotics are not required, the affected horse will benefit from a prolonged natural immunity approximately 75 percent of the time.

If the horse is experiencing other signs of illness, is depressed, or fever is prolonged, antibiotics may be warranted even after the abscesses have drained. A number of antibiotics may be recommended, including penicillin, ceftiofur and trimethoprim-sulfdiazine, or sulfamethoxazole.

HOW SERIOUS IS IT? In most cases, strangles will resolve without complications. Yet it is serious because of the high risk of its spreading from horse to horse, resulting in a widespread outbreak. If a horse becomes ill with strangles, measures to control its spread are essential, including strict isolation of a sick horses and strict hygiene in the barn. The organism can survive in the environment for as long as 55 days. But, if shedding from infected or carrier horses can be eliminated, it is possible to completely clear the environment of the organism if proper disinfection measures are taken.

Ideally, sick horses will be housed in completely separate buildings to avoid affecting other horses. At minimum, sick horses should be maintained in enclosed stalls with solid walls at the end of a barn aisle where there is no routine traffic of horses or handlers. Manure and other wastes should be disposed of in a remote location, so no contamination of "clean" areas with waste materials will occur. Burning bedding and manure after cleaning is a good practice to consider.

Infected horses should be handled only after all the other horses have been handled, and handlers should maintain rigorous sanitation procedures. This would include wearing coveralls and shoe covers when handling sick horses, and using a foot bath containing an appropriate disinfectant such as a quarternary ammonium (Roccal®-D) or phenolic based disinfectants (Lysol® or Pine-Sol®). (*Note: Although bleach is an effective disinfectant against most viruses and bacteria, it is inactivated by organic material, making its efficacy less than ideal in a barn situation.*)

Once infected, a horse may harbor the organism for at least 6 weeks after he appears fully recovered and should be considered a potential source of infection for that amount of time. Three pharyngeal wash samples taken at weekly intervals after clinical signs have resolved are necessary to demonstrate that a horse is no longer shedding the organism and capable of spreading the disease. These samples should be tested in the lab using both PCR (polymerase chain reaction) and culture, which tests for both genetic material of live or dead organisms and growth of viable organisms. If the results of all three of these washes are negative, the horse can safely be released from isolation.

POTENTIAL COMPLICATIONS. Metastatic abscesses (abscesses that form in other parts of the horse's body) and a rare but severe autoimmune problem known as purpura hemorrhagica may be complications. Purpura leads to significant edema, or swelling of legs, skin and internal organs, and can result in large areas of sloughed skin, organ failure, or even death.

Rarely, a horse will become a chronic carrier of the disease when the *Strep equi* organism takes up residence in his guttural pouches. Chronic carriers may be responsible for repeated outbreaks of the disease in facilities where they reside, making the existence of a carrier horse at a facility a serious problem. In a barn where repeated outbreaks have occurred, it is necessary to identify and treat carrier horses that might be living on the property. This requires performing the same series of pharyngeal washes described above on every horse at the site, and treating those horses with positive results—an indication that they may be harboring the organism. In an active outbreak, this testing must be performed a minimum of thirty days after horses experiencing strangles are clear of clinical signs. Treatment may require lavage (washing) of the guttural pouch with an antimicrobial in addition to systemic (oral or intramuscular) antibiotics.

Influenza

WHAT IT IS. A viral respiratory disease that commonly affects younger horses between the ages of 1 and 3 years. It has a very short incubation period of 1 to 3 days and is easily spread from horse to horse by aerosol transmission (through the air). As a consequence, this infection can spread rapidly through barns, resulting in a severe outbreak.

A horse infected with influenza will have a very high fever (103 to 105 degrees F) that begins 3 to 5 days following exposure to the virus. The virus attacks the lining of the respiratory tract and causes serious damage to the respiratory defense mechanisms, which results in the characteristic symptom of a severe, deep, repetitive cough.

DIAGNOSIS. Influenza may be suspected if a number of horses in a herd have a high fever and a severe cough. Blood work will show a low white blood cell count typical of a viral infection.

Isolation of the influenza virus may be difficult and impractical since the virus is only shed by the horse during the first 24 to 48 hours of infection. A test is available that identifies the virus from a nasal discharge during this period, and although it is expensive it does offer the advantage of an immediate diagnosis when there is concern about an outbreak.

Influenza infection can also be confirmed by measuring antibodies in the blood against the virus at the time of illness, and again 21 days following the onset of symptoms. Antibodies will increase by approximately four times over this time period as the horse's immune system responds to the virus. However, this test does not provide a specific diagnosis until long after the horse is recovering—meaning its only value would be for future management decisions.

The Horse's Body: Health and Disease

TREATMENT. Treatment for influenza is good management, including rest in a well-ventilated stall. Avoidance of stress is a part of the treatment. Non-steroidal anti-inflammatory medications may be recommended to reduce the fever or help keep the horse comfortable. The horse should be monitored carefully for a secondary bacterial infection that might lead to pneumonia, which would require treatment with antibiotics. As a rule of thumb, a horse experiencing influenza should be given one week of rest for every one day he had a fever.

HOW SERIOUS IS IT? For a number of reasons, influenza is the most serious of the respiratory viruses that affect horses. Because the virus causes extensive damage to the respiratory tract, an affected horse may require up to 3 months of rest for full recovery before going back to work. In addition, its short incubation period means rapid spread, and large numbers of horses are likely to be infected before the outbreak is controlled. Finally, damage caused by the virus makes the horse more susceptible to complications.

POTENTIAL COMPLICATIONS. Influenza can put the horse at risk for secondary bacterial infections such as pneumonia or pleuropneumonia due to damage to the lining of the respiratory tract. Inflammation of the airways may also predispose the horse to developing inflammatory airway disease or COPD (heaves).

Rhinopneumonitis

WHAT IT IS. Rhinopneumonitis is a respiratory disease caused by the equine herpes virus (EHV). This virus has two subtypes that can cause respiratory disease, EHV-1 and EHV-4. Although it can infect horses of any age, respiratory disease due to this virus is most common in young horses between the ages of 4 and 8 months of age. The virus can cause a very low-grade infection, and may be passed in nasal discharge for up to 3 weeks following infection. It has a 2- to 10-day incubation period, and during an outbreak, it will move through a barn very slowly.

A horse infected with this virus will have a fever, nasal discharge, and cough, but because the respiratory lining is less damaged, will not be as ill as a horse infected with the influenza virus.

DIAGNOSIS. As with influenza, antibodies against the rhino virus can be measured in the bloodstream and a rise in antibody levels between the time of onset of the disease and 3 weeks into the recovery period will help identify EHV as the causative virus. However, because this disease causes less severe signs, it may not be recognized immediately, making it difficult to obtain samples at the right time. It is also possible to identify the virus in a nasal discharge for up to one week following infection. In most cases, the vet will not attempt to specifically identify the virus in a horse experiencing signs typical of EHV because the disease is mild and most horses recover with minimal complications.

TREATMENT. The treatment recommended for rhinopneumonitis is similar to that for influenza: good management, including rest in a well-ventilated stall, and avoidance of stress. Nonsteroidal anti-inflammatory medications may be prescribed to reduce the fever or help keep the horse comfortable. The rule of one week off for each day the horse had a fever applies to this respiratory virus as well.

HOW SERIOUS IS IT? Respiratory disease due to EHV is generally mild and self-limiting.

POTENTIAL COMPLICATIONS. EHV can cause abortion in pregnant mares. In addition, there is always the risk of secondary bacterial infection leading to pneumonia or pleuropneumonia due to damage to the respiratory tract, although these risks are less with EHV than with influenza.

Minimize Risk of Respiratory Disease

Many respiratory conditions are closely linked, and are often related to airway inflammation due to an allergic response or simply because of ongoing irritation. You can take the following steps to help minimize irritation to your horse's airways in order to reduce his risk for respiratory disease:

- Clean the barn. Minimize the horse's exposure to dust and other potential irritants by sweeping or blowing out the barn daily. Move the horse out before cleaning begins to help keep him away from stirred-up dust.

- Provide turnout. An open field is a better environment for a horse with sensitive airways, because irritants are less concentrated in the open air. If turnout isn't possible, make sure the barn is well ventilated and keep the horse stalled as close to an open door or window as possible.

- Protect from arena dust. Avoid stabling in a barn where stalls are attached to an arena where dust is in the air while horses work. Water arena surfaces regularly to keep the dust down.

- Water-down feed. Hay is a huge potential source of respiratory irritants. To minimize the horse's exposure, wet hay by soaking it in a large bucket of water before feeding time.

- When hauling, make sure trailers are well ventilated, with all vents kept open. Avoid bedding on trailer floors that can be a source of irritants in the air.

- Maintain a regular schedule of routine vaccinations to protect the horse against viral respiratory infections. What starts as a simple "cold" can progress to a chronic airway disease. (See pages 147–148 for information.)

TABLE 7.1

Guide to Respiratory Symptoms

If your horse has symptoms of respiratory disease, this information chart will help you determine what they mean.

SYMPTOM	INDICATES WHAT?	POSSIBLE DIAGNOSIS
Nasal discharge— one nostril	Inflammation or infection is causing mucous and inflammatory cells to accumulate. The problem most likely originates from the front of the horse's head, before the two nasal passages join at the back of the pharynx.	Sinusitis (often has a foul odor). Guttural pouch empyema. Guttural pouch mycosis.
Nasal discharge— both nostrils	Inflammation of infection is causing mucous and inflammatory cells to accumulate. The problem most likely originates from the pharynx or lower airway.	Pharyngitis. Pneumonia. Inflammatory airway disease. COPD. Influenza. Rhinopneumonitis.
Nasal discharge— bloody	Bleeding is occurring somewhere in the respiratory tract.	EIPH. Guttural pouch mycosis. Ethmoid hematoma.
Cough	Inflammation results in irritation or accumulation of discharge that triggers a cough as a defense mechanism to expel offending irritants.	Pharyngitis. Inflammatory airway disease. COPD. Pneumonia. Pleuropneumonia.
Fever	The immune system is most likely responding to an infection— either bacterial or viral.	Pneumonia. Pleuropneumonia. Influenza. Rhinopneumonitis. Miscellaneous respiratory viruses.
Breathing noise when exercising	There is a structural abnormality causing a disruption of airflow, usually of the laryngeal area.	Laryngeal hemiplegia. Arytenoid chondritis. DDSP. Epiglottic entrapment.
Difficulty breathing at rest	The horse is experiencing difficulty moving air in and out of the lungs.	Pneumonia. Pleuropneumonia. COPD.

Your Horse has a "Cold." What Should You Do?

You throw your horse his hay ration, and hear him coughing in his stall. On closer inspection, you notice mucous in both nostrils. He seems fairly alert, and he's eating dinner with his normal enthusiasm. Should you panic? Call the vet immediately? Or just take a deep breath and wait until morning? The following steps will help you decide what to do:

STEP 1. Take his temperature. In most cases it will be normal or slightly elevated. If it's higher than 102 degrees F, call your veterinarian for advice. You may be advised to administer a dose of a nonsteroidal anti-inflammatory medication such as phenylbutazone or flunixin meglumine to help lower his temperature and make him feel better. Most respiratory viruses start with a fever that can last from 1 to 3 days. If your horse does have a fever, you should take his temperature twice daily until it drops to normal and stays there for at least 48 hours. If your horse's fever is very high (i.e., 104 degrees F or higher), your vet may want to examine him and perform blood work. If it stays elevated for longer than 3 days or your horse seems very ill, you should also schedule a visit. Your horse may have a bacterial infection that should be treated with antibiotics. Just like in humans, the majority of colds are caused by viruses that won't be helped by antibiotics. However, your vet will prescribe antibiotics if he believes bacteria are involved because of a high or persistent fever or high white blood cell count.

STEP 2. Give him a break. If your horse's temperature is normal or only slightly elevated, he probably has a minor virus that will resolve with rest and a little tender loving care. Cancel any rides or training sessions you have planned for a week or so, and give him a chance to recover. Remember the rule of thumb: a week of rest for every day his temperature is elevated.

STEP 3. Count the days. Most typical respiratory viruses will resolve completely within 10 to 14 days. If your horse has a nasal discharge that persists for longer than this amount of time, he may have developed a secondary bacterial infection. In this circumstance, the population of normal bacteria living in your horse's respiratory tract takes advantage of his compromised state and begins to overgrow, resulting in a persistent nasal discharge and cough. Although this situation is different from a true bacterial infection, your veterinarian may still prescribe antibiotics to help clear the bacteria.

STEP 4. Back to work. Once your horse is symptom free for at least 3 days he should be ready to go back to work. Allow a minimum of a full week of rest even with a minor cold that lasts more than a day or so.

CHAPTER 8

The Nervous System

THEN AND NOW

In the 1800s, Edward Mayhew, an English veterinarian, recognized that tetanus enters the horse's body through a wound, and leads to muscle spasms that cause the jaw to lock, preventing the animal from eating. He developed a technique for passing a flexible tube through the horse's nostrils into the stomach, in order to administer nutrition in the form of a linseed gruel. With this treatment, along with darkness, quiet, and gentle care, some horses survived this common, often fatal disease.

Today, tetanus is rarely seen due to the effectiveness of tetanus vaccination. When tetanus does occur, treatment is much the same as it was nearly two centuries ago. This is with the addition of the tetanus antitoxin to help combat the circulating toxins and antibiotics to kill the responsible bacteria. Nasogastric intubation remains a common technique that's used in every area of veterinary care.

THE NERVOUS SYSTEM, THE HORSE'S CONTROL CENTER, is divided into two portions, central and peripheral. The central nervous system is made up of the brain and spinal cord and is the primary processing center for information. The peripheral nervous system consists of the nerves that detect stimuli, relay information to the central nervous system, and return instructions to the various organs of the body.

The following describes the basic structures of the nervous system.
FIGURE 8.1

Brain

The brain is protected by the skull, and is composed of three primary parts, the cerebrum, the cerebellum, and the brain stem. The cerebrum, the largest part of the brain, is responsible for functions of intelligence and memory, in addition to controlling the senses—sight, smell, hearing, touch, and taste. The cerebellum, located at the back of the cerebrum, is responsible for balance and muscular coordination. The brain stem (also called the medulla oblongata) is at the upper end of the spinal cord where it meets the brain, and is responsible for involuntary activities such as circulation, breathing, and regulation of body temperature.

The outer layers of the brain, called the meninges, help protect it from damage. These three layers are the dura mater (outer layer filled with capillaries, or small vessels carrying blood and nutrients), arachnoid mater (middle layer filled with protective fluid called cerebrospinal fluid, or CSF), and the pia mater (thin, inner protective layer).

Spinal Cord

The spinal cord is enclosed in the spinal column for protection. It is further protected by outer connective tissues, and is bathed in a layer of cerebrospinal fluid. The five sections into which the spinal cord is divided correspond to the portions of the spine surrounding it: the cervical, thoracic, lumbar, sacral, and coccygeal. Each of these five sections sends out and receives signals that control specific areas of the body.

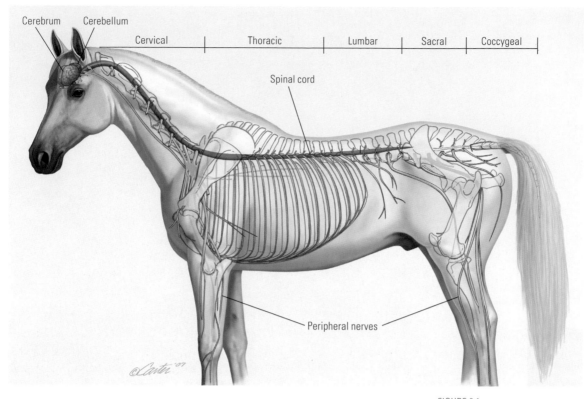

Cerebrum Cerebellum

Cervical　　　Thoracic　　　Lumbar　　Sacral　　Coccygeal

Spinal cord

Peripheral nerves

FIGURE 8.1.
The nervous system.

The spinal cord is comprised of individual nerve cells that are bunched together within the spinal cord—similar to the way individual wires make up a telephone line. These nerve cells consist of long cord-like portions called axons, which transmit messages through one or more message centers called dendrites.

Peripheral Nerves

These nerves are small bundles of nerve cells that branch off from the spinal cord to various areas of the body. They receive and relay messages to the brain and spinal cord (afferent nerves), and then send instructions back to the body (efferent nerves). Twelve pairs of cranial nerves extend directly from the brain to supply structures in the head, including those that control vision, hearing, and smell. The remaining peripheral nerves extend out from the spinal cord like the branches of a tree.

How the Horse Processes Information

Messages are transmitted throughout the nervous system by chemical messengers called neurotransmitters. These chemicals are released from the end of one nerve cell and travel across a small gap called a synapse, where they are detected by the next nerve cell in line. All of the functions of the horse's body are controlled through this same basic method of message transmission in various parts of the nervous system.

　　　　　　　　　　　　　　　　　　　The Horse's Body: Health and Disease

The Neurological Examination

In many cases neurological problems cause similar symptoms. The veterinarian will begin the neurological examination by trying to localize the problem within the nervous system. Does the problem involve the central or the peripheral nervous system? If central, is it from the brain or the spinal cord? If the spinal cord is suspected, what section of the cord is affected? If it is peripheral, which nerves are involved? These are the questions the vet must answer by taking the following steps:

History

The history of the symptoms is important for diagnosing many neurological conditions. For example, a history of trauma with a sudden onset of signs might help identify a specific injury, whereas a history of a slowly progressive onset of signs might point toward a tumor or other slowly developing condition.

Physical Examination

The physical examination of the nervous system involves a systematic evaluation of the function of the brain, spinal cord, and peripheral nerves. The vet will usually begin at the head, and gradually work his way backwards along the horse's body. The following describes abnormalities the veterinarian will be looking for as a part of the neurological exam.

- Behavioral changes such as depression, aggression, walking in circles, or the horse pressing his head against solid objects such as a stall wall, mean that the neurological abnormality most likely involves the brain. Seizures are also an indication of brain involvement.

- Blindness, a lack of a menace response, or lack of a pupillary light response may indicate injury to the optic (second cranial), oculomotor (third cranial), or facial (seventh cranial) nerves.

- Abnormal eye movement when the head is moved may indicate damage to the oculomotor (third cranial), trochlear (fourth cranial), and trigeminal (fifth cranial) nerves.

- Loss of sensation to the face or drooping of the muzzle, ears, or eyes may indicate an injury to the trigeminal (fifth cranial) or facial (seventh cranial) nerves.

- Difficulty eating or swallowing or noises when breathing may point toward injury to the glossopharyngeal (ninth cranial), vagus (tenth cranial) and accessory (eleventh cranial) nerves which all supply the pharyngeal and laryngeal area.

- A protruding tongue or the inability to retract the tongue when it is pulled out of the mouth may indicate injury to the hypoglossal (twelfth cranial) nerve. This sign can also be seen with brain injury.

- Loss of coordination (called ataxia), general weakness and loss of proprioception (the horse has difficulty placing his limbs appropriately) generally indicate a spinal cord abnormality. The horse might stumble sideways, lean against a wall for support or, in extreme cases, be unable to stand. The vet will test the horse's coordination by moving him in small circles to evaluate movement, asking him to negotiate hills or other obstacles, and asking him to back up.

  If signs of ataxia and weakness are more pronounced in the hind limbs than in the forelimbs, the injury is most likely toward the top of the cervical (neck) area. If these signs are more pronounced in the fore limbs than in the hind limbs, the injury is most likely in the lower cer vical area or at the beginning of the thoracic (chest) area. If only the hind limbs are affected, the injury is most likely behind the second thoracic vertebra.

  If the horse is down and unable to raise his head, the injury can be localized to the upper three cervical vertebra. If he can lift his head and neck, the injury is behind the third cervical vertebra, and if he can dog-sit, the injury is most likely behind the second thoracic vertebrae.

- The cutaneous trunci reflex, exhibited when the horse twitches the skin on his body when pinched with a small hemostat or clamp (his natural "shoo-fly" mechanism), may also be lost with a spinal cord injury. The point where this reflex disappears can help define the most forward point of the injury.

- Abnormalities of movement that involve a single limb may indicate an injury to a specific peripheral nerve. A good example is the dragging forelimb commonly seen with an injury to the radial nerve.

  Once the veterinarian has completed his examination, further tests might help to specifically pinpoint a neurological disease or injury.

Radiographs

Radiographs of the skull and spinal column may help to identify abnormalities of these skeletal structures that could be affecting the brain and spinal cord. In some cases, a myelogram will be recommended. This procedure involves injecting a contrast material (a liquid containing iodine, which appears bright white on a radiograph in contrast to the darker soft-tissue structures) into the CSF (fluid surrounding the spinal cord). This will allow the veterinarian to see things like a malformation of a vertebra or a tumor pressing against the spinal cord and causing neurological symptoms.

CSF Tap

Cerebrospinal fluid may be collected with a needle and examined for abnormalities such as blood, increased protein levels (indicating inflammation), signs of parasites or infection, or any other abnormalities that might help pinpoint a diagnosis.

The Horse's Body: Health and Disease

Advanced Diagnostics

MRI, CT scans, and nuclear scintigraphy are all diagnostic tools that might prove useful for diagnosing a neurological condition, and are becoming increasingly available at referral veterinary centers. In addition, measurement of electrical activity in muscles (electromyography) and in portions of the nervous system (nerve conduction studies or electroencephalography) can help identify the source of nervous system disorders.

WHEN THINGS GO WRONG

The following are the most common conditions likely to be diagnosed in a horse exhibiting neurological symptoms.

Meningitis

WHAT IT IS. Inflammation of the tissues surrounding the brain and spinal cord caused by infectious organisms including bacteria, viruses, or fungi, or due to a reaction of the immune system. A wide variety of signs may be observed, often those pointing toward brain involvement, such as behavioral changes, head pressing, and circling.

DIAGNOSIS. Diagnosis can be difficult, and depends on suspicion of a neurological problem based on symptoms. A horse with meningitis may have a fever, and blood tests might show a high white blood count with bacterial meningitis, low white blood count with viral meningitis, or very high fibrinogen due to inflammation. In many cases, a definite diagnosis will be made from an analysis of cerebrospinal fluid. Viral causes of meningitis may be identified through measurements of antibodies against the virus in the horse's bloodstream. These would include Eastern, Western, and Venezuelan encephalitis, or sleeping sickness. A definitive diagnosis in a case of meningitis will be made during a postmortem examination.

TREATMENT. The key to successful treatment is determining the underlying cause and treating it appropriately. For example, if a bacterial meningitis is identified, a suitable antibiotic will be necessary. Sometimes anti-seizure medications will be a part of the treatment. Anti-inflammatory medications are usually needed, and intravenous fluids or fluids with DMSO may be administered to control inflammation and swelling of nervous tissues. The three forms of sleeping sickness can be prevented with vaccination.

HOW SERIOUS IS IT? The prognosis depends on the underlying cause, but is generally guarded to poor. Many cases are fatal.

POTENTIAL COMPLICATIONS. Even if a horse recovers from meningitis, it is possible that he will continue to show neurological signs because of damage to his nervous system.

Epilepsy

WHAT IT IS. Epilepsy is a brain disorder that leads to recurrent seizures with no other underlying cause. Seizures occur when the electrical activity of the brain is disrupted. A full seizure causes the horse to become unconscious, go down, and become rigid (tonic phase). This is followed by a period of rapid contraction and relaxation of muscles (clonic phase). During a seizure, a horse may urinate, defecate, sweat, clamp his jaws, or roll his eyes. Partial seizures can occur with a variety of different symptoms, including limb twitching, facial or eyelid twitching, and chewing motions. Following a seizure, the horse will enter a period called the "postictal" phase, where he'll be depressed and may appear blind for a period of several hours.

A syndrome of juvenile epilepsy has been reported in Arabian foals with a sudden onset of seizures prior to 12 months of age. Rarely does epilepsy occur in older horses.

DIAGNOSIS. A diagnosis of epilepsy depends on eliminating all other possible causes of seizures. (See Table 8.1.) This may require extensive diagnostic tests, including blood work, analysis of cerebrospinal fluid, skull radiographs, and perhaps even an MRI examination of the brain.

TREATMENT. If other causes for seizures have been ruled out, treatment with anticonvulsant medications such as phenobarbital may be recommended. For foals with juvenile epilepsy, phenobarbital treatment is recommended for 6 months following the initial seizure, or until the foal reaches 12 months of age. In affected foals, seizures will usually stop at this time, with no increased risk for seizures to occur in their adult years. Blood tests to monitor blood levels of phenobarbital may be suggested during the period of treatment.

Treatment to control a seizure at the time it is occurring may not be recommended. Most seizures are self-limiting and short-lived (average of one minute), and administration of medications can be extremely dangerous. In rare cases, the veterinarian may administer an anticonvulsant medication such as diazepam (Valium®) to control a prolonged seizure. It's important to keep in mind, however, that a seizure causes more distress to owners and handlers observing the event than it does to the horse experiencing it.

In instances of adult epilepsy, specific events such as feeding time or the estrus cycle in a mare may trigger the onset of seizures. In such cases, management changes may help limit seizure incidence. Increased turnout time or free access to forage may limit stress associated with feeding, and treatment with progesterone to control estrus may help eliminate the trigger for in-heat mares.

HOW SERIOUS IS IT? Juvenile epilepsy in Arabian foals is usually self-limiting with no adverse effects on the horse once the disorder has been outgrown. Epilepsy in adult horses can have serious consequences, including danger to a rider if the horse is to continue in work. In general, a horse known to have a seizure disorder should not be ridden.

POTENTIAL COMPLICATIONS. Seizures can be dangerous to both the affected horse and his handlers, resulting in significant injuries.

Narcolepsy

WHAT IT IS. A brain abnormality that causes uncontrolled episodes of deep sleep that are accompanied by a loss of muscle tone and may cause the horse to suddenly collapse. A narcoleptic episode may be stimulated by a number of different things, including petting or stroking of the head, feeding time, or simply periods of quiet stall rest.

DIAGNOSIS. Narcolepsy will be suspected if a horse is observed to buckle at the knees and stumble, collapse, or fall repeatedly. The first sign of narcolepsy is usually evidenced by many small injuries that occur during the night in the stall when no other source of injury is likely. Blood tests and examination of cerebrospinal fluid are usually normal. A diagnosis can be confirmed by administering a dose of a medication called physostigmine salicylate, which will stimulate a narcoleptic attack in horses with the condition.

TREATMENT. The medication imipramine may help control narcolepsy in severely affected horses. In many cases, however, treatment is not practical.

HOW SERIOUS IS IT? Narcolepsy can affect the usefulness of a horse if the condition is severe. If the horse were to collapse when being ridden the rider could be injured. Although it is generally not advisable to ride a horse affected with this condition, many mildly affected horses with predictable episodes that occur in the stall will continue being used for riding, and even for high-level performance.

POTENTIAL COMPLICATIONS. Trauma secondary to collapsing episodes.

Cerebellar Abiotrophy

WHAT IT IS. A disease seen in the Arabian breed that involves abnormal development of the cerebellum. Affected foals between the ages of 2 and 4 months begin to show signs that include loss of coordination and spastic movements accompanied by a head tremor when attempting to move the head and neck.

DIAGNOSIS. Diagnosis is made based on typical clinical signs.

TREATMENT. No treatment is available.

HOW SERIOUS IS IT? Cerebellar abiotrophy often results in euthanasia because affected foals are unable to function adequately and may be dangerous to themselves and handlers. Some reports indicate that improvement can occur as foals mature.

POTENTIAL COMPLICATIONS. Injuries due to lack of coordination.

Rabies

WHAT IT IS. A viral disease carried by wild animals that causes neurological symptoms and usually leads to death within 3 to10 days.

DIAGNOSIS. A diagnosis can be confirmed with a test for antibodies against the virus in either the blood or cerebrospinal fluid.

TREATMENT. No effective treatment exists. Rabies can be prevented with vaccination.

HOW SERIOUS IS IT? Rabies is always fatal.

POTENTIAL COMPLICATIONS. The rabies virus can be transmitted to humans and is a fatal disease in all species. For this reason, if a diagnosis of rabies is suspected and confirmed, euthanasia is recommended.

Nigropallidal Encephalomalacia

WHAT IT IS. Degeneration of portions of the brain called the substantia nigra and the globus pallidus due to toxicity from eating the yellow star thistle plant (found in California, Oregon, Australia, and Argentina) or the Russian knapweed plant (found in Colorado, Utah and Washington). Muscles of the head become rigid, causing the lips and muzzle to retract and the tongue to protrude. The horse will be unable to eat. It is common for horses affected with this condition to submerge their heads in water buckets or troughs as they attempt to drink.

DIAGNOSIS. Diagnosis is based on symptoms and exposure to the plants known to cause the condition.

TREATMENT. No treatment is available.

HOW SERIOUS IS IT? Horses affected with this toxicity will usually dehydrate or starve to death. In most cases the horse will be euthanized.

POTENTIAL COMPLICATIONS. None.

Brain Trauma

WHAT IT IS. An injury to the head that causes swelling and potential damage to the brain. Symptoms may include loss of consciousness, behavioral changes, or seizures, in addition to outward signs such as bleeding or soft-tissue damage.

DIAGNOSIS. A diagnosis will be made based on a history of trauma to the head, accompanied by neurological symptoms of brain injury. The vet might recommend further diagnostic steps such as radiographs if a fracture is suspected.

TREATMENT. Initial treatment is focused on minimizing swelling that could lead to increased pressures within the brain and subsequent brain damage. This would involve administration of anti-inflammatories including corticosteroids, intravenous therapy with DMSO to reduce inflammation, and diuretics to limit fluid accumulation and resulting pressure within the skull. If a fracture has occurred, antibiotics will be recommended to reduce the chance of meningitis developing due to a

The Horse's Body: Health and Disease

bacterial infection. If the horse is seizuring, anticonvulsant medications might also be administered.

HOW SERIOUS IS IT? A head injury that results in brain damage can be very serious, and may even be rapidly fatal, if severe. Immediate treatment is critical for the best outcome, and any head trauma in a horse should be considered an emergency.

POTENTIAL COMPLICATIONS. Persistent seizures or other signs of brain damage such as changes in behavior can occur. Meningitis can occur if bacterial contamination accompanies the injury.

Spinal Cord Trauma

WHAT IT IS. An injury that affects a portion of the spinal cord, resulting in neurological symptoms depending on the location of the trauma. The extent of damage could range from soft-tissue swelling to spinal fractures.

DIAGNOSIS. A history of trauma accompanied by the onset of neurological symptoms consistent with spinal cord injury provides a suspected diagnosis. Radiographs will likely be recommended when a fracture is suspected.

TREATMENT. Similar to cases where brain trauma is a concern, initial treatment for spinal trauma is focused on minimizing swelling and fluid accumulation that could cause further injury to the spinal cord. This would involve administration of anti-inflammatories including corticosteroids, intravenous therapy with DMSO to reduce inflammation, and diuretics to limit fluid accumulation and resulting pressure within the spinal canal

HOW SERIOUS IS IT? The severity of a spinal injury is highly variable, and ranges from short-term swelling around the spinal cord that causes symptoms that will cease once swelling is resolved, to permanent damage to the spine and spinal cord that can be life threatening.

POTENTIAL COMPLICATIONS. Permanent damage to the spine can result. Meningitis can occur if bacterial contamination accompanies the injury. A horse that is down and unable to rise may develop deep sores that require extensive nursing care.

Cervical Vertebral Malformation (CVM, or "Wobblers")

WHAT IT IS. A malformation of a vertebra in the neck that puts pressure on the spinal cord, and causes neurological symptoms attributed to the spinal cord. There are a number of different subcategories of this condition depending on the exact nature of the malformation, its location, and how it developed. It can occur as a developmental abnormality in young horses, usually identified between 6 months and 3 years of age, or as a narrowing due to development of arthritis in older horses. CVM in young horses has been linked to developmental orthopedic disease, and may have both hereditary and nutritional components.

DIAGNOSIS. CVM may be suspected based on typical clinical signs, including ataxia (loss of coordination) and weakness. A definite diagnosis depends on radiographs of the vertebrae of the neck, and may also require a myelogram to confirm.

TREATMENT. In young horses, dietary adjustment and treatment with anti-inflammatories may help minimize signs and slow development of the condition. In older horses, surgical fusion of the vertebrae may be recommended.

HOW SERIOUS IS IT? CVM is performance-limiting in many cases, depending on its severity. Approximately 70 percent of horses treated surgically will improve, although only 50 percent are likely to be able to perform in athletic disciplines.

POTENTIAL COMPLICATIONS. Severe ataxia can increase chances for traumatic injury.

Equine Protazoal Myeloencephalitis (EPM)

WHAT IT IS. A disease caused by the protozoa known as *Sarcocystis neurona* that affects the brain and spinal cord. A second protozoal organism, *Neospora hughesi*, has recently been implicated as a possible cause. The protozoa is carried by opossums, and passed to horses when they ingest anything contaminated with feces from infected opossums. It may also be carried by armadillos, skunks, raccoons, and domestic cats, although these animals, known as "intermediate hosts," do not spread the organism directly to horses.

The organism can affect any part of the central nervous system, meaning it can cause a wide variety of neurological symptoms. These include ataxia (loss of coordination), generalized weakness, hind limb lameness that can't be pinpointed to a specific skeletal structure, or back pain. If the brain is involved, signs of brain disease or abnormalities associated with the cranial nerves may be seen. Many cases of EPM appear to be asymmetrical—one side of the body is more severely affected than the other.

DIAGNOSIS. An accurate diagnosis of EPM is complicated and controversial. As many as 60 percent of horses in many areas have been exposed to the organism, yet never show signs of the disease. Horses that have been exposed will all have antibodies in their bloodstream against the organism, making a blood test for antibodies worthless for confirming a diagnosis. However, a negative test of antibodies in the blood can be helpful in ruling out EPM as the cause of neurological symptoms.

Diagnostic tests for EPM require collection of CSF. The vet can collect this fluid with the horse standing and sedated, using a long needle placed into the spine through the space between the lumbar vertebrae and the sacrum. Alternatively, the vet may opt to put the horse down under a short-acting anesthetic to sample CSF from the space between the first vertebra and the skull.

CSF can be tested for antibodies (known as a Western blot test) or for genetic material of the actual organism (polymerase chain reaction or PCR test). Although these tests can be useful for helping to confirm a diagnosis, there can still be a large number of false positive results—meaning that the test is positive even though EPM is not the true cause of the horse's symptoms.

Because of these challenges to accurate testing for EPM, many veterinarians believe that a response to treatment is the best confirmation of the diagnosis. If the horse is exhibiting signs typical of EPM, analysis of CSF is positive for the organism, and the horse improves when appropriate treatment is started, that's good evidence that the protazoa is truly the cause of the horse's troubles.

TREATMENT. There are two primary treatments available for EPM. The first is a combination of the antimicrobial medications pyramethamine and trimethoprim-sulfonamide, which has been used to treat this disease since it was first identified. This treatment, which is usually recommended for a period of at least 6 months, can have adverse effects, including anemia.

Recently, the anticoccidial medication ponazuril (Marquis™) has been approved by the FDA for treatment of EPM, with a recommended treatment course of 28 days. (Similar medications, diclazuril and toltrazuril, are available in Canada.)

In addition to these medications used to kill the protazoa, nonsteroidal anti-inflammatory medications, corticosteroids, or DMSO may be needed to control inflammation of tissues during the early stages of the disease. Vitamin E therapy may also be recommended, both for its antioxidant properties that might protect tissues against damage and for its ability to boost the horse's immune system to help him combat the organism.

HOW SERIOUS IS IT? EPM can cause very serious signs, be difficult to diagnose, and be even more difficult and expensive to treat. Even after treatment some horses will have remaining symptoms because of permanent damage to the brain or spinal cord.

POTENTIAL COMPLICATIONS. Relapse is common following treatment for EPM, and may occur in as many as 10 to 20 percent of cases. If CSF testing can be performed and a negative result obtained prior to discontinuing treatment, the chances for relapse are greatly diminished.

Equine Herpes Virus (EHV-1, or Rhinopneumonitis)

WHAT IT IS. A viral disease caused by one form of the equine herpes virus. It attacks the nervous system and is passed from horse to horse by saliva, respiratory secretions, or even feces. Symptoms of the disease will appear approximately 6 to 12 days following exposure. The horse will begin to show signs of ataxia (loss of coordination), which may become severe enough to cause him to go down and be unable to rise. Loss of bladder function is a common characteristic of EHV-1 infection.

DIAGNOSIS. A specific diagnosis of EHV-1 can be difficult. The disease will be suspected if there is an outbreak of horses with neurological disease. Measurement of antibodies in the bloodstream can be helpful, especially if the number of antibodies increases between the time the horse first becomes sick and several weeks into his recovery. Genetic material from the virus can be identified in respiratory secretions to confirm a diagnosis.

TREATMENT. Treatment for this viral disease is supportive and might include anti-inflammatories, intravenous fluid therapy to ensure the horse does not become dehydrated, and nursing care of wounds or bedsores that can occur if the horse goes down. If the bladder is paralyzed, the vet may place a catheter into the bladder to empty it several times a day. Although vaccination protects the horse from other forms of EHV, it is not labeled for protection against the neurological form of the disease. Recent evidence suggests, however, that the modified live form of the vaccine may offer a degree of protection and use of this vaccine should be considered.

HOW SERIOUS IS IT? As many as 90 percent of exposed horses may become ill, meaning large outbreaks are common. And although horses that are mildly affected may recover without complications, fatality rates are as high as 40 percent in some outbreaks.

POTENTIAL COMPLICATIONS. Some horses recovering from EHV-1 infection will have permanent gait alterations or permanent loss of bladder function.

West Nile Virus Encephalitis (WNV)

WHAT IT IS. A viral disease that affects the brain and spinal cord, and leads to neurological signs including ataxia, hind limb paralysis, seizures, and coma. Many horses with this disease will have tremors around their noses and lips. The disease, which is carried by birds and spread by mosquitoes, was first introduced to the East Coast of the United States in 1999, and has rapidly spread west.

DIAGNOSIS. WNV will be suspected when a horse shows typical clinical signs in an area where WNV is known to occur. The diagnosis can be confirmed with a blood test that measures specific antibodies against the virus. This test can distinguish between an actual infection and vaccination because it looks for a specific type of antibody that is not found in vaccinated horses. The actual virus can also be isolated from blood or CSF.

TREATMENT. There is no specific treatment available. Nonsteroidal anti-inflammatory medications can help minimize signs and discomfort in mild cases.

HOW SERIOUS IS IT? WNV was fatal in 35 percent of infected horses when first introduced to the United States. As vaccination becomes more widespread, the fatality rate has diminished significantly.

POTENTIAL COMPLICATIONS. None.

TABLE 8.1

Causes of Seizures

CAUSE	REASON	HOW DIAGNOSED
Brain trauma	Swelling or damage to the brain alters brain function.	History or evidence of recent trauma to the head.
Brain tumors	Pressure on the brain alters brain function.	Skull radiographs, CT or MRI.
Electrolyte disturbances	Changes in electrolyte balance alter chemical signals within the brain.	Blood tests.
Epilepsy	A disruption of the normal electrical activity of the brain.	Recurrent seizures with no other identifiable cause.
Equine protozoal myelitis	Migration of protozoa through brain tissues alters brain function.	Tests of CSF and/or a positive response to treatment.
Intracarotid injection	Substance injected into the carotid artery travels directly to the brain and affects brain function.	Seizure immediately following an injection intended to enter the jugular vein.
Liver disease	Toxins normally cleared by the liver build up in the horse's system and alter brain function.	Blood tests or liver biopsy.
Rabies	Virus attacks brain tissues.	Tests of blood or CSF.
Toxicity	Alterations in chemical signals of the brain.	Exposure to toxins including bracken fern, organophosphates, moldy corn, lead, arsenic, and mercury.
West Nile virus	Virus attacks brain tissues.	Tests of blood or CSF.

Tetanus (Lockjaw) FIGURE 8.2

WHAT IT IS. A fatal disease caused by a toxin released from the bacteria *Clostridium tetani*. This organism is present in the soil everywhere and enters the horse's body through a wound. Horses are one of the most susceptible species to this toxin, which affects the nervous system by interfering with the function of neurotransmitters. An affected horse will first become stiff, and the stiffness gradually progresses to a rigidity of the entire body. His lips will be pulled back, nostrils will flare, and he'll be unable to chew due to rigidity of his jaw muscles (hence the term "lockjaw").

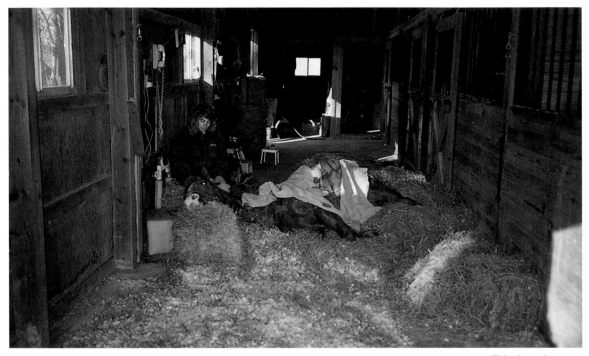

DIAGNOSIS. A diagnosis of tetanus would be based on a history of a wound with no record of vaccination in a horse showing typical symptoms.

TREATMENT. If tetanus is suspected, antitoxin (a direct source of antibodies against the organism) can be administered in large amounts. In addition, penicillin will kill the bacteria. If muscle rigidity is severe, sedative and anticonvulsive medications such as diazepam (Valium) might be helpful. Vaccination is protective against this disease and should be a part of every horse's routine medical care.

HOW SERIOUS IS IT? With dedicated nursing care in a quiet environment to minimize stimuli that might lead to muscle spasms and seizures, it is possible for a horse to survive a tetanus episode. However, the disease can be rapidly fatal in many cases, and euthanasia is often recommended in severe cases.

POTENTIAL COMPLICATIONS. Wounds or other injuries can occur due to the horse's inability to stand and function normally.

FIGURE 8.2. **This down horse is severely affected with tetanus, to the point where he is unable to stand. Although he may recover over time with good nursing care, vaccination to prevent this deadly disease is a much better alternative.** (Photo courtesy of Jan Palmer, DVM, Diplomate ACVS)

Equine Degenerative Myeloencephalopathy (EDM)

WHAT IT IS. A degenerative condition of the nervous system most commonly seen in young horses. Signs are usually first seen at approximately 6 months of age. They include weakness and a loss of coordination (ataxia) that is usually more pronounced in the hind limbs than the forelimbs. The exact cause is unknown, but appears to involve vitamin E and copper deficiency and may have a hereditary component.

DIAGNOSIS. Like many neurological diseases, EDM is difficult to diagnose while the horse is still alive. The only way to confirm a diagnosis is with a postmortem examination of portions of the brain and spinal cord under a microscope. A diagnosis will be presumed in a horse showing typical signs that improve with vitamin E supplementation where other diseases such as CVM or EPM have been ruled out.

TREATMENT. A horse with suspected EDM will be given dietary vitamin E supplementation at a rate of 6000 IU/day. In severe cases, injections of vitamin E may be recommended.

HOW SERIOUS IS IT? EDM can be a progressive condition that does not improve with treatment. Many horses with this disease are euthanized.

POTENTIAL COMPLICATIONS. None.

Stringhalt   FIGURE 8.3

WHAT IT IS. A condition where the horse exhibits involuntary flexion of one or both hind legs. In many cases, this abnormality is linked to ingestion of multistemmed dandelions, with symptoms commonly appearing after periods of very dry weather.

DIAGNOSIS. A diagnosis of stringhalt is made based on the horse's clinical appearance. Exposure to the plants that have been associated with the condition may increase suspicion of plant toxicity as the underlying cause.

Other conditions that have been linked to stringhalt-like symptoms include polysaccharide storage myopathies (see chapter 4) and EPM (see page 166). These conditions would be diagnosed via muscle biopsy (PSM) or analysis of cerebrospinal fluid

TREATMENT. Removing the horse from pasture and away from the potential toxin is recommended, and many horses will spontaneously recover within a period of days to weeks. Severely affected horses will continue to show signs for as long as 12 to 18 months, and some may never return to normal. Although a variety of different medications have been tried, none have proved very effective for treating the condition.

In cases where another underlying cause can be identified such as polysaccharide storage myopathy or EPM, treatment of the underlying condition is necessary.

HOW SERIOUS IS IT? When any attempt at movement is made, severely affected horses may be unable to negotiate around even a small stall or paddock due to extreme flexion of both hind legs.

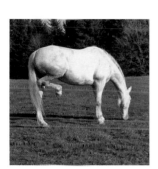

FIGURE 8.3. **The hyperflexion of this horse's hind legs is typical of stringhalt, a disease that can be associated with ingestion of multistemmed dandelions in parts of North America.**
(Photo courtesy of Lindsey Moneta)

POTENTIAL COMPLICATIONS. If symptoms persist, damage to the hind feet or joints of the hind limbs can occur because stress has been placed on them due to abnormal movement. A severely affected horse may fall down repeatedly when attempting to move.

Shivers

WHAT IT IS. A neurological disorder seen in draft and heavy breed horses such as warmbloods where the hind legs are suddenly jerked up off the ground and flexed toward the belly when the horse is asked to back up. Severely affected horses will be unable to move backward.

DIAGNOSIS. Because shivers has such unique symptoms and is most common in very specific types of horses, it can usually be diagnosed based on a clinical examination. Symptoms are likely to become more severe when the horse is excited or nervous.

HOW SERIOUS IS IT? There is no effective treatment, and the condition is often slowly progressive, making it a disease with serious consequences for affected horses.

POTENTIAL COMPLICATIONS. None.

Radial Nerve Paralysis

WHAT IT IS. Injury to the radial nerve that runs across the front of the horse's shoulder and controls extensors of the forelimb, causing the nerve to stop functioning effectively. A horse with radial nerve paralysis will drag the affected forelimb and be unable to extend the leg out in front of his body. In most cases he will be able to weight-bear normally. However, if the affected leg is placed underneath his body, the opposite forelimb can be picked up.

DIAGNOSIS. The movement pattern observed with a radial nerve paralysis is very typical and is usually enough to make a diagnosis of nerve damage. Known trauma to the front of the shoulder from a kick or fall will help confirm the suspicion of an injury.

TREATMENT. A radial nerve injury should be treated aggressively as soon as possible following the trauma to control inflammation and minimize swelling. Ice, cold-hosing, and nonsteroidal anti-inflammatory medications such as phenylbutazone or flunixin meglumine will be recommended. In more severe cases, initial treatments with corticosteroids such as dexamethasone will be helpful for minimizing inflammation.

HOW SERIOUS IS IT? Most cases of radial nerve paralysis will resolve completely with early and aggressive treatment. Rarely, a severe injury to the nerve can lead to permanent dysfunction.

POTENTIAL COMPLICATIONS. Fractures of the elbow area can easily be mistaken for uncomplicated radial nerve injuries. If the horse is unable to bear weight on the affected limb, is in a lot of pain with palpation and manipulation of the limb, or fails to respond to initial treatment, radiographs should be taken to rule out the possibility of fracture.

Suprascapular Nerve Injury ("Sweeny") FIGURE 8.4

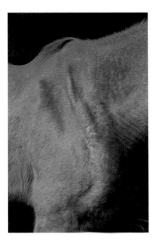

FIGURE 8.4. **An injury to this horse's shoulder area has caused damage to the suprascapular nerve, leading to this extreme muscle atrophy over the horse's scapula, or shoulder blade. This condition is commonly known as sweeny.** (Author photo)

WHAT IT IS. Damage to the suprascapular nerve, which extends out from under the horse's shoulder blade (scapula) and runs across the front edge of the shoulder. This nerve supplies the supraspinatus and infraspinatus muscles that are on the surface of the scapula to help support the fore-limb against the horse's body. Injury to this nerve can occur with direct trauma where the nerve passes across the front of the scapula or be due to stretching of the nerve secondary to a sudden backward movement of the leg. When this nerve is damaged, the horse will be unable to advance the leg forward, pull the leg in toward the body (abduct the leg), or support the shoulder blade. A typical "popping" motion of the shoulder can be seen with every step. In long-standing cases, the supraspinatus and infra-spinatus muscles will atrophy (shrink or become smaller), which can be easily observed over the outer surface of the scapula. Over time, the spine of the scapula becomes very prominent as the muscles become smaller and smaller.

DIAGNOSIS. A diagnosis of sweeny can be made with observation of the typical movement pattern, along with the atrophied appearance of the shoulder.

TREATMENT. If the injury is identified early, aggressive treatment with ice, cold water, and anti-inflammatories including phenylbutazone, flunixin meglumine, and/or dexamethasone will be recommended to minimize swelling and ongoing damage. Complete stall rest will also be recommended. With this condition, the shoulder "pop" that occurs with every step can lead to ongoing nerve injury due to nerve stretching. If the horse can be kept completely immobile, this damage can be minimized. As the condition progresses, the nerve can also become entrapped in scar tissue, which prevents regeneration. If this is suspected, a surgical procedure can be performed to relieve this entrapment.

HOW SERIOUS IS IT? Because of the instability of the shoulder associated with this condition, it is extremely difficult to eliminate ongoing stress to the suprascapular nerve to allow for complete healing and regeneration. The condition tends to be progressive, with chronic muscle atrophy and related loss of function.

POTENTIAL COMPLICATIONS. None.

Idiopathic Headshaking

WHAT IT IS. A fairly common problem that has a variety of possible causes and can be extremely difficult to diagnose. Horses affected with this condition will twitch, flick, or toss their heads, often suddenly and quite violently. Typically, the head tossing occurs in an up-and-down direction, and may be accompanied by the horse rubbing his face against his legs or other objects.

One popular theory is that pain associated with the trigeminal nerve, one of nerves that supplies the head, can be quite sudden and sharp, resulting in a violent flick, nod, or twitch-like movement. Headshaking syndrome can progress over time, with signs becoming more and more frequent and severe.

DIAGNOSIS. A thorough evaluation of headshaking involves a number of different diagnostic tests to help determine whether there is a specific cause. The following diagnostic tests are recommended:

- Skull radiographs to evaluate the sinuses, teeth, and other bony structures within the head that might be causing pain or discomfort.

- Endoscopic evaluation of the nasal passages to evaluate for signs of inflammation, foreign bodies, or other potential abnormalities. In some cases, tissue samples taken from the nasal passages might be examined for signs of allergies or other inflammatory problems.

- Thorough examination of the ears for mites or ear infections that could be causing pain. If middle ear problems are suspected, the vet might recommend obtaining a sample for laboratory testing to determine if antibiotic treatment is advisable.

- Blood tests to check for evidence of herpes virus infections (rhinopneumonitis) that can be associated with nerve pain.

If no specific underlying cause can be identified through these diagnostic steps, the horse may fit into the category of "idiopathic headshaking syndrome." Such a horse will exhibit the headshaking behavior for no apparent reason. In many cases, the twitching occurs most frequently during exercise, when weather conditions are extremely hot, or in bright light conditions. Sometimes, the behavior can be eliminated or reduced simply by outfitting the horse in a UV-blocking mask or specially designed contact lenses. Face masks that block airflow into the nostrils seem to reduce the behavior, perhaps by minimizing irritation to the nasal passages that might cause pain.

TREATMENT. A number of different medications have been used in headshaking horses, with variable success. The two most commonly recommended medications are cyproheptadine (an antihistamine-type medication used to control cluster headaches in humans) and carbamazepine (an antiepileptic drug). In addition, headshaking can be treated with UV-blocking masks, contact lenses, or face masks that block airflow into the nasal passages, if these measures are effective.

HOW SERIOUS IS IT? Headshaking may not be a life-threatening condition, but it can certainly be frustrating and may compromise performance or limit a horse's usefulness for riding. A horse that responds to medications may still be used for pleasure riding, although the medications used are prohibited for competition in many disciplines.

POTENTIAL COMPLICATIONS. No serious complications are likely to occur.

CHAPTER 9

The Reproductive Tract

THEN AND NOW

In the late 1800s, horse breeders believed that the mare was infused with the blood of the stallion as the fetus developed within the womb. After foaling, this blood was thought to remain circulating in her veins, meaning that she would pass his characteristics on to future foals—even those he didn't sire. In fact, the term "bloodline" that's still widely used today was derived from this belief.

Now we know that characteristics of the mare and stallion are passed to the foal through chromosomes or "genes" that are contributed by the egg of the mare and the sperm of the stallion and multiply during development. The mare and stallion contribute equally to the characteristics of their shared offspring—and each breeding is completely independent.

TOGETHER, THE REPRODUCTIVE SYSTEMS of the mare and stallion function to produce a foal. This chapter outlines those basic systems and describes the common problems likely to adversely affect the reproductive organs of the mare and stallion.

Reproductive Anatomy of the Mare   FIGURE 9.1

The following organs make up the reproductive tract of the mare.

Vulva

The vulva, the opening to the reproductive tract, lies just below the mare's rectum under her tail. At the lower portion of the vulva a small pouch or fold surrounds the clitoris, which is exposed when the mare demonstrates signs of estrus known as "winking."

Vagina

The vagina is the cavity between the vulva and the uterus. The cervix, which leads into the uterus, is at the front of the vaginal area.

Cervix

The cervix is a tubular structure approximately 5 to 7 centimeters long that forms the entryway to the uterus. It is surrounded by a wall of very elastic muscle fibers that relax or tighten according to the hormonal influences of the mare's estrus cycle. When the mare is in heat, the cervix softens to allow sperm access. When she's not in heat or when she's pregnant, the cervix tightens and closes off the uterus.

Uterus

The uterus consists of the uterine body and two horns that extend forward within the pelvic canal. A ligamentous structure, called the broad ligament, suspends and holds the uterus in place. The uterus has several

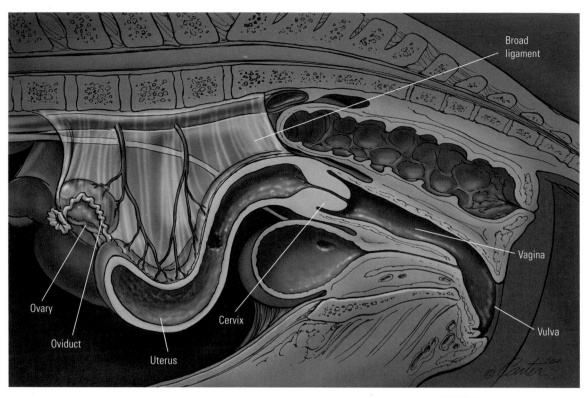

FIGURE 9.1.
**Reproductive tract
of the female.**

layers of tissue, including the innermost "endometrium" that contains glands essential for supporting a developing fetus.

Oviducts

The oviducts are long (10 to 20 centimeters) twisting tubes that extend from the tips of the uterine horns up to the ovaries. The oviducts are surrounded by muscle and have an inner layer of folds at the ovarian end to protect the egg and fragile embryo immediately after fertilization.

Ovaries

The ovaries, kidney-bean shaped structures approximately 5 centimeters in diameter, are attached to the oviducts. The ovaries are surrounded by blood vessels and contain tissue at their center where eggs are stored and released.

The Estrous Cycle

Reproductive function of the mare is heavily dependent on hormones controlled by glands associated with structures of the brain. These glandular structures include the hypothalamus and pituitary gland. What follows summarizes the hormonal events that control the mare's normal reproductive function.

The mare is considered seasonally polyestrous, meaning she has regular heat cycles during certain parts of the year, but does not cycle year-round. The natural breeding season extends from late spring to early summer, and is influenced by the lengthening daylight hours. As daylight increases, the hormone melatonin is released. Melatonin stimulates the release of another hormone, the gonadotropin-releasing hormone (GnRH), from the hypothalamus, which in turn stimulates the release of the follicle-stimulating hormone (FSH) from the pituitary. FSH acts on the mare's ovaries to encourage follicle development, the first step toward the release of an egg.

As the follicle develops, the hormone estrogen is released from the ovaries. Estrogen causes heat behavior to begin, including the behavioral signs of squatting to urinate repeatedly, winking the vulva, and turning the hindquarters in the direction of any interested stallion or gelding. Those external behavioral signs of heat are accompanied by changes within the reproductive tract, including a softening and opening of the cervix, and uterine contractions that help move sperm toward the egg if the mare is bred.

As the estrous cycle continues, a surge of lutenizing hormone (LH) eventually stimulates the follicle to ovulate, or release the egg, making it available for fertilization. The ruptured follicle then forms the corpus luteum, a structure that releases the progesterone necessary to maintain an early pregnancy. If no pregnancy occurs, prostaglandins are released from the uterus to cause the rupture of the corpus luteum, and a new cycle begins.

The average estrous cycle is approximately 21 days long, including 15 days of diestrus ("not in heat") and 6 days of estrus ("in heat"). When the mare is in heat, she will show the external behavioral signs described above, including raising her tail—especially in the presence of a stallion. If she kicks, pins her ears, squeals, or strikes at the stallion, she's most likely in her diestrous period.

Examination of the Mare

A number of different diagnostic procedures will be used to evaluate the reproductive tract of the mare. These procedures play an important role in the day-to-day management of the broodmare, and can evaluate problems of the reproductive tract in any mare.

Rectal Palpation

The vet examines the mare's cervix, uterus, and ovaries by placing a gloved hand into her rectum, which lies just on top of the reproductive tract. With this examination the vet can determine the tone and size of her uterus, the size of her ovaries, and the activity of her ovaries.

Ultrasound

An ultrasound probe is passed into the mare's rectum to allow visualization of her uterus and ovaries. This procedure makes it possible to accurately determine where the mare is in the sequence of her heat cycle, and whether there are any abnormalities present, such as uterine cysts or fluid.

Vaginal Speculum

The vet inserts a sterile tube into the mare's vagina in order to examine her vagina and cervix. Redness, abnormal discharge from the cervix,

Managing the Mare in Heat

If breeding isn't a part of the plan, a mare's heat cycles can be a source of frustration and complications for the mare owner. Pinned ears and squeals can make dealing with an in-heat mare unpleasant, but her well-placed kicks can be dangerous on the trail or in the show ring. An owner can choose from among a number of different options to help control heat cycles if they become too much to handle.

Option 1: Daily oral progesterone

WHAT IT IS. The synthetic progesterone Regu-Mate® is administered daily, either on the feed or directly through an oral dosing syringe.

PROS. This is an extremely reliable and safe method for controlling heat cycles in the performance mare and does not appear to have any significant long-term ill effects.

CONS. Daily Regu-Mate® administration is expensive and a hassle. Because this synthetic progesterone can be absorbed through the skin, extreme care must be taken during administration. Vinyl or plastic gloves should be worn for protection.

Option 2. Acupuncture staples

WHAT IT IS. A surgical staple is placed in the ears at an acupuncture point that has been demonstrated to reduce the intensity of heat-cycle behaviors.

PROS. This is a simple, inexpensive procedure to perform that has minimal risks. It can be reasonably effective in many mares for reducing the intensity of heat cycles.

CONS. Acupuncture staples won't stop a mare from cycling completely, and they may not have a strong enough effect to completely control heat-cycle related behavior problems.

Option 3: Uterine marble

WHAT IT IS. A glass marble approximately 1 inch in diameter is placed in the mare's uterus to stop her from cycling.

PROS. This simple, inexpensive procedure has minimal risks.

CONS. This is only effective in approximately 50 percent of mares.

pooling of urine within the vagina, or visible structural abnormalities are all indicators of potential problems.

Uterine Culture and Cytology

The mare's vulva and surrounding area are thoroughly cleaned. A long, sterile culture swab is passed through her cervix into her uterus to obtain a sample of cells, mucous, or other debris. The sample will be examined under a microscope, and swabbed onto a culture plate to attempt to grow bacteria or other microorganisms. This procedure will show whether the mare has significant inflammation or an infection within her uterus.

Option 4: Long-acting progesterone

WHAT IT IS. An injection of a long-acting progesterone formulation is given to stop the mare from cycling.

PROS. The injection can be very effective and is less expensive and less of a hassle than oral Regu-Mate®. The effect may last up to several weeks.

CONS. The formulations available are usually compounded, and do not have the reliability or safety guarantees that come with Regu-Mate®. They may act differently in different mares. Some formulations can cause local reactions (swelling, heat, and pain) at the injection site.

Option 5: Progesterone implants

WHAT IT IS. Progesterone-releasing capsules are placed under the mare's skin to stop her from cycling.

PROS. The implants may be effective for many months, eliminating the need for ongoing injections or daily oral medication.

CONS. These implants are made for cattle, and their long-term effects on horses are unknown. Research also indicates that they do not release enough progesterone to be effective, so they may not be reliable in every mare.

Option 6: Spaying

WHAT IT IS. The mare's ovaries are removed surgically to stop her from cycling.

PROS. This is a permanent solution that will stop heat-related problems forever in many mares.

CONS. Removing the ovaries means the mare can never be bred. It is major surgery, which can be costly and carries some risk. Some mares will continue to cycle even after being spayed due to the release of the hormone estrogen from other locations within the body.

Uterine Biopsy

This procedure is usually reserved for older mares, mares that have had a number of foals, and mares that have been difficult to get pregnant for several heat cycles. It may be recommended for a young healthy mare prior to breeding with very expensive or difficult-to-obtain frozen semen.

A small tissue sample is obtained by using a specially designed instrument that is inserted directly into the mare's uterus. This sample will be sent to a laboratory, where it will be examined under a microscope for signs of inflammation, scarring, or other abnormalities.

Hormonal Assays

Measurement of hormone levels in the blood can help identify abnormalities that produce abnormal hormone levels or help determine the cause of fertility problems.

Endoscopy

The mare's uterus can be directly visualized using an endoscope, an instrument for examining the inside of a hollow organ.

WHEN THINGS GO WRONG

What follows are the most common abnormalities likely to affect the mare's reproductive system.

Endometritis

WHAT IT IS. Inflammation of the uterus that may be accompanied by an infection with microorganisms.

DIAGNOSIS. Endometritis can be diagnosed by uterine culture and cytology to ascertain the presence of abnormal numbers of white blood cells, indicating inflammation, and/or bacteria or other organisms (such as yeast), indicating infection. Uterine biopsy can provide even more information about the degree and depth of inflammation. Affected mares will likely have fertility problems, may have abnormal (often frequent) heat cycles, and an ultrasound examination of the uterus may show fluid.

TREATMENT. Treatment usually consists of lavage (washing) of the uterus with fluids, and/or infusion of appropriate antimicrobial medication to kill organisms. The hormone oxytocin will be administered in small doses to help stimulate mild contractions to help clear material from the uterus.

HOW SERIOUS IS IT? Mares susceptible to endometritis are likely to have fertility problems, and may require repeated treatments if they are to be used for breeding purposes. Some mares will develop inflammation following breeding because their uterus is unable to respond appropriately to clear itself, and treatments will be required following every breeding.

POTENTIAL COMPLICATIONS. Endometritis can lead to pyometra.

The Horse's Body: Health and Disease

Pyometra FIGURE 9.2

WHAT IT IS. An infection of the uterus that results in the accumulation of large amounts of pus (up to 60 liters). Mares may show symptoms of fever and depression, there may be a visible discharge from the vulva, and heat cycles may be irregular.

DIAGNOSIS. Pyometra is identified with rectal palpation or by an ultrasound examination of the uterus in a mare showing typical signs. The vet may recommend a culture of the material in an attempt to identify a specific organism.

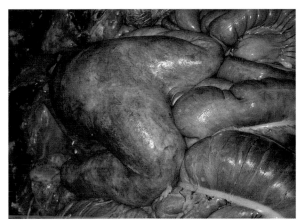

FIGURE 9.2. **This uterus, infected with pyometra.is distended with pus.** (Photo courtesy of Lisa Metcalf, DVM, Diplomate ACVT)

TREATMENT. Treatment involves emptying the uterine contents through lavage with large volumes of fluids, and may require treatment over a period of several days. Antimicrobials may be placed in the uterus to help kill organisms. In severe cases that are difficult to clear, removal of the uterus may be recommended.

HOW SERIOUS IS IT? Pyometra can be very difficult to treat effectively, may be recurrent, and will often result in permanent damage to the uterus that can affect fertility.

POTENTIAL COMPLICATIONS. Permanent infertility.

Urovagina

WHAT IT IS. An accumulation of urine in the vagina. The condition is most commonly found in older mares that have had multiple foals. The pooling of urine in the vagina causes irritation, and may drop through the cervix into the uterus to cause endometritis.

DIAGNOSIS. Urovagina will be identified when a pool of urine is observed in the vagina during a speculum examination.

TREATMENT. Surgery can be performed to extend the urethra toward the opening of the vagina to prevent urine from dropping back toward the uterus. This surgical procedure can be performed with the mare standing and sedated. It does not require general anesthesia.

HOW SERIOUS IS IT? If extensive damage to the uterus results, the mare may be infertile even after surgery is performed. The urine can be very irritating to the mare even if she is not to be used for breeding.

POTENTIAL COMPLICATIONS. Permanent infertility. Scalding of the vulva and hindquarters due to irritation from urine.

Mastitis

WHAT IT IS. Inflammation and infection of the mammary glands (udder). Mastitis is most common in lactating mares immediately following weaning of a foal, although it can occur in any mare at any time. A mare will have an enlarged udder that is hot and painful, and she may have a fever. Milk will usually have an abnormally thick, clotted appearance.

DIAGNOSIS. Mastitis will be suspected in a mare with typical symptoms, and can be confirmed with culture of the discharge obtained from the udder.

TREATMENT. The vet will recommend milking the mare to remove accumulated organisms and debris, as well as the insertion of an antimicrobial agent into the affected teat. Many mares will respond to this type of treatment alone. In more severe cases, oral or injectable antibiotics will be recommended. Anti-inflammatories will also be prescribed to reduce a fever and help the mare feel better.

HOW SERIOUS IS IT? Most cases of mastitis are easily treated.

POTENTIAL COMPLICATIONS. Though rare, chronic or recurring infections become difficult or impossible to eliminate.

Granulosa Cell Tumor   FIGURES 9.3–9.4

WHAT IT IS. The most common type of ovarian tumor seen in mares. Because they release the male hormone testosterone, they can result in stallion-like behavior.

DIAGNOSIS. The veterinarian will detect an enlarged ovary on rectal palpation that has a typical appearance when examined ultrasonographically. The other ovary may be smaller than normal due to the effects of hormones released by the tumor. A granulosa cell tumor will be suspected if the mare shows stallion-like behavior, and the diagnosis can be confirmed with blood tests that evaluate hormone levels, including the hormones testosterone, progesterone, and inhibin.

TREATMENT. Removal of the affected ovary will be recommended.

HOW SERIOUS IS IT? Granulosa cell tumors are easy to identify, and can be effectively treated with surgery. In a broodmare, loss of one ovary can affect fertility, although most mares will continue to ovulate normally from the remaining ovary. Rarely, granulosa cell tumors can affect both ovaries.

POTENTIAL COMPLICATIONS. The most significant complications are those associated with general anesthesia and surgery.

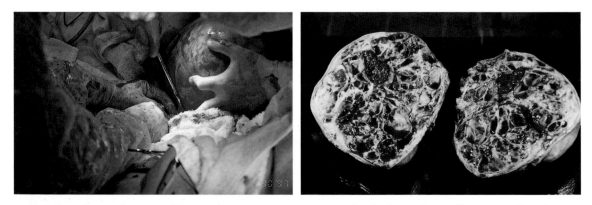

FIGURE 9.3. **Granulosa cell tumors will cause the mare to exhibit stallion-like behaviors due to release of the hormone testosterone. Surgical removal is recommended.** (Photo courtesy of Jan Palmer, DVM, Diplomate ACVS)

FIGURE 9.4. **A typical granulosa cell tumor consists of multiple cavities as seen here.** (Photo courtesy of Jan Palmer, DVM, Diplomate ACVS)

The Caslick's Procedure

The Caslick's procedure is a common, minor surgical procedure that involves suturing part of the vulva to correct a variety of conditions in mares, for example:

- Young, athletic mares prone to "windsucking," or drawing air into the vagina during exercise.

- Mares with tipped vulvar conformation (the top of the vulva tips forward toward the rectum) that are at risk for contaminating the vagina and uterus during defecation. This condition commonly occurs in older mares that have had multiple foals.   FIGURE 9.5

- Broodmares with a history of recurrent uterine infections.

The vet sutures closed the top portion of the vulva to prevent contamination. Sutures should then be removed prior to birth if the mare is bred.

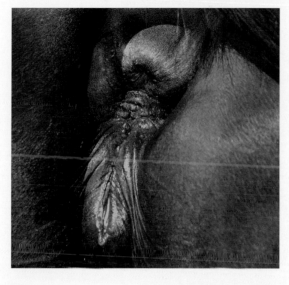

FIGURE 9.5. **The tipping forward of this mare's vulva puts her at risk for contaminating her uterus with fecal material. A Caslick's procedure would be recommended to close the top of the vulva and prevent this from occurring.**

Ovarian Hematoma

WHAT IT IS. Excessive bleeding into a follicle on the ovary after the egg has been released, resulting in a blood-filled sac that can be as large as 50 centimeters in diameter.

DIAGNOSIS. The veterinarian will feel an enlarged ovary on rectal palpation and can evaluate the typical appearance of a hematoma with an ultrasound examination. A mare with an ovarian hematoma will usually continue to cycle normally and will not exhibit the unusual behavior a granulosa cell tumor causes, a distinguishing factor in diagnosis.

TREATMENT. Most ovarian hematomas will resolve on their own within two to three heat cycles.

HOW SERIOUS IS IT? Most hematomas resolve without complications and without affecting fertility.

POTENTIAL COMPLICATIONS. Rarely, a persistent large hematoma will cause damage to the ovary due to pressure over a period of time.

Reproductive Anatomy of the Male FIGURE 9.6

The following organs make up the reproductive tract of the male. If he's been left intact (his testicles haven't been removed), he is a stallion. If he's been castrated (his testicles and their associated structures have been removed), he's a gelding. (See page 190 for information about castration.)

Scrotum

The scrotum is the sac of skin that houses the testicles and their associated structures. In the gelding, the scrotum shrinks down to a small, empty sac after castration has been performed.

Testicles

The testicles are paired structures that are egg-shaped, vary widely in size among individual horses, and are suspended inside the scrotum by the spermatic cord. The spermatic cord contains the veins, arteries, and

FIGURE 9.6.
Reproductive tract of the male.

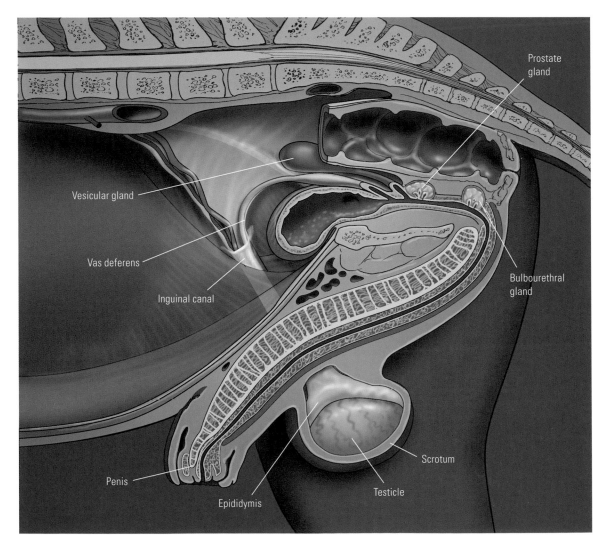

The Horse's Body: Health and Disease

nerves that supply the testicles, the cremaster muscle that lowers and raises the testicles within the scrotum to aid with temperature regulation, and the vas deferens. The spermadic cord is contained in a thin membrane called the tunica vaginalis, which extends from the lining of the abdominal cavity through the internal and external inguinal rings, or openings between the scrotum and the abdomen.

Epididymis

The epididymis is a long, curled tube that connects the testicles to the vas deferens. It nourishes and transports sperm from the testicles to the vas deferens.

Vas Deferens

The vas deferens is a tube that extends from the end of the epididymis to the urethra and is responsible for delivering sperm to the urethra so that it can be deposited in the mare during breeding.

Accessory Sex Glands

The accessory sex glands consist of the prostate gland, seminal vesicles, the bulbourethral gland, and ampullae and contribute to the seminal plasma, or liquid portion of the semen that helps support and nourish the sperm.

Penis

The penis is the organ of copulation (breeding), and is divided into three parts: the glans, the body, and the roots. The glans is the enlarged tip of the penis, where the end of the urethra sits just below a pocket of skin, or "diverticulum." The body is the elongated portion of the penis that becomes engorged with blood and erects to allow for breeding, and the roots join the penis to the bottom of the horse's pelvis.

Prepuce (Sheath)

The prepuce consists of large folds of skin that cover the penis when it is resting.

Reproductive Functions of the Stallion

The function of the male reproductive system includes both the production of sperm and the delivery of those sperm into the mare for conception. In the mare, winter anestrus involves a shutting down of her reproductive system, but the stallion's reproductive functioning lasts all year long. He continues to produce sperm throughout the winter months, although total numbers may be decreased.

The process of spermatogenesis, or sperm production, takes place in the seminiferous tubules within the testicles and takes approximately 55 days to complete. The newly produced sperm then mature and develop the ability to move forward on their own as they pass through the epididymis over a period of approximately 4 to 5 days. They then spend a variable amount of time (2 days to several weeks, depending on the amount of sexual activity of the stallion) at the end of the epididymis before they are either ejaculated or eliminated during urination.

The nervous system controls the actual breeding event, and when the right stimuli are detected (such as a mare in heat), there is increased blood flow to the penis in combination with decreased drainage to cause an erection. Ejaculation then occurs following appropriate stimulation of the penis, either by a mare or an artificial vagina. The average volume of ejaculate is between 30 and 100 milliliters.

The normal stallion will show interest in the mare in heat and drop his penis within 1 to 2 minutes of exposure to her. He mounts her within 3 minutes, completes between five and eight intravaginal thrusts, three to five short thrusts while he ejaculates and then flags his tail, relaxes, and dismounts.

Examination of the Stallion

Examination of the stallion involves the following steps.

Physical Examination of the External Genitalia

The vet will examine the stallion's testicles, scrotum, sheath, and penis both visually and with palpation. In order to fully evaluate the penis, the vet may ask for the stallion to be exposed to an in-heat mare. This not only allows the penis to be examined, but also helps evaluate whether the stallion's sexual response is appropriate. Usually measurement of scrotal width will be performed, as the size of the testicles often relates to the amount of sperm produced.

Ultrasound

If an abnormality is suspected, ultrasound of the scrotum and testicles might help identify the problem.

Endoscopy

Endoscopic examination of the urethra might help identify the source of bleeding if blood is detected in semen, or to detect a stricture (narrowing) of the urethra.

Culture and Cytology

Samples taken from the outside of the penis, the tip of the urethra, or the small diverticulum (sac) at the tip of the penis may be collected for evaluation under a microscope, and cultured to look for bacteria or other organisms that might be causing disease.

The Horse's Body: Health and Disease

Breeding Observation

The stallion's libido (sexual desire) and ability to breed a mare are best evaluated through observation of his breeding behavior. The veterinarian will observe the stallion's response to a mare in heat, as well as his ability to develop an erection, mount, and ejaculate either during a live breeding, or when semen is being collected with an artificial vagina.

Semen Analysis

The semen will be examined under a microscope for total volume, number (concentration) and structure (morphology) of the sperm, and activity and movement (motility) of the sperm.

WHEN THINGS GO WRONG

The following abnormalities are likely to affect a male horse's reproductive system.

Cryptorchidism (Retained Testicles)

WHAT IT IS. One or both of the testicles fail to drop into the scrotum. This should occur usually between the last 30 days of gestation and first 10 days following birth. In some cases, the testicles will drop into the inguinal rings and remain there for an extended time before they actually drop into the scrotum.

DIAGNOSIS. If testicles are not palpable in the scrotum by 4 to 6 months of age, cryptorchidism will be suspected. In an older horse with an unknown history, measurement of testosterone in the blood can help confirm cryptorchidism if it is suspected due to aggressive or stallion-like behavior in a gelding. For best accuracy, the vet may recommend a stimulation test with a hormone called human chorionic gonadotropin (HCG). Blood levels of testosterone and estrogen levels will increase five times above their base value following administration of HCG to a male horse if testicular tissue is present. If no elevation occurs, testicular tissue is absent and the horse is not a cryptorchid. Rarely, the vet may recommend rectal palpation or ultrasound to locate a testicle in the abdomen.

TREATMENT. Surgery will be recommended to remove testicles from a cryptorchid stallion. This is more than a routine castration because the surgery often involves opening the abdomen, similar to a colic surgery, to locate the testicles.

HOW SERIOUS IS IT? Cryptorchidism will limit the male horse's usefulness as a stallion. For a male horse intended to be a gelding, however, it is an easily solved disorder.

POTENTIAL COMPLICATIONS. Complications are possible secondary to surgery, which can be fairly invasive and requires general anesthesia. If a retained testicle is not removed, the apparent "gelding" can become very aggressive.

Inguinal and Scrotal Herniation

WHAT IT IS. The intestines of the stallion slip through the inguinal rings, dropping completely into the scrotum in some cases. These hernias can be congenital in foals (and are thought to be hereditary) or acquired in a mature stallion.

DIAGNOSIS. An inguinal or scrotal hernia may be detected due to an enlargement of the scrotum. In older stallions it will often be diagnosed because of a colic episode that might occur when the intestines become trapped. The presence of intestines in the scrotal sac will be confirmed with ultrasound examination.

TREATMENT. Surgery will be performed to reposition the intestines and close the inguinal rings. In cases where there is damage to the intestines, this may accompany colic surgery and removal of sections of damaged intestines.

HOW SERIOUS IS IT? Simple herniation is usually easy to correct. However, it can have serious consequences if it is not recognized early.

POTENTIAL COMPLICATIONS. One of the most serious complications will occur if castration is performed on a horse with an undetected inguinal hernia. In this situation, the intestines can actually drop out of the castration site following surgery, resulting in life-threatening consequences. It is also possible for intestines trapped in the inguinal ring or scrotum to become twisted or strangulated, leading to intestinal damage.

Torsion of the Spermatic Cord

WHAT IT IS. The testicles rotate within the scrotum. A rotation of 360 degrees can cause disruption of the blood supply and produce signs of acute pain.

DIAGNOSIS. The stallion may exhibit colic symptoms, and the affected testicle is often enlarged and surrounded by fluid. Torsion may be detected by palpation. If, however, the testicle has rotated 360 degrees, its orientation will still be normal and palpation can be deceptive. Ultrasound examination of the cord will help confirm a diagnosis.

TREATMENT. The affected testicle may need to be removed. In a valuable breeding stallion, it might be possible to correct the position of the testicle and surgically fix it into the proper position.

HOW SERIOUS IS IT? A torsion of the spermatic cord can cause severe colic symptoms and require major surgery to correct.

POTENTIAL COMPLICATIONS. In a breeding stallion, damage or loss of the affected testicle can occur.

Hydrocele/Hematocele

WHAT IT IS. An accumulation of fluid (hydrocele) or blood (hematocele) within the layers tunica vaginalis inside the scrotum. Either can occur secondary to trauma, or they may have an unidentified cause.

The Horse's Body: Health and Disease

DIAGNOSIS. The scrotum will appear swollen, and fluid or blood can be detected with ultrasound examination. Fluid can be removed and evaluated using a needle and syringe to confirm a diagnosis. A hematocele is more likely to be painful and may be associated with damage to other structures.

TREATMENT. Depending on the underlying cause, either of these conditions may resolve spontaneously. If trauma is severe, removal of the testicle that has been damaged may be necessary.

HOW SERIOUS IS IT? Either condition can affect spermatogenesis and fertility in a breeding stallion.

POTENTIAL COMPLICATIONS. Loss of the affected testicle.

Penile Prolapse (Paraphimosis)

FIGURES 9.7–9.8

WHAT IT IS. The penis becomes damaged and the gelding or stallion is no longer able to pull it back into the sheath. This can occur due to trauma, swelling of the penis secondary to some viral or bacterial diseases, or the administration of phenothiazine tranquilizers (acepromazine).

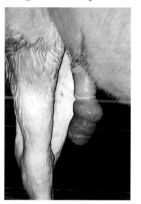

FIGURE 9.7. **This gelding's penis has become swollen to the point where he is no longer able to pull it back into his sheath, a condition known as penile prolapse, or paraphimosis.** (Photo courtesy of Jan Palmer, DVM, Diplomate ACVS)

DIAGNOSIS. This condition is easily identified by the condition of the penis.

TREATMENT. The penis should be manually replaced into the sheath, or if that is not possible, supported against the belly with a bandage to prevent additional swelling and damage. Nonsteroidal anti-inflammatory medications and exercise will be recommended to minimize swelling.

HOW SERIOUS IS IT? Penile prolapse can be a very serious condition that results in permanent damage to the penis, even with immediate treatment.

POTENTIAL COMPLICATIONS. Prolonged prolapse of the penis can lead to permanent paralysis and loss of breeding ability. (*An important point to remember is that the common tranquilizer acepromazine should never be administered to stallions due to the risk of this condition and the complications associated with it.*)

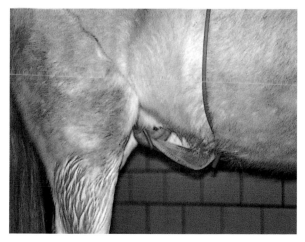

FIGURE 9.8. **Supporting the penis against the belly with a bandage may help prevent additional swelling and damage in hopes that it will return to normal.** (Photo courtesy of Jan Palmer, DVM, Diplomate ACVS)

Castration

If breeding won't be a part of a male horse's life, castration (removal of the testicles) is a procedure he'll most likely face sometime in his early years. Most owners of young male horses will schedule castration in the first year of life, although it's a procedure that can be performed at any time, even in a mature older stallion.

Prior to castration, the vet will want to confirm that the colt has two testicles that have descended into his scrotum. If the testicles haven't fully descended, he may be a cryptorchid and a more involved surgical procedure will be required to complete a castration. (See page 189.) It's also best if the colt is started on his initial vaccination series against tetanus prior to the procedure.

The vet will usually choose one of two methods for performing the castration, depending on his personal preference and the horse's temperament and manners. Some vets want to perform castrations "down," with the horse under a short-acting anesthetic, while others perform the procedure standing, using a sedative and a local anesthetic. Although the procedure may take a little longer from start to finish if the horse is laid down, proponents of this method believe it's safer for both the horse and veterinarian, particularly in cases where a complication might occur.

Either way, once the horse is prepared, an incision is made into the scrotum over one testicle. The testicle is pulled out of the sac, and an instrument called an emasculator is applied to the spermatic cord to seal the cord and crush the blood vessels. Sometimes a vet will tie the blood vessels off with suture material, although in most instances crushing is enough to adequately control bleeding. The same procedure is then carried out over the second testicle; the incision area is stretched and left open to allow for drainage.

Following the procedure, the most important part of facilitating recovery is to ensure the now-gelding gets plenty of exercise to encourage drainage from the surgical site. The veterinarian will usually recommend a period of quiet confinement for approximately 8 hours following surgery to ensure that all bleeding is controlled. After that time, turnout along with twice-daily exercise is recommended for a period of at least 10 days.

The most common complication following castration is that the surgical site seals closed prematurely, allowing fluid to accumulate. This can be avoided with adherence to the exercise schedule. If it does occur, the vet can simply manually reopen the incision to allow for drainage. Other possible complications include excessive bleeding, infection, or an inguinal hernia that might allow intestines to fall through the surgical site. The vet will tell you what to watch for, and what steps to take should signs of these complications occur.

Sheath Cleaning

FIGURES 9.9

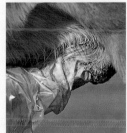

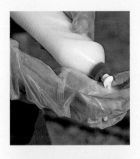

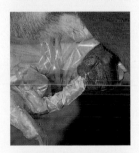

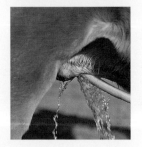

Sheath cleaning is a routine part of health care for the gelding or stallion that should be performed every 6 to 12 months. The sheath has a population of normal bacteria that help maintain a healthy balance. Therefore, a cleaning agent that does not have antimicrobial properties is recommended; either a commercially available sheath cleaner or a basic soap such as Ivory Liquid® is best.

Some stallions and geldings resent sheath cleaning, and sedation might be necessary. In any case, caution should be taken to avoid being kicked. Be prepared with a bucket of warm water, 20 to 30 paper towels, a cleaner, a long plastic glove, and an assistant to hold your horse. To clean the sheath, stand by your horse's left shoulder and reach down into his sheath with your gloved right hand and a handful of cleaner. Watch carefully for signs that your horse may kick, such as lifting his leg, or swishing his tail. If he does threaten to kick, take his warnings seriously and stop. Ask your veterinarian for advice.

If your horse tolerates your handling his sheath and penis, proceed by reaching up into the sheath and coating the inner surface with the cleanser. You should easily be able to feel the root of his penis at approximately elbow depth, even if he continues to hold the penis deep inside the sheath. Gently massage with your hand to loosen secretions and buildup along the shaft of the penis and the inside of the sheath, rinsing occasionally with a wet paper towel. Repeat the sudsing/rinsing cycles until the sheath's inner surface feels smooth to your touch, and the rinse water and towels appear clean.

The final step in cleaning your horse's sheath is to remove the "bean," an accumulation of thick, whitish material that forms in the pocket at the tip of the penis. This substance can become as large as a walnut, obstructing urine flow, and causing your horse discomfort. To remove the bean, gently run your index finger around the small pocket you can feel at the tip of his penis, and scoop out the clay like material. This step may be uncomfortable for your horse, so be careful—this is when he's most likely to kick.

When you've completed the cleaning process, give your horse's sheath a final rinse. This can be accomplished by inserting a hose 2 or 3 inches inside the sheath and simply allowing the water to flow for a minute or so, washing away any traces of cleaner or remaining debris.

FIGURE 9.9. **To clean your gelding or stallion's sheath, begin by putting a generous amount of a nonantimicrobial cleaner such as Ivory Liquid® into your gloved hand. Next, work your hand into his sheath, and apply cleaner around his penis as you reach deep inside. You should feel the root of his penis at approximately elbow depth. After you've cleaned the penis and inside surface of the sheath, remove the "bean" from the pocket at the tip of the penis. Gently run your index finger around the pocket to scoop out this material. To complete a final rinse, you can insert a hose 2 to 3 inches inside the sheath and allow a gentle flow of water until all of the cleaner is rinsed away.**

TABLE 9.1

Infectious Diseases of the Mare and Stallion FIGURE 9.13

A number of diseases involving bacteria, viruses, and protazoa can be passed between the mare and the stallion during breeding. The following chart outlines the most common of these diseases.

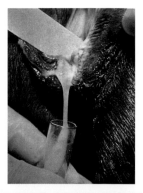

FIGURE 9.10. **This profuse discharge from the mare's vulva is due to contagious equine metritis, an infection that can be transmitted during breeding.** (Photo courtesy of Lisa Metcalf, DVM, Diplomate ACVT)

DISEASE	SYMPTOMS	SPREAD	DIAGNOSIS	MANAGEMENT	COMMENTS
Equine viral arteritis (EVA)	Fever and depression, with edema (swelling) of the belly and legs. Can cause abortion in mares.	Stallions can carry the virus without showing symptoms, and pass the virus to the mare in the semen, including fresh transported and frozen semen samples. Mares can pass the virus to other mares through respiratory secretions.	Virus can be isolated from semen. Blood tests for antibodies.	Stallions should be tested to identify carrier status. Vaccination is available for both stallions and mares. Any mare bred to a carrier stallion should be vaccinated prior to breeding.	None.
Coital Exanthema (Equine herpes virus type 3, or EHV-3)	Fever and depression. Round, pussy ulcers can form on the penis and vulva.	Affected stallions will pass the virus to mares during breeding when lesions are active.	This infection has a characteristic appearance. Diagnosis can be confirmed with virus isolation.	The disease is self-limiting in 2–4 weeks. Affected stallions and mares should be rested from breeding.	Depigmented (white) spots will remain on the penis and vulva after infection is resolved, but should not be cause for concern.
Dourine (*Trypanosoma equiperdum*)	Swelling and discharge from the penis and vulva. Large skin lesions. Anemia and profound progressive weight loss.	Transmitted during breeding.	Isolation of the protozoa from affected areas.	Treatment is usually not successful and can lead to a carrier state. Euthanasia is usually recommended.	Not seen in North America. Horses imported to the U.S. must test negative prior to being allowed entry.
Contagious equine metritis (CEM, *Taylorella equigenitalis*)	Stallions may not show symptoms but carry the bacteria. Vaginal discharge from mares.	Transmitted during breeding.	Culture and identification of the organism from the urethra and penis or uterus.	Can be treated with antibacterial washing of the penis and urethral fossa (pocket at the tip of the penis) of stallions, or lavage of the uterus of mares.	Not seen in North America. Horses imported to the U.S. must test negative prior to being allowed entry.

CHAPTER 10

The Skin

Horses used by teamsters to work the fields or haul heavy loads often suffered skin injuries where the harness rubbed them raw. A common remedy was to mix one cup of table salt with one gallon of water, and apply liberally to the problem areas every day in order to toughen the skin. The same wash was often recommended for use under the saddle and girth areas for ridden horses.

Modern science has had an enormous impact on the design and fitting strategies for all different kinds of tack. Saddles are made with adjustable air pillows to ensure there are no pressure points on the back. Computerized pads are even available that measure pressure underneath the saddle to help identify problem areas where adjustments might be recommended.

THE HORSE'S SKIN IS THE LARGEST ORGAN of his body, and ranges in thickness from 1 to 5 millimeters. Generally the skin is thickest over the back of the horse, becoming thinner as it extends toward his belly. The skin and its associated structures play a vital role as a protective barrier, temperature regulator, and surveillance mechanism to detect unwanted foreign invaders.

The following structures make up the skin. FIGURE 10.1

Epidermis

This outer surface of the skin consists of four layers: the horny cell layer, the granular cell layer, the prickle cell layer, and the basal cell layer. These layers are responsible for the actual physical protection the skin provides, and they also offer a base for other structures, such as cells involved with immune protection, hair follicles, and glands.

Dermis

This layer of skin is located between the epidermis and the underlying fat layer. The dermis consists of two layers, and provides strength to the overall structure of the skin, as well as a support for the blood vessels that supply the outer layers.

Subcutaneous Fat

This layer of fat rests between the dermis and deeper structures. It contains both fat cells and blood vessels, as well as the thin, flat panniculus muscle that allows the horse to twitch when a fly lands on him.

Hair

The hair follicles are continuous with the epidermis, and hold the root of each hair bulb that originates from the dermis. The hair follicles are closely associated with glands and small muscles (called the arrector pili) in addition to the hairs themselves.

Sebaceous (Oil) Glands

These glands are attached to the hair follicles and secrete sebum, a substance that consists of fats, proteins, and other matter that helps protect the skin.

Apocrine (Sweat) Glands

These glands are also attached to the hair follicles and secrete an element that consists of water, electrolytes, and metabolic waste products as well as substances that play a role in sexual attraction.

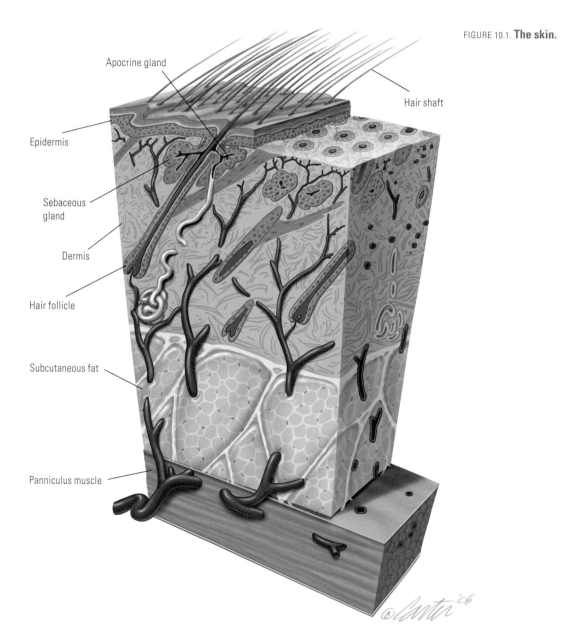

FIGURE 10.1. **The skin.**

Apocrine gland

Hair shaft

Epidermis

Sebaceous gland

Dermis

Hair follicle

Subcutaneous fat

Panniculus muscle

The Horse's Body: Health and Disease

Chestnut

A horny tissue growth that is located on the inside of all four limbs, just above the knees and hocks. Chestnuts are believed to be a remnant of the first digit, or "thumb," as the horse evolved from a multi-toed to a single-toed creature.

Ergot

This small (averaging 5 to 8 millimeters in diameter), horny tissue mass is located at the back of each of the horse's fetlocks. Similar to the chestnut, the ergot is believed to be a remnant of the fifth digit (baby finger or a toe).

Hooves

The hooves, covering the foot, are correctly classified as an extension of the horse's skin. (See chapter 4, "Musculoskeletal System," for a complete discussion of the horse's hooves.)

How the Skin Protects

The primary functions of the skin are to protect the horse from both trauma and invasion by foreign attackers, assist with temperature regulation, and help maintain the balance of fluids and electrolytes within his system. The physical protection provided by the skin is obvious—and thicker skin is present in more vulnerable areas such as the back, where predators are most likely to attack. Cells and blood vessels within the layers of the skin are also primed to recognize foreign threats such as bacteria or fungal organisms, and mount an immune response to fight off those threats.

The skin assists in maintaining body temperature in several ways. First, cells that produce pigments that color the skin (called melanocytes) are a key to protection against the sun. Because of these skin pigments, darker horses are better able to withstand the damaging effects of radiation than lighter ones. The hair also acts as insulation, complete with its small muscles that cause individual hairs to stand up under cold conditions in order to create an additional air layer. Finally, sweat glands provide one of the most critical means for temperature control. Sweat is produced when body temperature rises, and evaporation of sweat is the horse's primary cooling mechanism.

Shedding and replacement of hair is an important part of the skin's self-maintenance. Overall, the horse has ongoing cycles of hair loss where old hair shafts are continuously lost and replaced by new ones. However, during changes in season, shedding and hair replacement occurs in waves to help the horse adjust to changes in environmental conditions.

Examinations

History

A complete history of the horse's skin condition can be extremely important for determining a specific cause of skin problems. For example, a seasonally occurring condition may indicate an allergy—an important underlying cause of many skin problems. In addition, many skin conditions can be inherited, making information about bloodlines a potential key to making a diagnosis.

Visual Examination

Some conditions can be easily diagnosed with a thorough visual examination of the horse. For example, parasitic diseases can be diagnosed by observation of the parasites, such as lice, within the skin. It's also true that many skin diseases have a characteristic appearance, or pattern of distribution on the horse's body, that can give important clues toward making a diagnosis.

Scraping

Samples taken from the skin by scraping with a dull blade can reveal certain infectious organisms such as mange mites, bacteria, or even fungi, and may provide a diagnosis.

Cultures

Samples taken from the skin surface can be cultured in a laboratory in an effort to grow bacteria or fungi that may be at the root of a skin problem.

Histopathology

A small sample (called a biopsy) of the skin can be obtained and sent to a laboratory where it is examined under a microscope in order to determine the most likely cause of a skin condition. This microscopic evaluation might reveal infectious organisms (bacteria or fungi), inflammatory cells indicative of an allergy, or unusual changes in the skin structure that might help diagnose an unusual skin condition, such as an autoimmune disease where the body's immune system is attacking the skin cells.

Intradermal Skin Testing

If allergies are suspected as an underlying cause of a skin condition, intradermal skin testing can be performed to help determine precisely which allergens (allergy-producing substances) the horse is sensitive to. During this testing procedure, a small amount of a number of different allergens is injected into the skin. If the horse is sensitive to a specific allergen, a small swelling (wheal) will appear at the injection site. Allergens producing this reaction are recorded, and this information can be used to create a treatment plan using both avoidance and hyposensitization through a series of injections.

Skin diseases fall into a number of different categories, including infectious (caused by bacteria, fungi, or parasites), inflammatory (related to a reaction of the immune system), neoplastic or cancerous, hereditary, and traumatic. The following outlines the most common skin conditions diagnosed in horses.

FIGURE 10.2. **This horse is infested by lice, which cause extreme itching. If left untreated, his scratching behavior will lead to skin damage.** (Photo courtesy of Anthony Yu, DVM, Diplomate ACVD)

Infectious

Lice (Pediculosis)   FIGURES 10.2–10.3

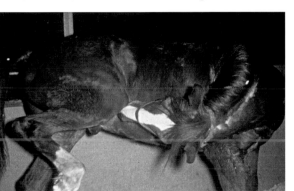

WHAT IT IS. Invasion of the skin by lice. Two species of lice affect horses, the sucking louse (*Haematopinus asini*) that feeds on blood and fluids and the biting louse (*Damalinia equi*) that feeds on dead skin and debris. Lice are likely to attack horses in poor condition or that have compromised immune systems, and are more common during winter months.

DIAGNOSIS. Lice lead to intense itchiness, which can result in scaling and hair loss when the horse scratches. In addition, they may cause severe weight loss if they go unrecognized and untreated. In most cases, lice can be seen with the naked eye to confirm a diagnosis.

TREATMENT. In general, lice infections are easily treated with a topical application of an insecticide. Oral ivermectin may also be effective against sucking lice.

HOW SERIOUS IS IT? If left untreated, lice can cause serious problems in a compromised horse. Once a diagnosis is made, however, they are easily treated.

POTENTIAL COMPLICATIONS. Severe weight loss and loss of condition can result in other significant diseases in an old or otherwise compromised horse.

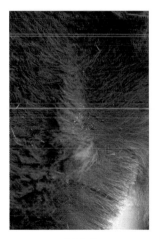

FIGURE 10.3. **Adult lice, eggs and scales of skin can usually be seen with the naked eye, making pediculosis easy to diagnose.** (Photo courtesy of Anthony Yu, DVM, Diplomate ACVD)

Mites (Mange)

WHAT IT IS. Invasion of the skin by mites, including *Psoroptes equi* (body mange) and *Chorioptes equi* (leg mange). These parasites can cause severe itching and resulting hair loss, skin damage, and crust formation. Draft breeds are particularly susceptible to *Chorioptes* mites, possibly due to the environment established under the thick feathering (hair) on their fetlocks.

DIAGNOSIS. Mange mites can be identified with skin scrapings examined under a microscope.

TREATMENT. Treatment with ivermectin is effective in most cases. Topical treatment with insecticides may also be recommended. (*Note: Amitraz, a common mange medication used in other species, should not be used in horses as it can cause depression, neurological symptoms, and gastro-intestinal upset.*)

HOW SERIOUS IS IT? Mange can lead to severe skin damage if it is unrecognized. However, once diagnosed it is usually responsive to treatment.

POTENTIAL COMPLICATIONS. Mange is an infectious condition that can spread to other horses within a herd. A quarantine period of 10 to 12 weeks is recommended to prevent spread.

Onchocerciasis FIGURE 10.4

WHAT IT IS. Roundworms live in connective tissues, resulting in a hypersensitivity (allergic-type) reaction. In North America, *Onchocerca cervicalis* is the most common culprit, and lives within the ligamentum nuchae—the long ligament that runs along the horse's neck. This parasite is carried by *Culicoides* ("no-see-um" gnats). Typical lesions consist of hair loss, ulceration, and crusts, as well as nodules that form from an accumulation of associated inflammatory debris. Lesions are most common along the face, neck, and belly.

DIAGNOSIS. The parasite larvae can be observed in biopsy samples taken from suspicious lesions. It is important to recognize, however, that the *Onchocerca* larvae may be found in normal horses, so they must be accompanied by a typical inflammatory reaction to confirm a diagnosis.

TREATMENT. Oral ivermectin is an effective treatment and should be administered along with an anti-inflammatory such as dexamethasone. Death of the parasite larvae following treatment can cause an acute inflammatory reaction, and dexamethasone helps minimize that response.

HOW SERIOUS IS IT? Because this problem involves a hypersensitivity reaction to this common parasite, affected horses are likely to have repeated problems that require ongoing treatment.

POTENTIAL COMPLICATIONS. None.

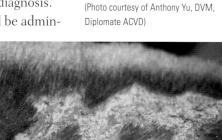

FIGURE 10.4. **The hair loss and crusting seen here is due to infection with *Onchocerca cervicalis*, a roundworm that lives in connective tissues.** (Photo courtesy of Anthony Yu, DVM, Diplomate ACVD)

Summer Sores (*Habronema*) FIGURE 10.5

WHAT IT IS. Roundworm infection of the skin, caused by worms that typically live in the horse's stomach (*Habronema muscae, Habronema majus,* and *Draschia megastoma*). Eggs and larvae are passed in the horse's feces, picked up by flies, and deposited on the horse's skin. They then cause open, non-healing wounds, often accompanied by excessive granulation tissue.

DIAGNOSIS. Larvae can be observed in biopsy samples taken from a non-healing wound.

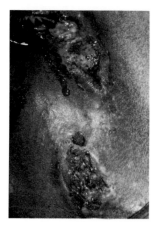

FIGURE 10.5. **These open wounds, called summer sores, are caused by *habronema* larvae that have been deposited on the horse's skin by flies.** (Photo courtesy of Anthony Yu, DVM, Diplomate ACVD)

TREATMENT. *Habronema* infections will often be surgically "debulked" (cutting away damaged tissue) and then treated with topical insecticides. Oral ivermectin may also be a part of the recommended treatment. In some horses, a hypersensitivity (allergic-type) reaction may contribute to the severity of the lesions, and treatment with corticosteroids might help minimize that response.

HOW SERIOUS IS IT? If summer sores go unchecked in sensitive areas, extensive tissue damage can result.

POTENTIAL COMPLICATIONS. Damage to tissues in close proximity to the lesions can occur.

Rain Rot (*Dermatophilus*) FIGURE 10.6

WHAT IT IS. A condition is caused by a bacterial organism called *Dermatophilus congolensis*. This organism thrives in wet conditions with a limited oxygen supply and is more likely to affect skin that's been damaged by insects, trauma, or chronic moisture. It most commonly causes problems in wet climates and is most likely to affect the horse's back or top of his hindquarters where water may accumulate.

DIAGNOSIS. Rain rot produces a skin condition characterized by thick crusts and matted hair that can easily be peeled away, leaving behind raw areas of sensitive skin. In climates where rain rot is common, the veterinarian can usually make a diagnosis simply by looking at the skin. The diagnosis is easy to confirm by submitting a sample of crust and hair to a laboratory for culture to identify the organism.

TREATMENT. Most cases of rain rot can be cured with topical treatment that includes thorough grooming to remove crusts and hair, followed by an antimicrobial shampoo such as chlorhexidine or benzoyl peroxide. Shampoo should be applied to the area, left in contact with the skin for 10 minutes, then rinsed and dried. A topical spray of dilute chlorhexidine (1:32 dilution) may be recommended following shampooing, and treatment should be repeated daily for a period of 5 to 7 days, then intermittently until the condition has resolved. More severe cases may require systemic antibiotic treatment.

HOW SERIOUS IS IT? Rain rot will resolve without complications once appropriate treatment is initiated. The condition can be prevented if moisture

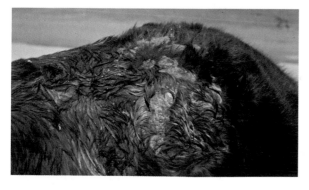

FIGURE 10.6. **These scabs and crusts are typical for the condition called rain rot, which is due to infection with the bacterial organism called *Dermatophilus congonlensis*.** (Photo courtesy of Anthony Yu, DVM, Diplomate ACVD)

is not allowed to accumulate on the horse's skin for extended periods of time. A rain sheet or other waterproof blanket may be appropriate for horses turned out for extended periods in rainy climates.

POTENTIAL COMPLICATIONS. Complications are unlikely. It is advisable, however, to dispose of crusts and hair collected from an affected horse to avoid spreading the bacteria in the environment and to minimize exposure of other horses.

The Skin

Dermatophytosis (Ringworm)

WHAT IT IS. Scaling and crusting of the skin due to infection with fungal organisms, including *Trichophyton equinum*, *Trichophyton verrucosum*, *Trichophyton mentagrophytes*, *Microsporum canis*, *Microsporum equinum*, and *Microsporum gypseum*. Initially, raised, circular swellings (wheals) will appear. Eventually, hair is lost and crusts and scales appear in affected areas. Hair may begin to regrow in the center of the lesions, resulting in the ring-like appearance that gives this condition its name. Ringworm is infectious. Symptoms will appear 1 to 4 weeks following exposure, and young, debilitated, or otherwise immune-compromised horses are most likely to be affected.

DIAGNOSIS. A diagnosis will be suspected based on the typical appearance of the lesions, especially if exposure to an infected horse is known or if multiple horses are affected. Culture of hair and scales in a substance designed to encourage fungal growth will confirm the diagnosis.

TREATMENT. Many cases of ringworm will resolve without treatment; however, an antifungal shampoo or topical rinse containing miconazole, ketoconazole, or chlorhexadine will shorten the duration of the disease and reduce its spread to other horses. A 0.5 percent solution of bleach sprayed on affected areas may also be effective. In general, treatment should be applied daily for 7 to 10 days, then twice weekly for 6 to 8 weeks, or for at least 2 to 4 weeks following resolution of all clinical signs.

The environment should also be disinfected, including tack, blankets, grooming equipment, stalls, and bedding. A 5 to 10 percent bleach solution is effective for most disinfection, although it will be inactivated by organic material so may not be the best choice for stalls and bedding. Other options are 5 percent lime sulfur or a 5 percent povidine/iodine solution.

HOW SERIOUS IS IT? In most instances, ringworm will resolve without much difficulty. Care should be taken to prevent it from spreading into the environment and causing an outbreak in other horses.

POTENTIAL COMPLICATIONS. Complications are rare with this disease. Ringworm may be spread to humans, especially young children.

Pastern Dermatitis (Mud Fever, Scratches, Grease Heel) FIGURE 10.7

WHAT IT IS. Lesions on the pastern area that range from crusts and ulcerations on the skin surface to extreme inflammation with reddening and swelling of the tissues, which can be very painful. Multiple causes of pastern dermatitis often combine to produce symptoms and may include bacterial infection, fungal infections, parasites, and severe inflammation. This condition commonly occurs in wet conditions, in horses that are turned out in muddy pastures or maintained in stalls with wet bedding. White legs are most likely to be affected.

The Horse's Body: Health and Disease

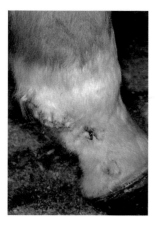

FIGURE 10.7. **The swelling of the lower leg accompanied by scabs and crusts seen here are due to pastern dermatitis, a severe skin condition with a wide variety of different underlying causes.** (Photo courtesy of Anthony Yu, DVM, Diplomate ACVD)

DIAGNOSIS. The general diagnosis of pastern dermatitis is based on the clinical appearance. A specific underlying cause may be identified with skin scrapings, culture, or biopsy.

TREATMENT. Initial treatment may be symptomatic and include broad-spectrum antimicrobial scrubs or topical ointments in combination with anti-inflammatory medications. In most cases, hair must be clipped away from lesions, and the horse should be maintained in a dry environment. Cases that don't respond to initial treatment may require specific diagnostic tests, such as culture, to identify an underlying cause, and treatment with systemic (oral or injectable) antibiotics may be necessary in addition to topical treatments.

HOW SERIOUS IS IT? Pastern dermatitis can cause extremely painful skin lesions accompanied by marked swelling. Some cases can be difficult to treat. In addition, many horses will experience recurrence of this condition even after it has been successfully resolved.

POTENTIAL COMPLICATIONS. Leg swelling can be difficult to eliminate once it becomes well established due to stretching and damage to the tissues.

Equine Papilloma (Warts)

WHAT IT IS. Small gray or pink growths that usually occur on the muzzle, nose, and mouth of young horses, usually between 6 months and 4 years of age. These warts, caused by a virus, will appear approximately 60 days following exposure.

DIAGNOSIS. Diagnosis is based on a very typical appearance.

TREATMENT. No treatment is necessary. Warts are self-limiting, and will regress approximately 3 to 4 months after they appear. Some veterinarians believe that physically crushing warts may stimulate the horse's immune response to help speed regression.

HOW SERIOUS IS IT? Not at all.

POTENTIAL COMPLICATIONS. None.

Aural Plaques   FIGURE 10.8

WHAT IT IS. Small white spots that appear on the inside of the ears due to trauma from flies. They can coalesce into larger white areas, and may appear raised above skin level.

DIAGNOSIS. Aural plaques can be diagnosed based on their appearance.

TREATMENT. No treatment is necessary.

HOW SERIOUS IS IT? Although unsightly, aural plaques generally do not cause any significant problems.

POTENTIAL COMPLICATIONS. None.

Insect Hypersensitivity   FIGURES 10.9–10.10

WHAT IT IS. Pruritis (itching) caused by an allergic reaction to insects, most commonly *Culicoides* ("no-see-um" gnats), and certain types of flies. The horse reacts to the itchiness by scratching, which in turn leads to hair loss,

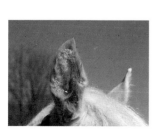

FIGURE 10.8. **These raised white areas on the inside of the ears are typical of aural plaques—a benign skin condition caused by flies.** (Photo courtesy of Mark Revenaugh, DVM)

The Skin

scaling, and crusting. The mane, tail, and belly are commonly affected, and in severe cases the horse will rub out all of the hair in these areas.

DIAGNOSIS. Insect hypersensitivities are seasonal, and typically occur during spring and summer months when insects are most active. The distribution of hair loss and thickened skin that accompany the problem are often enough for the vet to make the diagnosis. Allergy testing may confirm a sensitivity to insects—and even identify the specific culprits.

TREATMENT. Fly control is a critical component to controlling insect hypersensitivity. This may include body sprays with a 2 percent permethrin-based product, fly sheets, and fly-repelling ointments on the belly where flies attack. Avoiding turnout during dawn and dusk, when insects are most active, and removing standing water where insects breed from the horse's environment can also help.

Antihistamines such as diphenhydramine, hydroxyzine, or doxepin hydrochloride may be recommended to help minimize itching. In cases where antihistamines aren't effective, corticosteroids, including prednisolone or dexamethasone, may be prescribed. Topical treatment with antibiotic/cortisone ointments on the most severely affected areas may also help. For severe cases, especially if multiple allergies are involved, hyposensitization ("allergy shots") may be used. (For more details on equine allergies, consult chapter 5, "The Immune System.")

HOW SERIOUS IS IT? Insect hypersensitivity can be an extremely difficult and frustrating problem to control. If a horse experiences this problem, aggressive treatment early each season before insects become most active is necessary to minimize hair loss and trauma to the skin.

POTENTIAL COMPLICATIONS. Secondary bacterial (staph) infections may occur that require treatment with antibiotics. The horse can injure himself in his attempts to scratch, causing puncture wounds or lacerations.

Eosinophilic Granuloma
(Collagenolytic Granuloma, Nodular Necrobiosis)

WHAT IT IS. Nodules from 0.5 to 5.0 centimeters in diameter form under the skin in various parts of the horse's body. They are non painful and covered by normal hair. When tissues are examined, these nodules are composed of degenerating collagen surrounded by eosinophils (the white blood cells most commonly involved in allergic-type reactions). Although the cause is not completely known, a hypersensitivity or allergic response is most likely.

DIAGNOSIS. Diagnosis is based on a typical clinical appearance and can be confirmed with a biopsy.

TREATMENT. Treatment may not be necessary. If nodules are large or in a sensitive area, they may respond to systemic treatment or the injection of individual nodules with corticosteroids. Topical DMSO (dimethyl sulfoxide, a solvent material with anti-inflammatory properties) may also be beneficial, especially if combined with a corticosteroid.

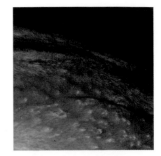

FIGURE 10.9. **Scabs such as these on the horse's belly are a sign of insect hypersensitivity, an allergic problem that causes extreme itching, which can lead to significant skin damage.** (Photo courtesy of Anthony Yu, DVM, Diplomate ACVD)

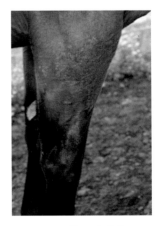

FIGURE 10.10. **Here, hair loss and skin trauma are evident where the horse has rubbed his legs due to an insect hypersensitivity.** (Photo courtesy of Anthony Yu, DVM, Diplomate ACVD)

The Horse's Body: Health and Disease

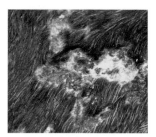

FIGURE 10.11. **These thick crusts are due to pemphigus foliaceus.** (Photo courtesy of Anthony Yu, DVM, Diplomate ACVD

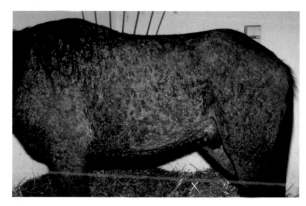

FIGURE 10.12. **In this severe case of pemphigus foliaceus, the horse's entire body has been affected.** (Photo courtesy of Anthony Yu, DVM, Diplomate ACVD)

HOW SERIOUS IS IT? Eosinophilic granulomas cause minimal problems unless they become large enough or are in a location where they interfere with tack. In those cases they can easily be removed.

POTENTIAL COMPLICATIONS. None.

Pemphigus Foliaceus   FIGURES 10.11–10.12

WHAT IT IS. Blisters form on the skin due to the horse's own antibodies attacking cells on the skin surface, which leads to the development of crusts, scales, and erosions.

DIAGNOSIS. Diagnosis is based on skin biopsy.

TREATMENT. To control this condition, the horse's immune system must be suppressed to prevent his antibodies from attacking his own tissues. Most commonly this treatment is accomplished through the use of corticosteroids such as dexamethasone or prednisolone.

HOW SERIOUS IS IT? Pemphigus is a serious, debilitating skin condition that will require lifelong treatment.

POTENTIAL COMPLICATIONS. Secondary bacterial or fungal infections can occur in damaged skin if the condition is not well controlled.

Melanoma   FIGURES 10.13–10.14

WHAT IT IS. A skin tumor that arises from dark skin pigment cells called melanocytes. Melanomas are extremely common in gray horses and in Arabians. It has been estimated that as many as 80 percent of gray horses over 15 years of age have melanomas.

DIAGNOSIS. Most melanomas are easily diagnosed based on their appearance. A cytology or biopsy sample can confirm the diagnosis.

TREATMENT. Where tumors are small, slow-growing, or in nonsensitive areas treatment is unnecessary. If they begin to grow they can be surgically removed, or reduced with cryosurgery (freezing) or treatment with a topical cauterizing agent. One study has demonstrated a decrease in size and number of melanomas following treatment with the medication cimetidine at a dose rate of 2.5 mg/kg 3 times daily for 3 to 4 months. This treatment may be useful for horses with large numbers of tumors that can't be treated individually. Another treatment that has been under investigation and has shown some success involves a vaccine created from surgically removed tumors. It works by stimulating the horse's own immune system to react against the tumors.

HOW SERIOUS IS IT? Small melanomas in a gray horse are generally not a cause for concern. Many will stay small and insignificant for years. If they begin to grow, become ulcerated, or involve sensitive areas then they can become a significant health issue.

POTENTIAL COMPLICATIONS. Seventy-five percent of all melanomas occur in the skin. They can metastasize to other organs, however, resulting in organ failure and death.

Sarcoid FIGURES 10.15–10.16

WHAT IT IS. One of the most common skin tumors seen in horses. In fact, sarcoids make up approximately one-third of all reported tumors in horses. It is believed that a virus called the bovine papilloma virus (BPV) plays a role in the development of sarcoids, and that these tumors are more likely to occur in a horse with a compromised immune system. They occur in horses under the age of 7, may have a hereditary component, and are most common in donkeys and mules, Appaloosas, Arabians, and Quarter Horses. There are four forms of sarcoids:

1. OCCULT (FLAT): appears as a flat or slightly bumpy area of hairless skin.

2. VERRUCOUS (WARTY): often mistaken for warts, with a raised, irregular, hairless appearance. Trauma can cause a verrucous-type sarcoid to become fibroblastic.

3. FIBROBLASTIC: a firm nodule that may be completely covered by skin with hair. This type is most likely to grow rapidly and may ulcerate and bleed.

4. MIXED VERRUCOUS-FIBROBLASTIC: firm nodules combined with raised, irregular, hairless wart-like masses.

DIAGNOSIS. Because these tumors are so common, a presumptive diagnosis can often be made based on their appearance. *(Note: Although a biopsy can confirm the diagnosis, it may be contraindicated for flat or verrucous sarcoids because it can cause as many as 50 percent of these slow-growing tumors to transform into the more aggressive fibroblastic type.)*

TREATMENT. Many occult or verrucous sarcoids are stable or slow growing, and will not metastasize to other areas. Treatment may not be recommended because of the risk of transforming these tumors into a more aggressive type. For aggressive fibroblastic sarcoids, treatment can be frustrating, and no one treatment is effective in all cases.

Surgical excision may be recommended, although additional treatment is often required to prevent reoccurrence. It's been theorized that reoccurrence is common, even if the tumor is completely removed, due to reseeding of the area with viral particles during suturing. A variety of different treatments have been suggested and used for sarcoids, including injection of the area with immune system modulators that are purported to stimulate the horse's immune system to attack tumor cells, injection with chemotherapy agents such as cisplatin that kill tumor cells, cryosurgery (freezing), and application of topical cauterizing agents to kill the tumors. Research is ongoing to evaluate more effective treatments for eliminating these common and often difficult-to-manage tumors.

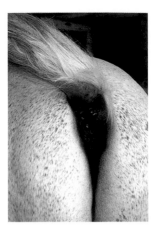

FIGURE 10.13. **Small melanomas under the tail are very common in gray horses. These melanomas often grow very slowly and cause minimal problems.** (Photo courtesy of Mark Revenaugh, DVM)

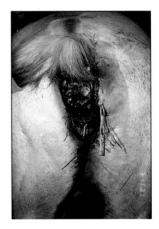

FIGURE 10.14. **If melanomas grow rapidly or are in sensitive areas, removal may be recommended.** (Photo courtesy of Jan Palmer, DVM, Diplomate ACVS)

The Horse's Body: Health and Disease

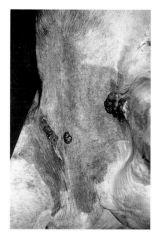

FIGURE 10.15. **These tumors are typical of mixed verrucous-fibroblastic sarcoids. They may grow rapidly, ulcerate, and bleed.** (Photo courtesy of Jan Palmer, DVM, Diplomate ACVS)

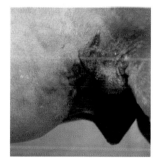

FIGURE 10.16. **The area of thickened, hairless skin in this horse's flank is typical of an occult sarcoid. It is associated with a larger mass under the skin that is likely to be a more aggressive type of this common skin tumor.** (Photo courtesy of Anthony Yu, DVM, Diplomate ACVD)

HOW SERIOUS IS IT? Although sarcoids don't metastasize to other organs, the fibroblastic type can be locally aggressive and cause problems in sensitive areas. A large tumor in the girth area, for example, may cause problems with the saddle, and tumors on the face can be unsightly.

POTENTIAL COMPLICATIONS. Sarcoids rarely have significant complications, except for problems associated with removal of large, aggressive tumors.

Cutaneous Lymphosarcoma

WHAT IT IS. Single or multiple isolated nodules that are usually completely covered by hair, but may enlarge and ulcerate as they progress. These nodules are composed of cancerous lymphocytes (immune system cells). Cutaneous lymphosarcoma may occur as the primary problem, or may be accompanied by lymphosarcoma of internal organs. If other organs are involved, the horse may show signs beyond simple skin lesions, including weight loss, depression, and diarrhea.

TREATMENT. Treatment involves corticosteroids, usually dexamethasone, administered long-term. Vaccines created from cells taken from the tumors themselves have been beneficial in some cases by stimulating the horse's own body to respond against the tumor cells.

DIAGNOSIS. A biopsy of the cells taken from the tumor is the most accurate diagnostic test.

HOW SERIOUS IS IT? Many horses diagnosed with cutaneous lymphosarcoma can survive for a number of years with ongoing treatment. The disease is usually progressive, though, and involvement of other organs is common.

POTENTIAL COMPLICATIONS. Laminitis is a possible complication of long-term dexamethasone administration.

Mastocytoma (Mast Cell Tumor)

WHAT IT IS. Mast cell tumors can occur in two forms: as solitary nodules that are likely to appear on the head and as a diffuse swelling of the lower legs with associated mineralization (deposits of hardened mineral-based substances such as calcium) of the tissues. Mastocytoma is due to an abnormal accumulation of mast cells, one of the cells of the immune system, and is five times more likely to affect males than females.

DIAGNOSIS. Biopsy of the nodule or affected area will confirm a diagnosis.

TREATMENT. Isolated nodules may be successfully removed surgically. Some tumors will respond to injection with cortisone, and some isolated tumors will regress on their own, especially in younger horses. Cases where cells are spread throughout the tissues, resulting in limb swelling and mineralization, may be difficult to treat.

HOW SERIOUS IS IT? Metastasis, or spread, is unlikely. Small isolated nodules are generally easy to manage. The more diffuse form of this condition can have very serious consequences, especially if mineralization results in tissue damage and subsequent lameness.

POTENTIAL COMPLICATIONS. Tissue damage due to extensive mineralization is the most significant complication of this condition.

Hyperelastosis Cutis   FIGURE 10.17

WHAT IT IS. A disease with autosomal recessive inheritance, meaning a horse may carry the gene without exhibiting signs. In an affected horse, the skin is extremely fragile, tears easily, and does not heal following injury due to a disruption in the connections between the two layers of the dermis. The skin may feel mushy or stretchy and does not appear to be attached over multiple areas of the body.

DIAGNOSIS. Diagnosis is based on the typical skin lesions in a horse with appropriate bloodlines. The gene for this disease has been traced to Poco Bueno/King bloodlines in the Quarter Horse breed, and may be found in related Paints, Appaloosas, or other horses carrying those bloodlines. Biopsy samples, using specialized techniques to preserve damaged areas of the skin, can be helpful for confirming a diagnosis in some instances.

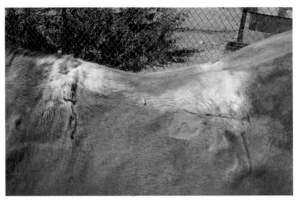

FIGURE 10.17. **Evidence of trauma where the saddle has been placed is typical for a horse with hyperelastosis cutis, a severe hereditary skin disease seen in certain lines of Quarter Horses.** (Photo courtesy of Anthony Yu, DVM, Diplomate ACVD)

TREATMENT. There is no known cure. Symptomatic treatment of wounds or skin damage can help affected horses to remain comfortable.

HOW SERIOUS IS IT? Severely affected horses may have debilitating skin lesions over much of their body. They often cannot be ridden because trauma from tack is enough to cause injury. In addition, because of the heritability of the disease, they should not be bred.

POTENTIAL COMPLICATIONS. None.

Linear Keratosis   FIGURE 10.18

WHAT IT IS. An inherited disease in Quarter Horses that appears between 1 and 5 years of age. It is characterized by linear bands of hair loss and hyperkeratosis (thickened skin), usually on the neck or side of the chest. These lesions don't itch, and are nonpainful.

DIAGNOSIS. The vet will suspect linear keratosis in a Quarter Horse that has lesions typical of the disease. A skin biopsy can confirm the diagnosis.

FIGURE 10.18. **This pattern of hair loss is due to linear keratosis, an inherited skin disease seen in Quarter Horses.** (Photo courtesy of Anthony Yu, DVM, Diplomate ACVD)

TREATMENT. In most cases, treatment is unnecessary. If small areas are affected, surgical removal may be curative. Topical vitamin A cream may help minimize skin thickening to help manage the condition.

HOW SERIOUS IS IT? The disease itself causes minimal problems beyond unsightly areas of thickened skin and hair loss. But, because it is inherited, affected horses should not be bred.

POTENTIAL COMPLICATIONS. None.

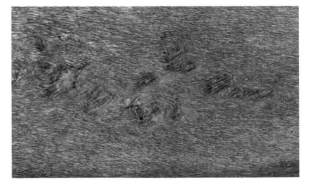

The Horse's Body: Health and Disease

Reticulated Leukotrichia FIGURE 10.19

WHAT IT IS. A skin condition seen in Quarter Horses, Thoroughbreds, and Standardbreds that is believed to be inherited. It begins with a lace-like linear pattern of crusting and hair loss over the horse's back. Areas of hair loss regrow with white hair, resulting in a characteristic lacy pattern.

DIAGNOSIS. Diagnosis is typically based on the clinical appearance, particularly after white hair has grown in the lesion area. Biopsy may help confirm a diagnosis when the lesions are first developing.

TREATMENT. None necessary.

HOW SERIOUS IS IT? The only significance of this problem is cosmetic. Due to the potential inheritability, affected horses should probably not be bred.

POTENTIAL COMPLICATIONS. None.

Cannon Keratosis ("Stud Crud")

WHAT IT IS. A disease that causes thick plaques of crusted skin and scales that form on the front of the hind cannon bones. Contrary to popular belief, this condition is not caused by urine splashing up onto the hind legs. It is actually a disorder in keratinization, or the development of the horny cell (outer) layer of the skin.

DIAGNOSIS. Cannon keratosis can often be diagnosed by its appearance. Although usually unnecessary, a skin biopsy will confirm the diagnosis.

TREATMENT. If a horse has cannon keratosis, it is not a condition that can be cured. It can be managed with regular grooming by using a soft rubber curry or grooming mitt to remove crusts, intermittent antiseborrheic shampoos (such as those containing benzoyl peroxide), and topical treatments including glucocorticoids or vitamin A.

HOW SERIOUS IS IT? Cannon keratosis is nothing more than an unsightly nuisance that can easily be kept under control with careful management.

POTENTIAL COMPLICATIONS. Because seborrhea, crusts, and scales can be secondary to other skin conditions such as dermatophilosis or dermatophytosis, it's important to make sure there isn't an underlying cause. The veterinarian may recommend diagnostic tests such as scrapings, culture, or skin biopsy if a potential underlying cause is suspected.

Trauma FIGURES 10.20–10.22

WHAT IT IS. Skin can be damaged by either blunt or sharp trauma, resulting in abrasions, bruising, lacerations, or punctures.

DIAGNOSIS. A traumatic event or accident is likely to precede an injury, which will be identified by simple observation. The vet may employ a number of different techniques to evaluate the seriousness of a wound. Initially, the injury will be examined and probed to determine how deep it is, what structures are involved, and whether a foreign body is present. Radiographs might be suggested if bone involvement is suspected. If the wound is near a joint, the vet may inject a sterile solution into the joint to

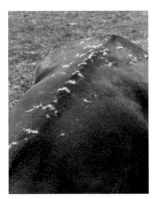

FIGURE 10.19. **This lace-like linear pattern of white hair is typical of reticulated leukotrichia. Lesions initially consist of crusting and hair loss over the back. Once healed, hair grows in white, resulting in this characteristic appearance.** (Photo courtesy of Anthony Yu, DVM, Diplomate ACVD)

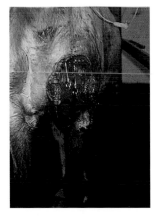

FIGURE 10.20. **This large wound on the chest may be a challenge to treat due to extensive damage to underlying tissues.** (Photo courtesy of Jan Palmer, DVM, Diplomate ACVS)

determine if it has been penetrated and potentially contaminated by observing whether or not the solution flushes back out of the wound. Joint involvement is critical to identify because an infection within a joint can be a life-threatening complication.

TREATMENT. Treatment will depend on the type and extent of the injury. Typically, it will include cleaning, flushing, and suturing unless the wound is a puncture type which is best left open to heal from within. Puncture wounds will be cleaned and flushed, but not sutured. Nonsteroidal anti-inflammatory medications will be administered and prescribed to help control swelling and damage from inflammation. Antibiotics will also be recommended. For wounds on the limbs, bandages, splints, or even casts may be applied to protect and stabilize the injury. Wounds on the upper body heal more easily and bandaging may not be necessary. (For a guide to wound treatment options, refer to the table on page 210.)

HOW SERIOUS IS IT? Skin trauma ranges from a mild, simple abrasion that requires no treatment to a life-threatening wound that involves a joint, tendon, or other critical structure.

POTENTIAL COMPLICATIONS. A number of complications can occur to challenge successful wound treatment. These include:

- INFECTION. An infected wound won't heal, and if antibiotics prescribed initially aren't adequate, a wound may require culturing in order to select an appropriate antibiotic. A sample from the wound is submitted to a laboratory so the bacteria can be identified, and their sensitivity to various antibiotics determined.

  In some cases, a wound may penetrate to bone, causing an osteomyelitis (bone infection) or a sequestrum (a small fragment of bone that is surrounded by infected material). Because the surface of a bone has a limited blood supply, this type of infection may require surgery to resolve. Antibiotics can also be distributed through the blood vessels to specific areas using a tourniquet to isolate circulation to the area.

  A joint or tendon sheath that becomes infected due to a wound can cause a life-threatening complication. Successful treatment of joint infections requires flushing with large volumes of sterile solutions and infusion of antibiotics, often performed under general anesthesia.

- TISSUE DEATH. If a wound is very large, treatment is delayed, or the orientation of the wound is such that the blood supply is compromised (for example, a flap with its base at the lower portion of the wound), it's possible that skin and underlying tissues will die and the wound will not heal by "first intention," meaning that the sutured edges knit together. In this case, the remaining defect in the tissues, once the dead tissues have sloughed off or have been cleaned away, must fill in with healing tissue known as granulation tissue, which can significantly prolong the healing time.

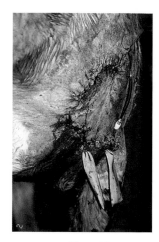

FIGURE 10.21. **The rubber tubing placed into the lower portion of the wound allows drainage, which minimizes the risk of suture loosening.** (Photo courtesy of Jan Palmer, DVM, Diplomate ACVS)

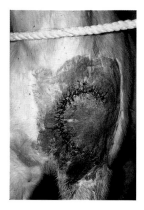

FIGURE 10.22. **After several days, the drain is removed and the sutures remain intact. Now the wound is expected to continue healing without complications.** (Photo courtesy of Jan Palmer, DVM, Diplomate ACVS)

The Horse's Body: Health and Disease

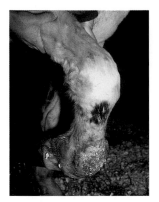

FIGURE 10.23. **This fleshy mass of tissue is known as proud flesh, or excessive granulation tissue.** (Photo courtesy of Jan Palmer, DVM, Diplomate ACVS)

• PROUD FLESH. Excessive granulation tissue is called proud flesh and it develops when normal mechanisms that control healing tissue fail, and fleshy masses of excess tissue bulge over the wound site. In order to control proud flesh, it must be trimmed until it is level with the wound edges in order to allow the skin to extend across the wound and complete healing. Topical treatment with cortisone can slow the granulation tissue and help keep it under control. Pressure bandages will be recommended as well. Wounds below the knees and hocks are most susceptible to proud flesh. This frustrating complication of wound healing rarely occurs on wounds of the upper body.   FIGURE 10.23

When to Call the Vet

You drag your horse in from the pasture when you notice the blood dripping down his right front leg. You think, "What's happened now?" The following step-by-step guide will help you evaluate your horse's injury and decide when it's time to call the vet.

STEP 1. Control bleeding: Wounds are often accompanied by bleeding. If blood is spurting from the wound in rhythm with the horse's heart-beat, it may indicate that an artery has been severed. Apply direct pressure with a gloved finger or small pad of gauze and call the vet immediately. If bleeding is more continuous in nature you can probably control it with a pressure bandage until the vet arrives. (See chapter 3, "Horse First-Aid.")

STEP 2: Is he lame? Lameness may indicate that a critical structure such as a joint, tendon, or ligament is involved. Call the vet.

STEP 3: Does he need sutures? As a general rule, wounds that should be sutured will heal best if sutured as soon as possible. If you are able to separate the edges of the wound by pulling gently with your fingers on the skin on either side, it should be sutured. Call the vet. Wounds below the knees or hocks, or on the face, are most critical.

STEP 4: Are any other critical structures involved? If you see yellowish, sticky fluid coming from a wound (typical of synovial or joint fluid), or can see whitish structures typical of a tendon or ligament, the wound may involve more than the skin. Call the vet.

STEP 5: Questions? Call the vet. It's always best to seek your veterinarian's opinion when your horse experiences an injury. A phone consultation may be all that's needed, but the vet is the person best equipped to help you make that decision.

TABLE 10.1

Home Treatment Guide

Your horse has a wound. He's not lame, you've talked to your vet and you've determined it's not serious enough to require sutures. The following guide will help you decide what home treatments to apply, and how to apply them.

TREATMENT	HOW IT HELPS	WHEN TO USE IT	HOW TO APPLY
Ice/cold-hosing	Reduces inflammation to minimize swelling and tissue damage. Cleans contaminated tissues.	Any time your horse has an abrasion or laceration.	Run cold water from the hose, or apply ice packs to the area for approximately 15 minutes.
Nonsteroidal anti-inflammatory drugs	Helps minimize swelling and tissue damage associated with the injury.	When you detect swelling or heat following an injury, indicating inflammation.	Administer phenylbutazone (4 mg/kg dose) or flunixin meglumine (1 mg/kg).
Flushing or irrigating	Cleans debris and microbial organisms from the tisues.	Any time your horse has an opening in the skin due to an injury.	Gently flush the tissues with a dilute antimicrobial solution, such as betadine and water in a 1:10 or less dilution (weak tea–colored).
Systemic antibiotics	Suppresses or kills bacteria contaminating a wound.	Your veterinarian should advise you about antibiotic administration.	Obtain the appropriate antibiotic and dosing instructions from your veterinarian.
Topical antibiotics	Suppresses or kills bacteria contaminating a wound.	Any time your horse has an opening in the skin due to an injury.	After the wound has been completely cleaned, apply a thin layer of an antimicrobial ointment directly over the wound. A good choice would be a triple-antibiotic ointment that contains bacitracin, neomycin, and polymyxin-B.
Bandaging	Protects the wound, helps minimize movement of the wound edges to promote healing, and helps control swelling.	Any time your horse has an opening in the skin, or you detect swelling of soft tissues due to an injury.	See chapter 3 for a complete guide to applying a pressure bandage. For small wounds without associated swelling, spray-on liquid bandage products may be useful to protect the wound.

CHAPTER 11

The Urinary Tract

THE HORSE'S URINARY TRACT is responsible for collecting and removing fluid wastes from his body. It is also involved with helping to maintain fluid balance by regulating the concentration of the urine. If the horse is dehydrated, the urine becomes more concentrated to preserve fluids. If he has plenty of fluids in his system, the urine will be more dilute.

The following structures make up the urinary tract.   FIGURES 11.1–11.2

Kidneys

Paired kidneys rest just under the back of the rib cage on either side of the spine. The larger, triangular right kidney is slightly in front of the bean-shaped left kidney. Both kidneys are held in place by two special layers of connective tissue, and are surrounded by fat.

Ureters

The ureters are short, muscular tubes that drain the urine produced in the kidneys out into the bladder.

Bladder

The bladder is the storage chamber for urine. It is a pear-shaped sac with muscular walls that become thinner and thinner as the bladder fills with urine. Once it has stretched to a certain point, receptors within the bladder wall are stimulated, causing the muscles to contract and lead to the emptying of the bladder.

Urethra

The urethra is the tube that receives urine from the contracting bladder to allow emptying. The urethra in the mare is very short, and empties into the floor of the vagina. The urethra in a gelding or stallion extends the full length of the penis.

THEN AND NOW

Acute kidney inflammation was recognized as a serious problem in the 1940s. The recommended treatment involved injecting boiled flaxseed into the rectum, applying a thin paste of ground mustard over the loins, and covering the area with a blanket saturated with hot water until the skin thickened and the hair stood up. Although it was recommended that the patient be encouraged to drink as much as possible, fluid therapy wasn't a realistic treatment option, and this condition often had a poor prognosis.

Now we know that the key to an acute kidney crisis is to administer intravenous fluids in order to flush the kidneys and prevent further damage. With early recognition and aggressive fluid therapy, a horse with acute kidney failure has a good chance for a full recovery.

How the Horse Processes Fluids

Blood flow through the kidneys is extensive. Although the kidneys represent approximately 0.3 percent of the body's mass, they receive approximately 20 percent of the total amount of blood circulating through the body. The majority (85 percent) of this flow of blood is to allow filtering through the kidneys for the elimination of waste materials. Only a small amount actually provides oxygen and nutrients necessary for kidney function to occur.

The blood is filtered through a serious of small tubules in the kidneys that help to remove waste products while returning nutrients and necessary fluids to the bloodstream. Urine concentration is regulated by the kidneys according to the horse's individual needs. An average horse produces between 1.5 and 8 liters of urine per day, depending on environmental temperatures, amount of waste products to be removed, and availability of water to replace fluid losses.

After urine is produced, it is passed through the ureters into the bladder for storage, and eliminated through the urethra.

Diagnosis

A diagnosis of problems associated with the urinary tract will likely involve the following steps:

Urinalysis

A urine sample is collected and submitted to a laboratory for analysis. In most situations, urine can simply be collected midstream when the horse is urinating. If a bacterial infection is suspected, however, the vet may prefer to collect a urine sample by passing a catheter through the urethra into the bladder. Bacterial contamination is more likely in a voided sample, and catheterization avoids this potential confusion.

Normal horse urine ranges in color from pale to deep yellow and often appears cloudy due to large amounts of calcium carbonate crystals and mucous. The laboratory portion of the urinalysis involves measurement of specific gravity (degree of concentration), as well as evaluation of pH (degree of acidity), and identification of protein, red blood cells, white blood cells, bacteria, or other cells that are abnormal.

One of the most important features of the urinalysis is the specific gravity. If the kidneys are functioning properly, they should be able to concentrate the urine according to the fluids available in the horse's system. If the kidneys are failing, they will be unable to concentrate urine—even when the horse is dehydrated. A water deprivation test, where water is withheld from the horse for a period of time prior to the collection of urine, may be performed in order to assess the kidneys' ability to concentrate urine.

The Horse's Body: Health and Disease

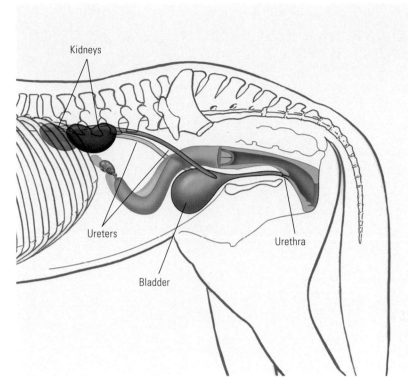

FIGURE 11.1. **Urinary tract of the female.**

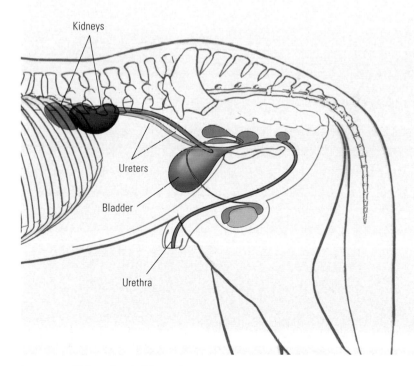

FIGURE 11.2. **Urinary tract of the male.**

Blood Work

Measurement of blood urea nitrogen (BUN) and creatinine are the two specific blood tests used to assess function of the urinary tract. However, these values will increase only when as much as 75 percent of the kidneys are no longer functioning—meaning a large amount of kidney damage may be present before kidney failure can be identified. Anemia and lowered chloride and sodium values may also accompany kidney failure.

Ultrasound

Ultrasound examination of both the kidneys and bladder can help identify and characterize abnormalities of the urinary tract. The kidneys can be examined for enlargement or shrinkage or other changes in their structure, as well as for the presence of kidney stones. The bladder can be evaluated for the presence of stones by a simple rectal palpation.

Endoscopy

Endoscopy of the bladder allows for direct visualization using fiber-optic or video technology via a tube that is passed through the urethra directly into the bladder. Through endoscopy, stones, cancer, or other abnormalities of the bladder may be identified.

Kidney Biopsy

When kidney failure has been identified, and nature of the damage can be specifically defined with a kidney biopsy. A sample of the kidney tissue can be obtained through the skin, using a specialized biopsy instrument.

WHEN THINGS GO WRONG

The following are the most common conditions likely to affect the horse's urinary system.

Acute Kidney Failure   FIGURE 11.3

WHAT IT IS. The kidneys stop working abruptly, often due to toxicity or severe dehydration. Acute failure may occur when chronic disease is present. Toxins that affect the kidneys may include medications such as antibiotics (e.g., gentamicin and amikacin) or anti-inflammatories (e.g., phenylbutazone and flunixin meglumine). Heavy metals (mercury) and some plants (e.g., red maple and oak) are also toxic to the kidneys. Products of muscle breakdown such as hemoglobin or myoglobin that are released into the bloodstream with muscle-related problems (e.g., exertional rhabdomyolysis, or tying-up) can also cause kidney damage. (See chapter 4, "The Musculoskeletal System.")

DIAGNOSIS. Diagnosis of kidney failure primarily depends on blood work. Signs of dehydration accompanying some other disease along with elevated blood urea nitrogen (BUN), which indicates that the kidneys are

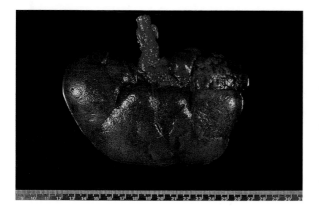

FIGURE 11.3. **This damaged kidney could be the underlying cause of depression and unthriftiness. If damage progresses to the point of kidney failure, death can result.** (Author photo)

failing to remove toxins adequately, and elevated creatinine, which indicates death of kidney tissue—all point toward a diagnosis of kidney failure. Urinalysis can also aid diagnosis.

TREATMENT. For a horse with acute kidney failure the administration of large volumes of intravenous fluids is critical. This helps correct dehydration, flush potential toxins, and encourages the kidneys to begin functioning. The medication dopamine may also be administered. Dopamine dilates blood vessels within the kidneys to aid blood flow to the tissues. In addition, the diuretic furosemide may be given to help stimulate the kidneys to begin producing urine. Any exposure to potential toxins should be identified and eliminated.

HOW SERIOUS IS IT? If acute kidney failure is identified early, treated aggressively, and chronic damage to the kidneys is not present, it can be successfully treated. Cases where kidney failure is primarily due to dehydration are usually completely reversible.

POTENTIAL COMPLICATIONS. Chronic kidney damage is the most common and significant complication.

Chronic Kidney Failure

WHAT IT IS Failure occurs when damage to parts of the kidneys has occurred, hampering the kidneys' ability to remove wastes and regulate fluid balance. Chronic damage can occur following an acute kidney crisis, due to long-term exposure to potential toxins, or secondary to many other conditions affecting the urinary tract.

DIAGNOSIS. The symptoms of chronic kidney failure are often vague, and include loss of appetite, weight loss, and weakness. A decline in performance may be the first thing detected in an athletic horse. Lab work will be used to confirm a diagnosis, with increased BUN and creatinine levels the most consistent abnormalities. Many horses will have electrolyte abnormalities in the blood, including lowered sodium and chloride levels, and increased calcium levels. Urinalysis may show that the urine is dilute because the kidneys have lost their ability to concentrate urine and preserve electrolytes. Proteins are also commonly seen in the urine, reflecting protein loss. Ultrasound of the kidneys and a biopsy may be recommended to determine the extent and nature of the damage to the kidney structure.

TREATMENT. Chronic kidney failure cannot be cured, although treatment can help minimize signs, protect the kidneys from further damage, and prolong the horse's life. Initial treatment involves identifying any condition such as an infection that would require antibiotics, eliminating the horse's exposure to any potential toxins, and giving oral or intravenous fluids to minimize kidney injury or damage. Once the kidneys are stabilized, the vet is likely to recommend routine monitoring with blood tests to assess various changes that can occur in the horse's system due to the kidneys' loss of function. The following strategies may be employed in the management plan for dealing with chronic kidney damage.

- Avoid NSAIDS medications and exposure to other potential kidney toxins.

- Feed a diet composed primarily of grass hay, and avoid alfalfa. The protein levels of the diet should be maintained below 10 percent to minimize the protein load on the kidneys. In addition, avoiding alfalfa will limit the amount of calcium that the kidneys are required to process.

- Due to changes in metabolism, horses in kidney failure may become acidotic (a state of lowered pH, or more acid-like conditions in the bloodstream). Sodium bicarbonate may be recommended as a dietary supplement if this occurs.

- Horses with chronic kidney failure are likely to become anemic. The vet may recommend a variety of supplements, including B vitamins or iron, to help combat this problem.

- Fresh, clean water must be available at all times to avoid dehydration, which can cause the kidneys to experience acute failure.

HOW SERIOUS IS IT? Chronic kidney failure is a very serious condition that may progress and threaten the horse's life. With careful management, however, a horse can live for many years and may even continue to perform in athletic disciplines.

POTENTIAL COMPLICATIONS. Chronic kidney damage puts the horse at risk for acute failure that may be life threatening.

Pyelonephritis

WHAT IT IS. An infection of the kidneys due to bacterial invasion.

DIAGNOSIS. Pyelonephritis may be an underlying cause of kidney failure. If a horse in kidney failure has a fever, and a high white blood cell count indicating infection, pyelonephritis would be suspected. Bacteria seen in a kidney biopsy would confirm the diagnosis.

TREATMENT. Antibiotics would be required in addition to treatment necessary to control kidney failure.

HOW SERIOUS IS IT? Pyelonephritis can be life threatening.

POTENTIAL COMPLICATIONS. Acute kidney failure. Pyelonephritis may also lead to the formation of kidney stones.

Bladder Stones   FIGURES 11.4–11.6

WHAT IT IS. Hard mineral matter that forms in the bladder, causing irritation to the bladder wall and difficulties with urination.

DIAGNOSIS. Bladder stones will be suspected based on typical clinical signs of straining during urination, blood in the urine, and the inability of the horse to urinate a full stream. Many bladder stones can be identified on

The Horse's Body: Health and Disease

rectal palpation alone, although ultrasound is often used to confirm the diagnosis. Endoscopic examination will allow for direct visualization in cases where a more definite diagnosis is needed.

TREATMENT. In most cases, surgical removal of the stones will be recommended. Lithotripsy, or breaking apart of stones using a variety of different mechanical devices, may allow the horse to pass stones out through the urethra or will make removal through endoscopic techniques possible, thus avoiding surgery.

HOW SERIOUS IS IT? Surgery to remove bladder stones usually requires general anesthesia and is a major surgical procedure. Most bladder stones can be removed successfully, with minimal long-term adverse effects. It has been reported that stones reoccur in as many as 40 percent of cases.

POTENTIAL COMPLICATIONS. Complications related to major abdominal surgery and anesthesia are the primary cause for concern when bladder stones have been diagnosed.

FIGURE 11.4. **Bladder stones can be surgically removed, a surgery that's most commonly performed under general anesthesia with an incision into the horse's abdomen to reach the bladder.** (Author photo)

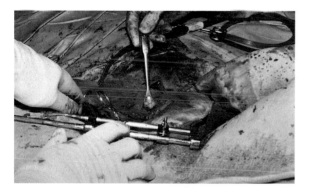

Nephrolithiasis (Kidney Stones) or Urolithiasis (Stones in the Ureter)

WHAT IT IS. Mineralizations that occur in the kidneys or ureters. These stones may form secondary to infection (pyelonephritis) or as a primary condition related to inflammation.

DIAGNOSIS. These stones are likely to be accompanied by chronic kidney failure or an episode of acute kidney failure. The initial signs observed are usually due to poor kidney function. Stones may be identified during an ultrasound examination performed to pinpoint the cause of kidney failure.

TREATMENT. Although surgery is possible, it is rarely performed. Prognosis is extremely guarded in most instances due to underlying kidney damage.

HOW SERIOUS IS IT? Stones in the kidneys or ureters are often a life threatening condition.

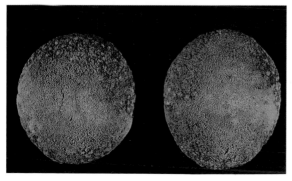

FIGURE 11.5. **A horse with this large bladder stone would strain to urinate, urinate small amounts, and be likely to have blood in his urine.** (Author photo)

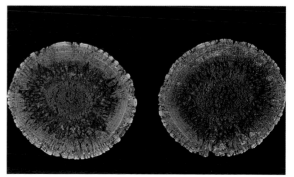

FIGURE 11.6. **A slice through the middle of the stone shows how it forms in layers that produce rings, similar to the rings of a tree stump.** (Author photo)

POTENTIAL COMPLICATIONS. Kidney failure.

Cystitis FIGURE 11.7

WHAT IT IS. An inflammation of the bladder that may or may not be accompanied by an infection. The condition may be due to trauma or be secondary to a factor that causes the bladder to become paralyzed (possible with neurologic problems). A horse with cystitis will urinate frequently, strain during urination, and may have urine leakage.

DIAGNOSIS. A urinalysis will confirm a diagnosis of cystitis. Urine samples should be obtained using a catheter to insure accuracy. White blood cells indicating inflammation will be seen, and bacteria may be present.

TREATMENT. When infection is present, the administration of an appropriate antibiotic will be required. If the cystitis is secondary to trauma or a condition causing bladder paralysis, treatment of the underlying cause will be necessary to encourage normal bladder function.

HOW SERIOUS IS IT? Cystitis due to a bacterial infection is usually treatable. Otherwise, success of treatment depends on the ability to deal with the underlying problem.

POTENTIAL COMPLICATIONS. Long-standing infections of the bladder may put the horse at risk for pyelonephritis and potential kidney failure.

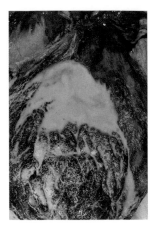

FIGURE 11.7. **The yellowish discharge and reddened appearance of the bladder lining is evidence of a severe case of cystitis, or bladder inflammation.** (Author photo)

Psychogenic Polyuria and Polydipsia (PU/PD)

WHAT IT IS. The horse begins to drink inordinate amounts of water due to boredom, associated with a lifestyle that involves confinement to a small area such as a stall. As a result of this excessive water drinking, the horse urinates excessively. Because of the large amounts of fluids passing through the kidneys, the normal balance of electrolytes within the kidneys is diluted or "washed out," compromising the horse's ability to concentrate his urine. So he drinks even more—and a vicious cycle begins.

DIAGNOSIS. A horse with psychogenic PU/PD will have no evidence of kidney failure in blood work, yet his urine specific gravity may be low due to the kidneys' electrolyte imbalance and subsequent inability to concentrate the urine. Urine concentration may still fail to appear even if water is withheld for 24 hours. However, if water is provided at a rate of 40 ml/kg/day for up to 4 days, the electrolyte balance will be restored, and the kidneys will regain their ability to concentrate the urine.

TREATMENT. The key component to solving this problem is to change the environment to minimize boredom. Increased turnout and a more frequent feeding schedule may be effective measures. Water intake can be restricted to 40 ml/kg/day for the average horse except when the demands of exercise or hot weather require more be given.

HOW SERIOUS IS IT? Psychogenic PU/PD is a management hassle, but should have no serious effects on the overall health of the horse. Once recognized, it should be fairly easy to control.

POTENTIAL COMPLICATIONS. None.

The Horse's Body: Health and Disease

CHAPTER 12

The Endocrine System

THEN AND NOW

Hormones weren't even discovered until the early 1900s, meaning diseases of the endocrine system weren't recognized or treated until recent years. In fact, veterinary textbooks from as late as the 1940s make no mention of the endocrine system except to say that diseases are rare, with symptoms little understood.

These days, Cushing's disease is recognized as one of the most common problems seen in older horses. The ability to diagnose and treat Cushing's is perhaps one of the primary contributors to the health of geriatric horses in today's world.

THE HORSE'S ENDOCRINE SYSTEM is comprised of a set of endocrine glands that release substances known as hormones, the body's basic regulators. In this chapter, we'll review the hormonal pathways working in the horse's body, what they are, how they work, and what happens when things run amok.

The endocrine system is very complex, and involves many different structures and hormones. The following comprise the most important components of the horse's endocrine system that are likely to be involved in an endocrine disease.

FIGURE 12.1

Hypothalamus

The hypothalamus located just above the pituitary gland, is the part of the horse's brain that regulates function of many of the glands within the body. It is the source of various "releasing hormones" that activate hormones in other glands. It is also the site of the thirst center that detects changes in hydration and stimulates the horse to drink as well as the release point for neurotransmitters that stimulate heating and cooling mechanisms to help maintain normal body temperature.

Pituitary Gland

The pituitary is a small structure that is attached at the base of the horse's brain. The pituitary is the source of many of the "stimulating hormones" or controllers of other endocrine glands. Some of the most common and clinically relevant are the thyrotropin stimulating hormone (TSH), which controls the thyroid; the luteinizing hormone (LH) and the follicle stimulating hormone (FSH), which control ovarian function in the mare; and adrenocorticotropic hormone (ACTH) which controls the release of glucocorticoids (stress hormones) from the adrenal glands.

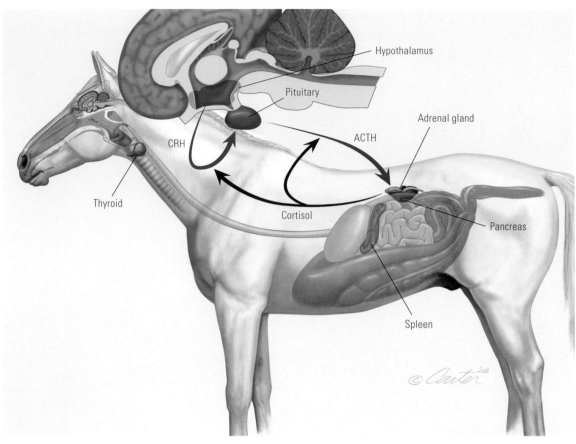

FIGURE 12.1. **The endocrine glands. Hormones function with a classical negative feedback mechanism as depicted here.**

Adrenal Gland

An adrenal gland is embedded in fat at the front of each kidney. These glands secrete glucocorticoids, which are released during periods of stress, as well as epinephrine and norephinephrine, the hormones that regulate the horse's "fight or flight" response.

Thyroid Gland

The thyroid lies on either side of the horse's neck, just below the throat-latch area. It can be palpated externally, and is approximately as big as a flattened golf ball. The thyroid releases two primary hormones: tri-iodothyronine (T3) and tetraiodothyronine (T4). These hormones regulate iodine that's absorbed from the intestines. Iodine is an important controller of synthesis and release of many hormones. The thyroid also produces another horomone called calcitonin, which is responsible for maintaining the balance of calcium.

Pancreas

The pancreas, a triangular organ, is situated in the horse's abdominal cavity, just below the kidneys. It is surrounded by the stomach and small intestines. The pancreas secretes the hormone insulin, as well as

The Horse's Body: Health and Disease

glucagon and somatostatin, which help regulate blood sugar levels within the body. In basic terms, the pancreas responds to high blood sugar (glucose) levels by releasing insulin, which then helps facilitate metabolism and storage of glucose needed for the body's functioning.

How the Endocrine System Functions

The endocrine system is principally responsible for the regulation of the body's other organ systems. The central office (the brain) detects signals from the outside world as well as from within the horse's body. These signals are then processed through one major regulatory center—the hypothalamus. This part of the brain sends out messengers (releasing hormones) to many satellite offices (glands) distributed throughout the body. These glands send out more messages (hormones) that direct activities in many remote locations, and communicate with one another through a series of feedback loops.

An illustration of this: The vet approaches the horse with a needle, prepared to give an injection. The horse's brain says "STRESS," which stimulates the release of the corticotrophin-releasing hormone (CRH) from the hypothalamus. CRH takes this message to the pituitary gland, which then releases the adrenocorticotropin-releasing hormone (ACTH). ACTH acts on the adrenal cortex to stimulate the release of cortisol—the stress hormone. When cortisol is released, it sends messages back to both the pituitary and the hypothalamus to stop releasing CRH and ACTH— a classic negative feedback loop. At the same time, the cortisol stimulates a range of different responses within the horse's system to help him respond to the stressful event he's facing.

Hormonal Testing

Most health problems associated with endocrine or hormonal disorders produce certain classic clinical signs. For example, a horse with Cushing's disease (a common hormonal abnormality of older horses due to a pituitary tumor that causes increased release of glucocorticoids) will have a very typical appearance that includes a long, curly hair-coat, excessive sweating, and abnormal fat deposits over his body. He may also begin to behave aggressively toward handlers and other horses. These factors make a thorough physical examination and history of the horse's behavior and condition an extremely important part of making a diagnosis.

If a hormonal problem is suspected, blood tests are generally used to confirm a diagnosis. These tests may include measurement of specific hormones circulating in the bloodstream, or stimulation tests that measure the body's response to the administration of specific stimulating hormones. Because of the feedback loops that control most endocrine function, stimulation tests are the most accurate when they are available. For example, hypothyroidism would be most accurately diagnosed by using a thyroid-stimulating hormone (TSH) test. For this test, thyroid levels would be measured, a hormone known as TSH would be administered, and the effect of the TSH on the thyroid levels would be evaluated. Unfortunately, stimulation tests are often difficult or impossible to perform due to the unavailability of essential chemicals such as TSH, making diagnosis of hormonal problems complicated and often frustrating.

WHEN THING GO WRONG

The following are the most common diseases that involve the horse's endocrine system.

Cushing's Disease

WHAT IT IS. This disease of older horses is the result of an adenoma (benign tumor) in the pituitary gland that causes the excessive release of a hormone called adrenocorticotropin (ACTH). The ACTH in turn stimulates an increase in the amount of cortisol hormones released from the adrenal glands into the bloodstream. This increase in circulating cortisol leads to clinical signs that include a long, curly hair-coat that doesn't shed during summer months (seen in 85 percent of affected horses), abnormal fat deposits over parts of the body (commonly observed in the depressions above the horse's eyes), increased sweating, loss of muscle tone accompanied by a pendulous abdomen, increased drinking and urinating, and increased susceptibility to infections and laminitis. It's theorized that some of the clinical signs of Cushing's disease are the result of pressure on the hypothalamus by the tumor, in addition to the actual functional effects of the tumor itself.

The average age of affected horses is between 19 and 21 years. Ponies may be more susceptible than full-sized horses, and some studies indicate that mares are more likely to be affected than geldings or stallions.

DIAGNOSIS. The vet will often suspect Cushing's disease simply because of the clinical signs and appearance of a horse. A variety of blood tests may be used to confirm the diagnosis.

Initially, a basic chemistry panel is likely to be recommended, and a higher than normal blood sugar (glucose) measurement is strongly suggestive of Cushing's disease in a horse exhibiting the usual clinical signs.

The most reliable test for diagnosis of this disease is the low-dose dexamethasone suppression (LDD) test. To perform this test, the veterinarian will measure the horse's resting cortisol levels in the blood, and will then administer a dose of the corticosteroid medication called dexamethasone. In a normal horse, administration of dexamethasone will suppress the normal release of cortisol, resulting in a lowered ("suppressed") resting cortisol measurement. In a horse with Cushing's disease, the normal feedback mechanisms that control cortisol release will not respond to the dexamethasone administered, and the resting cortisol levels will remain normal.

Because laminitis is a potential complication of dexamethasone administration, and horses with Cushing's disease often experience laminitis that is severe and nonresponsive to treatment, many veterinarians are reluctant to perform the LDD test on a horse that is already experiencing symptoms of laminitis for fear of making the condition worse. In these cases, a number of different blood tests can be used to help confirm the diagnosis. The most common is measurement of ACTH levels in the blood. ACTH levels in horses with Cushing's disease have been reported to be approximately six times higher than those measured in normal horses. This test requires very careful handling of blood samples, and although it may not be as reliable a diagnostic test as the LDD test, it is useful to help confirm a diagnosis of this disease in horses experiencing symptoms of laminitis.

TREATMENT. The chief component of a treatment plan for a horse with Cushing's disease is good basic care that includes clipping the hair-coat during hot summer months or when the long, curly hair typical of this disease becomes matted or unhealthy. Regular dental care is especially important, as Cushing's horses may be more prone to dental problems because of their inability to fight infections. Finally, regular foot care and special attention to any early sign of laminitis are necessary to minimize the chance of this complication.

At the present time two medications can help treat Cushing's disease. One is pergolide mesylate (Permax®, now also available as a generic). Although there's not a lot of solid scientific data about the specific effects of pergolide on the horse, nevertheless it has proven to be effective in controlling Cushing's symptoms. The vet may opt to test the efficacy of this medication by monitoring the horse's blood sugar levels, or response to the LDD test. Dosages are then adjusted as needed to achieve optimal results.

Cyproheptadine is another medication that may be recommended for a horse diagnosed with Cushing's disease. This medication is less effective than pergolide for controlling Cushing's symptoms, yet it has been shown to be useful in approximately 35 percent of cases. In some circumstances, pergolide and cyproheptadine will be used in combination for maximum effect. Specifically, some horses seem to develop a resistance to pergolide after a period of 2 to 3 years, and adding cyproheptadine to the treatment plan can help control symptoms once that resistance occurs.

HOW SERIOUS IS IT? In many cases, Cushing's disease is a fairly benign condition that causes few problems and can be easily managed. In cases where laminitis becomes a significant component of the disease, it can become life threatening.

POTENTIAL COMPLICATIONS. The most serious complication of Cushing's disease is laminitis, an extremely painful condition that can be difficult to control. If the horse has Cushing's, the laminitis that accompanies it is often resistant to treatment and can spiral out of control.

Susceptibility to infection resulting from the high levels of circulating cortisol in the horse's system can also lead to complications. In particular, skin infections that are exacerbated by the long hair-coat and excessive sweating that accompanies Cushing's may require extra attention. And infections in the periodontal tissues that lead to dental problems, including tooth loss and sinus issues, can be cause for concern.

Equine Metabolic Syndrome (Peripheral Cushing's Syndrome) FIGURE 12.2

WHAT IT IS. This recently recognized condition is described as an obesity-associated insulin insensitivity. If a horse has EMS, tissues become nonresponsive to insulin, which is essential for regulating blood sugar levels, and glucose (sugar) intolerance develops. Because the tissues aren't responding, the horse's pancreas continues to release more and more insulin, resulting in extremely high circulating insulin levels.

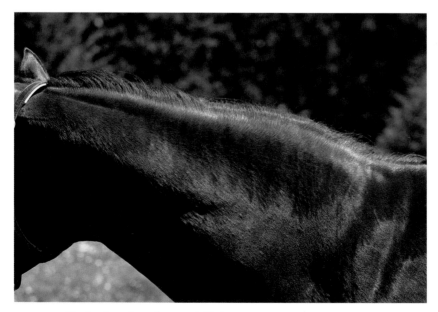

FIGURE 12.2. **The fat deposit on the top of this horse's neck gives him a cresty appearance, typical of many endocrine abnormalities, including both Cushing's disease and equine metabolic syndrome.**

Commonly seen in horses between 8 and 18 years of age, this metabolic disease looks very much like Cushing's disease. Horses with EMS typically have a cresty neck, as well as fat deposits in other areas such as the rump and back. Geldings may appear to have a "swollen sheath" due to fat deposits in that area.

DIAGNOSIS. Diagnosis of EMS is primarily based on the physical appearance of the horse, and a very high circulating insulin level. Because horses with Cushing's disease have a similar appearance and may also have high insulin levels, an LDD test may be necessary to differentiate between the two diseases. Unfortunately, this test cannot always be safely performed on these horses because of the risk of causing laminitis.

TREATMENT. The only really effective management tools for EMS are weight control and increased exercise. However, it can be difficult to manage weight in a very easy-keeping horse. Other experimental treatments include supplementation with trace minerals containing chromium and magnesium, which are believed to help regulate insulin metabolism.

HOW SERIOUS IS IT? EMS can be extremely frustrating and difficult to manage. If laminitis results, it can even be life threatening.

POTENTIAL COMPLICATIONS. The most serious possible complication of EMS is laminitis. It's theorized that the increased risk of laminitis is due to the effect of insulin on the cardiovascular system which leads to a disruption of blood flow within the laminae of the horse's feet. (*Note: It's interesting that EMS, Cushing's disease, stress, and the administration of corticosteroids such as dexamethasone in high dosages all share this risk for laminitis, and all result in increased levels of circulating insulin in the horse's body through different mechanisms.*)

Hypothyroidism

WHAT IT IS. True hypothyroidism is extremely rare. In fact, most experts believe that it is not really a disease entity in horses. However, low circulating thyroid hormone levels are fairly common, often secondary to other chronic diseases. This condition, known as "sick euthyroid syndrome," is usually associated with both Cushing's disease and equine metabolic syndrome, among other diseases. Administration of the nonsteroidal anti-inflammatory medication phenylbutazone can also lower circulating thyroid levels.

In horses whose thyroid glands have been removed, signs of hypothyroidism include a lack of appetite, dull hair-coat, lowered body temperature, and increased sensitivity to cold. It's interesting that neither obesity nor laminitis occurs in these horses, two conditions commonly identified as typical of hypothyroidism. This may be explained by the fact that many horses identified as "hypothyroid" actually have one of the other common endocrine diseases associated with obesity and laminitis, with low thyroid levels a strictly secondary problem.

True hypothyroidism has been documented in foals and is related to either excessive or inadequate iodine intake. These foals may have enlarged glands (goiter) and will be weak and uncoordinated. They may have musculoskeletal disorders, including a lack of development of the small bones in the knees and hocks, and ruptures of the common digital extensor tendon.

DIAGNOSIS. It is extremely difficult to accurately diagnose hypothyroidism, making this one of the most incorrectly, overdiagnosed conditions in horses. Measurement of circulating levels of the thyroid hormones T3 and T4 is commonly recommended. However, because much of the thyroid hormone in the horse's body is bound to protein rendering it inactive, these measurements are often misinterpreted. Even though a normal total T3/T4 measure does rule out hypothyroidism, a low total T3/T4 measurement is not an accurate diagnostic test. The only really meaningful test is measurement of free (unbound) T4, and the most accurate measurement technique is one called equilibrium dialysis. (*Note: The commonly used radio-immunoactivity or RIA method for measuring the thyroid is considered inaccurate by many testing laboratories.*)

To truly diagnose primary hypothyroidism in horses would require a thyroid stimulation test, which is generally impractical due to a lack of available TSH necessary to perform the test.

TREATMENT. Most hypothyroidism identified in horses is secondary to another disease, such as Cushing's disease or EMS. Therefore, effective treatment depends on treating the primary problem. In rare cases, thyroid supplementation may be beneficial—most commonly when treatment of the primary problem is not successful and lowered thyroid hormone levels persist. In these situations, L-thyroxine may be recommended at a dosage rate of approximately 10 mg daily for a 1000-pound horse. If thyroid supplementation is initiated, it is highly recommended that free T4 levels be monitored.

HOW SERIOUS IS IT? The seriousness of hypothyroidism mainly depends on the principal problem contributing to the lowered thyroid levels.

POTENTIAL COMPLICATIONS. Again, complications of hypothyroidism primarily depend on the underlying condition. Laminitis is a common, serious complication of the metabolic diseases associated with low thyroid levels.

Thyroid Adenoma   FIGURE 12.3

WHAT IT IS. A thyroid adenoma is a benign enlargement of one or both sides of the thyroid and is commonly seen in older horses.

DIAGNOSIS. Most veterinarians will recognize a thyroid adenoma simply based on its appearance. Rarely, a biopsy may be recommended to ensure the enlarged thyroid is not due to an aggressive type of cancer.

TREATMENT. None required.

The Horse's Body: Health and Disease

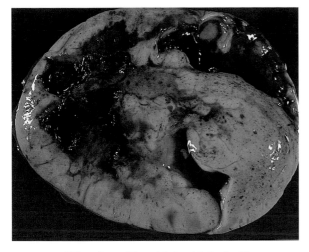

FIGURE 12.3. **This enlarged thyroid gland is typical for a thyroid adenoma, a common, benign condition seen in older horses.** (Author photo)

HOW SERIOUS IS IT? Although unsightly, a thyroid adenoma is not a cause for concern.

COMPLICATIONS. None.

Pheochromocytoma

WHAT IT IS. Pheochromocytoma is a tumor of the adrenal gland that results in increased secretion of catecholamine hormones (epinephrine and norepinephrine).

DIAGNOSIS. This very unusual condition might be suspected if the horse exhibits signs of increased sweating and anxiety, a racing heart, an elevated respiratory rate, and twitching or "fasiculation" of muscles. Some horses will exhibit signs of colic, and may have elevated potassium levels on routine blood tests. If the vet suspects a pheochromocytoma based on these signs, the diagnosis can be confirmed through measurement of norepinephrine in the horse's bloodstream. Most cases of pheochromocytoma are only identified during a postmortem examination.

TREATMENT. The only effective treatment is removal of the affected adrenal gland, which is an extremely difficult and complicated surgery to perform.

HOW SERIOUS IS IT? The prognosis for a horse with pheochromocytoma is extremely poor. Symptoms can be severe, and practical treatment is unavailable.

POTENTIAL COMPLICATIONS. These tumors have a tendency to bleed, and may rupture within the horse's abdominal cavity, resulting in death.

Anhidrosis

WHAT IT IS. Anhidrosis is the inability of the horse to sweat under appropriate conditions. It is most common in extremely hot geographical areas. Although the precise cause of this disease is unknown, it is believed to be related to an endocrine imbalance. Horses with anhidrosis tend to have higher levels of circulating epinephrine, which is believed to "turn off" the functioning of the sweat glands.

DIAGNOSIS. A diagnosis of anhidrosis is suspected in a horse that fails to sweat even during hot conditions or with hard work. A very rapid respiratory rate and prolonged cool-out time might also support a diagnosis of anhidrosis because the affected horse has lost his primary cooling mechanism. Administration of a medication called terbutaline, which stimulates receptors on the sweat glands, can help confirm a suspected diagnosis; terbutaline will cause a normal horse to sweat, but a horse affected with anhidrosis will not.

TREATMENT. The only reliably effective treatment for this condition is to move the horse to a cooler environment. Often, electrolyte supplements containing sodium and potassium may help stimulate sweat production.

HOW SERIOUS IS IT? Anhidrosis can be a very serious problem in horses required to exercise in hot areas. In some cases, the only solution is to move the horse to a cooler area if he must continue to work.

POTENTIAL COMPLICATIONS. Because a horse suffering from anhidrosis has lost his primary cooling mechanism, he is at increased risk for heat exhaustion and heat stroke, which can be a serious, even life-threatening condition when it is severe.

CHAPTER 13

The Eyes

T HE HORSE'S EYE IS MADE UP of a complex system of light regulators and reflectors that allow him to see objects and movement, and translate what he sees to his brain for processing.

The following structures make up the horse's eye.   FIGURES 13.1–13.2

Eyelids (Ocular Adnexa)

Upper and lower lids extend from the skin on his face to protect his eye. The lids have long hairs that act as feelers, allowing him to detect an object coming close so he'll know to close his eyelids and protect his eye from injury. Eyelashes on the upper and lower lids provide further protection by preventing foreign material from reaching the eye. Strong muscles in the eyelids allow them to open and close.

Third Eyelid (Nictitating Membrane)

This flesh-colored flap of tissue sits at the inside corner of his eye for added protection. Its job is to aid in the removal of foreign bodies by sweeping across the corneal surface.

Nasolacrimal Duct

This very narrow tube runs between the horse's eye and his nose, with openings at the inside corner of the eye and in the nostril. The nasolacrimal duct system drains secretions from the eye out into his nose to avoid a buildup of fluids on his face.

Conjunctiva

This membrane lines the eyelids and covers the back of the eyeball. The conjunctiva protects, carries blood to the eye, and helps support the eyelids and other structures of the eye.

Cornea

This clear outer layer at the front of the eye allows light through so the horse can see.

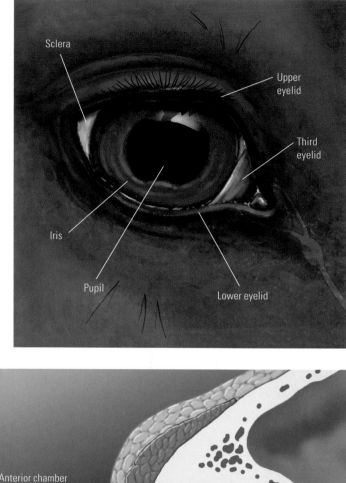

FIGURE 13.1. **External structures of the eye.**

Sclera

Upper eyelid

Third eyelid

Iris

Pupil

Lower eyelid

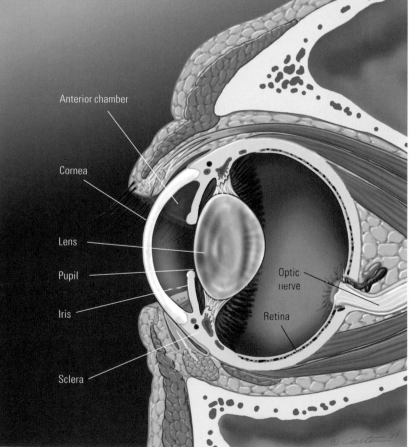

FIGURE 13.2. **Internal structures of the eye.**

Anterior chamber

Cornea

Lens

Pupil

Optic nerve

Iris

Retina

Sclera

The Horse's Body: Health and Disease

Iris/Pupil

The iris, the membrane inside the eye behind the cornea, has an opening (the pupil) at its center to let light through. Small muscles control the iris to allow the pupil to open or close depending on how light or dark it is.

Sclera

The thick, white outer layer of the eyeball that's covered by the conjunctiva at the back of the eye, and is continuous with the cornea in front. The sclera is what makes the eye a "ball" because of its shape and thickness.

Lens

A clear structure that's curved at front and back, and is located behind the iris and the pupil. The lens controls the direction of light passing through the eye to help form the images the horse sees.

Retina

A shiny, reflective layer of tissue at the back of the eye. The retina receives and processes the information that's passed through the other structures of the eye and allows the horse to see.

Optic Nerve

This nerve attaches at the back of the eye, and carries messages from the eye to the horse's central nervous system so he can interpret what he sees.

How the Horse Sees

The horse's vision is designed to help him survive as a prey animal in his natural environment. That means he's especially dependent on his ability to see in different light conditions, is more sensitive to moving objects than stationary ones, and has a wide field of view.

The horse's light sensitivity is excellent, both at night and in bright light. His lens has yellow pigments that filter out short wavelengths—similar to the way in which yellow-tinted sunglasses reduce glare in bright light. A small, darkly pigmented mass called the corpora nigra at the top of his pupil acts like a visor to shade the eye from direct light. At night, the horse's large cornea allows a lot of light into the eye. A highly reflective area on the back of the eye, the tapetum lucidum, reflects light back to the retina and gives photoreceptors a second chance to aid with dim-light vision. Finally, his pupil dilates very wide to allow more light in during darker conditions, and its slit-like shape allows more complete closure during bright-light conditions.

Your horse may not notice the flag that's hanging by your barn—at least not until a gust of wind causes it to flap. Next thing you know, he's halfway across the arena in full-blown flight mode. Although your horse may have poor visual acuity when it comes to stationary objects (from 20 feet away, the horse can distinguish details that a human with normal vision could distinguish at 30 to 60 feet), his vision is extremely sensitive to motion. After all, he doesn't need to read the fine print, but in his natural environment his motion sensitivity allows him to detect a predator the minute it makes a move.

The position of the horse's eyes give him an excellent visual range, which is at its best when his head is raised. His head-up reaction to any threatening stimuli gives him a 350-degree sphere of vision, with blind spots the width of his head directly behind him, directly below his nose, and just above and straight in front of his forehead. There's very little crossover between his two eyes, meaning he has primarily monocular vision and minimal depth perception. He uses monocular cues to detect depth, such as light and shadows, contour and motion.

Evaluation

The Eye Exam

A basic eye examination is performed using an ophthalmoscope to visualize the cornea, iris, pupil, lens, and retina. Depending on the horse's temperament, sedation may be required. If the horse's eye is very painful, causing him to squint or hold his eye completely closed, the vet may need to deaden the nerves that supply the powerful muscles of the horse's eyelids in order to hold them open for a complete evaluation. Additionally, drops that cause the pupils to dilate may be needed to allow for a thorough evaluation of the back of the eye.

Most basic eye exams also include staining of the cornea with a dye called flourescein. This stain will be taken up by damaged areas of the cornea, resulting in a bright green color highlighting a scratch or ulcer on the corneal surface. If the veterinarian suspects an infection or other corneal abnormality, swabs or scrapings of the eye surface may be performed for laboratory tests, including culture (to grow bacteria, fungi, or other organisms) and cytology (to look at cells under a microscope that might help diagnose a specific problem).

Vision Testing

Two simple tests are used to evaluate the horse's vision: a menace test and a test of his ability to negotiate obstacles or a maze.

A menace test involves rapidly moving your hand toward the horse's eye, taking care not to touch the sensitive feeler-hairs on his eyelids or to create a rush of air that he might feel. If your horse sees, he'll react to your approaching hand by flinching or moving his head away. Don't try this test on your newborn foal, however. A menace response is learned, and won't appear until approximately 2 to 3 weeks of age.

You can also assess your horse's ability to see by asking him to negotiate obstacles, either while you're leading him or when he's free in an

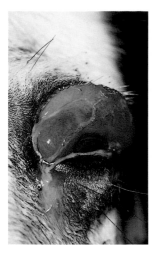

FIGURE 13.3. **Severe trauma can result in extreme swelling of the conjunctiva and a thick discharge from the eye. This horse has fractured the bones surrounding the eye.**
(Photo courtesy of Paul Scherlie, DVM, Diplomate ACVO)

enclosed area such as an arena or paddock. If your horse easily walks over poles on the ground (or stops and spooks at them!) and is able to navigate around barrels, buckets, or other objects in an enclosure, that's good evidence he sees. To evaluate his night vision, try this test in dark conditions.

WHEN THINGS GO WRONG

Eye problems can arise in any of the various structures that make up the eye, and can range in severity from minor irritations to major, vision-threatening diseases. The following are the most common problems you're likely to encounter with your horse's eyes.

Eyelid Trauma   FIGURES 13.3–13.5

WHAT IT IS. Given his "act now, think later" instincts, your horse's eye is especially susceptible to trauma. If he sees or hears something that frightens him, he may swing his head to flee the scene and bang his eye. His eyelids will swell, and he may suffer an eyelid laceration.

DIAGNOSIS. Swelling or a laceration will be easily visible. The vet will also examine the cornea and deeper structures of the eye with an ophthalmoscope to ensure there is no further damage.

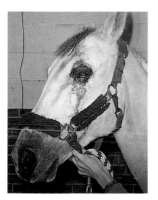

FIGURE 13.4. **Here the deformity of the horse's face, along with a bloody nasal discharge, are easily seen.**
(Photo courtesy of Paul Scherlie, DVM, Diplomate ACVO)

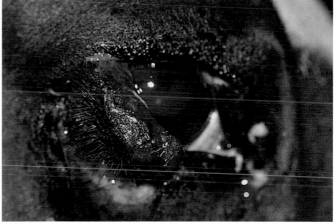

FIGURE 13.5. **This laceration of the lower eyelid, accompanied by extreme swelling, would require immediate suturing in order to maintain the integrity of the lids and preserve the normal protective mechanisms of the eye. The underlying structures of the eye itself appear to have been unaffected.**
(Photo courtesy of Paul Scherlie, DVM, Diplomate ACVO)

TREATMENT. Ice and anti-inflammatories (such as phenylbutazone or flunixin meglumine) to minimize pain and swelling. If a laceration is present, suturing will be necessary to protect the eye if the integrity of the eyelid is at risk.

HOW SERIOUS IS IT? In most cases, a "shiner" will resolve without complications even when the lids are extremely swollen. Very extensive eyelid lacerations will also heal well because of the large blood supply to the area.

POTENTIAL COMPLICATIONS. A strong blow can cause inflammation to the cornea or deeper structures in the eye, leading to a bout of uveitis (see page 236). Abrasions or ulceration of the cornea can occur. Fractures of the facial bones are possible. Lacerations that require suturing can heal with permanent disfigurement of the lids that may simply be cosmetic, or can compromise the lid's ability to protect the eyeball.

Conjunctivitis

WHAT IT IS. Inflammation of the conjunctiva because of irritation from dust or flies. May become infected with a bacterium or virus.

DIAGNOSIS. Discharge from the eyes along with redness and swelling of the conjunctiva will be visible. The veterinarian will examine the cornea and deeper structures of the eye with an ophthalmoscope to ensure there's no other underlying cause of these abnormal signs.

TREATMENT. Protection from the irritation (i.e., a fly mask), anti-inflammatories, saline eyewash to relieve irritation, treatment with antibacterial or antiviral ointments if infected.

HOW SERIOUS IS IT? Most cases of conjunctivitis resolve without complications. If your horse is prone to this problem, preventative measures such as regular use of a fly mask would be advisable.

POTENTIAL COMPLICATIONS. In most cases, conjunctivitis alone is an easily managed problem with few complications. Nasolacrimal duct blockage can occur.

Nasolacrimal Duct Blockage

WHAT HAPPENS? The nasolacrimal duct becomes blocked, preventing eye discharge from draining out into your horse's nose. Secretions build up on your horse's face underneath the corner of his eye.

DIAGNOSIS. The veterinarian may place a dye in your horse's eye, and watch for it to drain out in his nose. If it doesn't appear within several minutes, the duct may be blocked. Alternatively, the vet may opt to flush the duct. If discharge appears when the duct is flushed, blockage was present.

TREATMENT. Your veterinarian can pass a small tube through the nasolacrimal duct to flush it and clear out the blockage. Underlying conjunctivitis should also be treated if present.

HOW SERIOUS IS IT? More of a nuisance than anything. A blocked duct won't result in any serious problems with your horse's eye.

POTENTIAL COMPLICATIONS. If the duct has been blocked for an extended period of time, it may be impossible to flush and become permanently blocked. The buildup of secretions on your horse's face can irritate the underlying skin.

Corneal Abrasion/Ulcer FIGURES 13.6–13.8

WHAT HAPPENS. Trauma to the cornea results in a disruption of the cells at the surface. With an ulcer, an obvious round defect is present on the outer layer of the cornea.

DIAGNOSIS. Symptoms may include swelling, discharge, and squinting. There may be a visible cloudiness on the surface of the cornea. The vet will stain the eye with a dye that allows him to see where cells have been disrupted and fully evaluate the size and shape of a scratch or ulcer.

TREATMENT. Antibiotic ointments to prevent infection, atropine ointment to dilate the pupil and relieve painful spasms of the small muscles of the iris, and anti-inflammatories (phenylbutazone or flunixin meglumine) to relieve pain.

HOW SERIOUS IS IT? In most cases, corneal damage repairs on its own, usually within a week to 10 days. However, complications can be extremely serious, even resulting in loss of the eye.

POTENTIAL COMPLICATIONS. If an ulcer or abrasion becomes infected and does not respond to treatment, it can become a very serious problem and may result in loss of the eye. In some cases, a non-healing erosion can occur because the edges of an ulcer won't adhere to the underlying cornea. Additional treatment (including possible "cautery," or chemical burning of the edges) will be necessary to encourage healing.

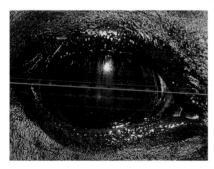

FIGURE 13.6. **This small, superficial ulcer is typical of a puncture-type injury to the cornea. Note the whitish appearance of the surrounding cornea—an indicator of fluid accumulation or swelling within the corneal tissues.** (Photo courtesy of Paul Scherlie, DVM, Diplomate ACVO)

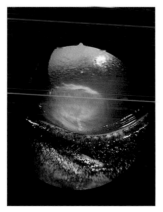

FIGURE 13.7. **This large corneal ulcer is also superficial. In spite of its dramatic appearance, it should heal without complications if appropriate treatment is applied.** (Photo courtesy of Paul Scherlie, DVM, Diplomate ACVO)

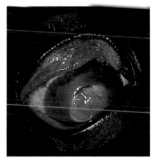

FIGURE 13.8. **This ulcer has become infected, a potentially serious complication. Note the volcano-like appearance of the defect and associated swelling and irritation of the surrounding tissues. Appropriate treatment with anti-microbial medications is essential in order to save this eye.** (Photo courtesy of Paul Scherlie, DVM, Diplomate ACVO)

Cataract FIGURE 13.9

WHAT IT IS. A defect in the lens that can inhibit or prevent light from passing through the eye and compromise your horse's vision.

DIAGNOSIS. Cloudiness may be visible deep within the eye. The veterinarian can see a cataract within the lens by using an ophthalmoscope.

TREATMENT. Although surgical removal is possible, it is expensive and often unsuccessful. No other treatment is available.

HOW SERIOUS IS IT? Many cataracts are congenital (present since birth) or the result of trauma to the eye. If the defect isn't extensive enough to affect your horse's vision, it may not be a problem. However, cataracts are a common finding in a horse with uveitis, in which case problems with your horse's eye are likely to progress to eventual blindness.

POTENTIAL COMPLICATIONS. A cataract can cause your horse's vision to be compromised if it's large enough to obstruct passage of light through the eye. See below for complications that can occur if uveitis is a factor.

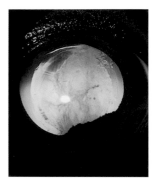

FIGURE 13.9. **This congenital cataract would appear as a cloudiness deep within the horse's eye. Because it affects most of the lens, it may negatively impact this horse's ability to see.** (Photo courtesy of Paul Scherlie, DVM, Diplomate ACVO)

Equine Recurrent Uveitis (ERU, or Moon Blindness)

FIGURES 13.10–13.11

WHAT IT IS. An autoimmune disease (antibodies in your horse's system begin attacking the tissues in his eyes) that causes many different problems. Inflammation in the cornea causes a painful buildup of fluid, which makes the eye appear cloudy. Blisters can form on the corneal surface and rupture, causing ulcers. Cataracts can occur. Products of inflammation, including white blood cells and protein deposits, can accumulate in the fluid inside of the eye itself. When your horse is experiencing a painful uveitis episode, muscles controlling the pupil can spasm, causing the pupil to become very small (called miosis). Typically, uveitis flares up intermittently, with attacks becoming more frequent and more severe over time.

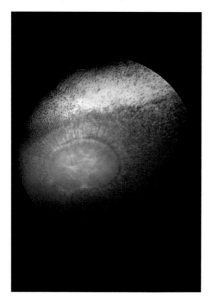

FIGURE 13.10. **Although the eye may appear completely normal from the outside, this abnormal "butterfly lesion" on the retina is a typical finding in a horse with equine recurrent uveitis.** (Photo courtesy of Paul Scherlie, DVM, Diplomate ACVO)

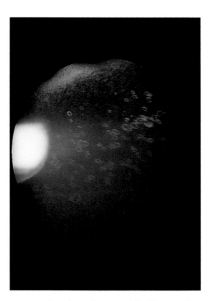

FIGURE 13.11. **Another abnormal finding on the horse's retina, these "bullet hole" lesions might only be detected by a vet through careful examination using specialized equipment.** (Photo courtesy of Paul Scherlie, DVM, Diplomate ACVO)

The Horse's Body: Health and Disease

ERU may be difficult to diagnosis initially because of the many different symptoms that can occur. Recurrent episodes can help to establish a diagnosis. In addition, a veterinarian skilled in equine ophthalmology, using specialized equipment, may be able to pinpoint signs of damage deep within the eye, even when the eye is quiet.

TREATMENT. The disease cannot be cured. It can be managed with anti-inflammatories to minimize discomfort and damage due to inflammation, atropine ointment to relax the pupil and relieve pain, and antibiotic ointments when necessary if corneal ulcers occur. Usually treatment is required on an intermittent basis in the initial stages. The disease is likely to progress to the point where ongoing consistent management is required.

HOW SERIOUS IS IT? Very. Uveitis is a chronic disease that is likely to cause your horse a lot of pain and eventually lead to blindness.

POTENTIAL COMPLICATIONS. Uveitis can lead to almost any complication imaginable, ranging from large cataracts that are likely to interfere with your horse's vision to infected corneal ulcers that can cause the eye to completely collapse.

Neoplasia   FIGURES 13.12–13.14

WHAT IT IS. Cancer affecting your horse's eyelid or conjunctival tissues.

DIAGNOSIS. A biopsy, or sample of tissue, may be submitted to a laboratory for analysis in order to determine the specific type of cancer. The most common types likely to affect your horse's eye include squamous cell carcinoma and equine sarcoid.

TREATMENT. Treatment depends on the specific type of cancer identified and how extensive it is. Surgical removal may be recommended. Radiation therapy, chemotherapy, or other more advanced cancer treatments

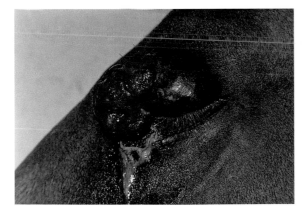

FIGURE 13.12. **This equine sarcoid on the horse's upper eyelid would be difficult to remove surgically due to its location and extent. Chemotherapy or other more advanced cancer treatments would be required.** (Photo courtesy of Paul Scherlie, DVM, Diplomate ACVO)

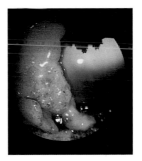

FIGURE 13.13. **This example of squamous cell carcinoma has extended into the actual corneal tissues. Removal of the eye may be required to treat this condition.** (Photo courtesy of Paul Scherlie, DVM, Diplomate ACVO)

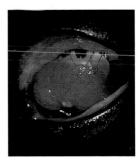

FIGURE 13.14. **Here another squamous cell carcinoma has invaded the surface of the cornea.** (Photo courtesy of Paul Scherlie, DVM, Diplomate ACVO)

may be recommended, depending on the aggressiveness and extent of the tumor.

HOW SERIOUS IS IT? Extremely variable. Some individual tumors will resolve completely with surgical removal or other treatment, while others will require multiple, extensive treatments.

Table 13.1

Symptom Checklist

SYMPTOM	WHAT YOU SEE	WHAT IT'S CALLED	WHAT IT MEANS	POSSIBLE PROBLEMS	WHEN TO CALL THE VET	HOME TREATMENT
Eyelid swelling	Tissues beneath lid appear to protrude. Swollen eye may remain closed.	Eyelid edema.	Fluid accumulated in eyelids due to leakage from blood vessels that occurs during inflammation.	Lid trauma, Conjunctivitis. Uveitis.	Can wait until morning if no other signs. May resolve in 12–24 hours without treatment.	Ice eye, flush with saline, administer anti-inflammatories.
Squinting	Horse keeps his eyelids closed; strongly resists attempts to open them.	Blepharospasm.	Horse contracts strong muscles in eyelids to close his eye and protect deeper structures. Usually a pain response.	Corneal abrasion. Corneal ulcer. Uveitis.	Can wait until morning, but call vet if not resolved within 12–24 hours.	Flush with saline, apply antibiotic ointment, administer anti-inflammatories.
Red eye	Enlarged blood vessels and general reddening of the conjunctiva and/or sclera.	Erythema.	Inflammation causes blood vessels to swell and become more prominent.	Trauma. Conjunctivitis. Uveitis.	Can wait 2–3 days if no other signs. May resolve on its own or with protection from dust, flies.	Flush with saline, apply antibiotic ointment, administer anti-inflammatories.
Clear discharge	Watery fluid coming from corner of eyes.	Epiphora.	Irritation or inflammation causes increased production of lubricating fluid, or blockage of nasolacrimal duct prevents drainage of normal fluid from nose, causing it to accumulate around the eye.	Trauma. Conjunctivitis. Blocked nasolacrimal duct. Corneal abrasion/ulcer. Uveitis.	Can wait 2–3 days if no other signs. May resolve on its own.	Flush with saline.

POTENTIAL COMPLICATIONS. Equine sarcoid, although locally aggressive, is unlikely to metastasize (spread to other body tissues); squamous cell carcinoma may metastasize, resulting in life-threatening disease. Disruption of the eyelids can compromise protection of your horse's cornea.

SYMPTOM	WHAT YOU SEE	WHAT IT'S CALLED	WHAT IT MEANS	POSSIBLE PROBLEMS	WHEN TO CALL THE VET	HOME TREATMENT
Cloudy discharge	Thick whitish, yellowish or greenish fluid from corner of eyes.	Mucopurulent discharge.	May have same causes as clear discharge, but can also indicate infection.	Trauma. Conjunctivitis (possibly bacterial). Blocked nasolacrimal duct. Corneal abrasion/ulcer (possibly infected). Uveitis.	Not an emergency if no other signs, but call vet tomorrow.	Flush with saline, apply antibiotic ointment.
Cloudy cornea	Whitish or bluish tinge to cornea. May be in small area or involve entire cornea.	Corneal edema.	Inflammation results in fluid leakage and buildup between cells of cornea.	Corneal abrasion/ ulcer. Uveitis.	Call right away. Vet can help you determine whether horse should be seen immediately or if it can wait until morning.	Flush with saline, apply antibiotic ointment, administer anti-inflammatories.
Constricted pupil	Pupil very small, even in a dark barn or stall, no reaction when bright light is shined in eye.	Miosis.	Spasms of tiny muscles that control iris cause pupil to shrink. Usually a pain response. Normal response to bright light.	Corneal abrasion/ ulcer. Uveitis.	May be normal if no other signs. Call vet for advice if accompanied by other signs, including blue/white cornea, squinting, or discharge.	Administer anti-inflammatories.

How-to Home Treatment

These four home treatments can be helpful in managing your horse's eye problem.

Ice the eye

WHY IT HELPS. If your horse's eye is swollen, ice will help to shrink the leaky blood vessels that cause the swelling.

TO APPLY. Wrap a bag of crushed ice, refreezable ice pack, or bag of frozen vegetables in a soft towel. Hold gently in place over the eye for 15 to 20 minutes.

Flush with saline

WHY IT HELPS. Your horse's eye may be irritated by dust or some foreign material. Saline will help cleanse the eye, remove foreign matter, and soothe the tissues.

TO APPLY. Ask a friend to help you restrain your horse. Using a bottle of saline with a gentle spray, spray directly into your horse's eye for several seconds. Most horses will tolerate this procedure, but if your horse objects to the direct spray, fill a syringe with saline and apply drop-by-drop to the inside of his lower eyelid. (*Note: You can purchase saline with a very gentle spray in the contact lens department of a grocery store or pharmacy. Make sure you purchase straight saline, not a more complex contact lens solution.*)

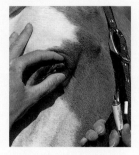

FIGURE 13.15. **To apply medication to your horse's eye, place your index finger and thumb on the top and bottom lids, and apply just enough pressure so that the lids evert, or turn themselves inside out.**

Administer anti-inflammatories

WHY IT HELPS. Reduces inflammation that causes the pain and discomfort associated with many eye problems.

TO APPLY. Administer either phenylbutazone or flunixin meglumine in a dosage appropriate for your horse's size (see medication guide on page 319).

Administer antibiotic ointment FIGURES 13.15–13.16

WHY IT HELPS. Will help cure a bacterial infection, or prevent one from occurring.

TO APPLY. Squeeze approximately ¼ to ½ inch of antibiotic ointment onto the inside of your horse's lower lid. If you're not comfortable applying the ointment directly from the tube, you can put it on a clean finger and then place it on the lid.

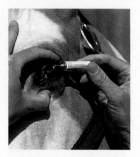

FIGURE 13.16. **With the medication in your opposite hand, squeeze approximately ¼ to ½ inch of ointment onto the inside of the lower lid. When you release the lids, the medication will come into contact with the cornea. If applying drops or saline instead of ointment, follow the same procedure. Simply drop or spray the liquid onto the inside of the lower lid and release.**

WARNING: Before you reach for that tube of ointment in your grooming box, STOP! Do you know what that ointment is? You could cause your horse's problem to become much more severe than it already is by using the wrong medication. For example, if the ointment you have on hand contains a steroid (such as dexamethasone or hydrocortisone), it could delay healing and promote infection in a corneal ulcer, causing a minor problem to become a potentially eye-threatening one. If you're not sure what the ointment is, DON'T USE IT!

CHAPTER 14

The Teeth

THEN AND NOW

During Renaissance times, advanced dental techniques involved surgical cutting of the lip of the horse to better accommodate the bit. Of course, the bits used then were usually quite large and complicated in design.

These days, bits are designed with the horse's mouth structure in mind. When a young horse starts training he'll have his wolf teeth removed, and a bit seat created at the front of his molars to ensure the bit has a comfortable place to rest. Fortunately, no surgical manipulation of the lips is needed for modern-day bits to fit properly.

THE HORSE'S DENTAL STRUCTURE and function are designed to accommodate a lifestyle of grazing and chewing forage all day long. The following describes the horse's teeth and jaws.

FIGURE 14.1

- The horse has between 36 and 44 permanent teeth. If he's a gelding or stallion, he has 44 permanent teeth. A mare has 36 to 40 permanent teeth.

- The front teeth, called incisors, are designed to shear off grasses and other forage in the pasture. The horse has 6 upper and 6 lower incisors.

- The back teeth, called molars, are designed to grind his food into a digestible form. The horse has 12 upper and 12 lower molars.

- The gelding or stallion has 2 upper and 2 lower canine teeth, leftover "fighting teeth" once used by his ancestors for protecting the herd. These teeth sit in the gap between the incisors and the molars. This gap is known as the bars of the mouth. Mares rarely have canine teeth.

- Most geldings and stallions and some mares have 2 small upper wolf teeth, remnants of molars that no longer serve a useful function. These small teeth sit just in front of the molar arcades of the upper jaw. Rarely, wolf teeth will also be present in the lower jaw. In some horses, they may be buried underneath the gum surface.

- The upper (maxilla) and lower (mandible) jaws are joined by the temporomandibular joint (TMJ), a joint that allows the mouth to open and close, as well as to move in the circular pattern required for chewing.

- Just like humans, horses also have two sets of teeth throughout their lifetime. The deciduous, or "baby teeth" (called "caps"), should all be replaced by permanent teeth by about 5 years of age.

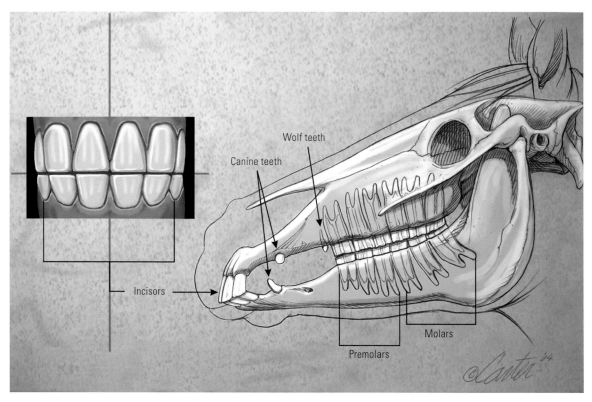

FIGURE 14.1. **Dental structure**

How He Chews

When the horse takes a bite, he begins by filtering things through his sensitive lips—that's how he can clean up every bit of grain, and carefully leave that crushed-up medicine or supplement at the bottom of his bucket. If he's grazing in the pasture, he uses his tongue to orient the grass, then his incisor teeth to grasp and tear. Once the food enters his mouth, he uses his tongue to push it against the teeth on one side, and then the lower jaw is moved from side to side against his upper jaw to grind. The horse's temperomandibular joint is very tight, meaning he has little front-to-back motion when he chews. He can only chew on one side at a time, but may alternate sides with every bite. Ideally, he'll distribute chewing evenly between both sides.

Once he's mature, he has a 10- to15-degree angle between the occlusal (grinding) surface of his molars. This angle develops because of the powerful grinding that's required for chewing hay, and is essential in order for him to chew effectively. As he chews, he wads each mass of food into a cigar-shaped form, which mixes with saliva as he works it from front to back and prepares to swallow.

In order to ensure that the horse has plenty of grinding ability as he matures, his molars continue to erupt throughout his lifetime at a rate of

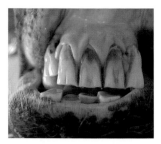

FIGURE 14.2. **Overgrowth of this horse's upper incisors has lead to abnormal wear and most likely has affected the function of the molars for chewing. This would have been preventable with regular dental work.** (Photo courtesy of David O. Klugh, DVM, FAVD, Equine)

about 2 to 3 millimeters per year. This rate of eruption matches the rate of grinding away you'd expect to see if he's fed a diet consisting primarily of hay and grass. The horse's incisors also continue to erupt throughout his lifetime, and in a natural grazing environment they'll be worn down as they're used to tear grass and other forage. However, a stall-kept horse won't use his incisors in this fashion, which can result in overgrowth. If the horse's incisors become too long, they'll actually prevent his molars from contacting one another, compromising his ability to chew effectively. FIGURE 14.2

The Dental Exam

The horse's teeth are out of sight—and easy to ignore. That's why it's especially important that they be examined regularly. The following steps comprise a thorough dental examination, and help to determine whether routine dental work is needed.

Watch Him Eat

If the horse drops a lot of food out of his mouth, turns his head sideways to chew, or shows any other signs of discomfort when he eats, good dentistry to correct imbalances in his mouth is definitely needed.

Evaluate Bit Comfort

If the horse tosses his head, opens his mouth, or champs constantly at the bit, he may be experiencing discomfort from his teeth. In particular, removing wolf teeth if he has them, and rounding off the front molars to create a place for the bit to rest (called a "bit seat") should make a noticeable difference. Obvious tooth marks on the bit itself can also indicate discomfort and the need for dental care.

Palpation

By running his fingers down the sides of the horse's head along the ridge created by his upper molars, the vet can determine whether sharp points have developed on the upper molars—potentially causing sores on the adjacent soft tissues. If the horse is sensitive to this pressure, he's in need of dentistry to smooth away sharp edges.

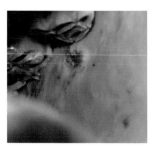

FIGURE 14.3. **Ulcers such as the one pictured here can easily occur if sharp points are allowed to form along the outer edge of the incisors, causing the horse a great deal of discomfort.** (Photo courtesy of David O. Klugh, DVM, FAVD, Equine)

Check Incisors   FIGURE 14.3

By lifting the horse's upper lip to see his incisors, the vet can assess incisor balance. If the incisors are at a slant (a cross-bite), curve into a smile (a ventral curvature) or a frown (a dorsal curvature), an incisor realignment would be in order. In addition, unbalanced incisors indicate that his molars are likely to need work.

Evaluate Molar Occlusion   FIGURE 14.4

The vet will attempt to slide the horse's lower jaw from side to side across his upper jaw. The incisors should stay closed until the lower jaw has slid no further than ½ to ¾ of a single tooth's width to either side. At that point, the molars should be in contact, and should cause a gap to occur between the upper and lower incisors if the lower jaw slides any further. If the lower jaw slides easily further than a full tooth width to either side of his upper jaw without creating a gap between the incisors, chances are his molars aren't meeting properly, and he's in need of dental work.

Visualization and Manipulation

Finally, the vet will sedate the horse and place him in a full-mouth speculum, a device designed to hold the mouth open for a thorough examination. Molars can be seen, each tooth can be felt individually for loosening, and the periodontal pockets between the teeth and soft tissues of the gums can be evaluated.

Radiographs

If problems are suspected, radiographs of your horse's teeth may be recommended. This allows visualization of the bones of the jaws, individual teeth, and tooth roots in order to identify potential abnormalities.

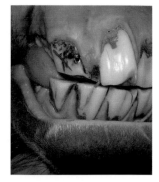

FIGURE 14.4. **This horse is missing an incisor due to a previous trauma—a situation that results in uneven stresses when he chews. With regular dental work the balance of his mouth can be preserved, however, so that he'll be able to chew properly.** (Photo courtesy of David O. Klugh, DVM, FAVD, Equine)

Preventative Dentistry

Even if the horse's teeth are in good shape, regular dental checkups should be scheduled every 6 to 12 months. Because his teeth continue to erupt at the rate of 2 to 3 millimeters per year, imbalances can become more and more pronounced if regular dental maintenance is not performed. Once the horse's mouth is properly balanced, a regular maintenance schedule will ensure it stays that way, and will allow your vet to identify problems before they become severe.

Dental Maintenance Techniques   FIGURE 14.5

Your vet will sedate the horse for routine dental procedures, and place him in a full-mouth speculum to hold his mouth open. Most modern dental procedures are performed using a combination of hand and power tools for maximum efficiency.

The first portion of the horse's mouth to be addressed is the front of the upper and lower molar arcade. The front edge of both rows of teeth will be rounded off to create a bit seat, and to ensure that hooks (enamel edges that hook

FIGURE 14.5. **Routine dentistry should be performed regularly. This requires sedation and a full-mouth speculum to allow the vet to examine all of the horse's teeth.** (Photo courtesy of David O. Klugh, DVM, FAVD, Equine)

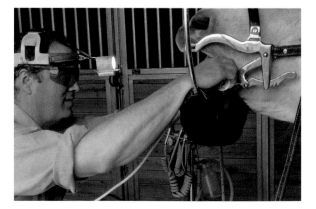

The Horse's Body: Health and Disease

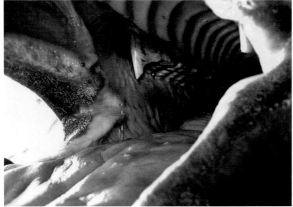

FIGURE 14.6. **This extremely large hook can not only cause damage to the gums on the opposite jaw, but will also make it difficult for the horse to chew properly.**
(Photo courtesy of David O. Klugh, DVM, FAVD, Equine)

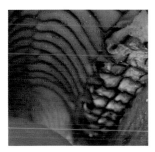

FIGURE 14.7. **The excessive ridges along the surface of this horse's molar arcade will prevent his molars from gliding effectively, therefore compromising his ability to chew. The veterinarian will smooth these ridges to the appropriate level to help correct the problem.**
(Photo courtesy of David O. Klugh, DVM, FAVD, Equine)

over the opposite tooth) or ramps (molars that take on the shape of "ski jumps" on the upper or lower teeth) don't push his molars out of alignment. These teeth will be rounded off to the gum line using either a hand file or a power-driven dremel tool. If the horse has wolfteeth, they will also be removed to ensure the bit has a comfortable place to rest. These small teeth will be elevated from the gum line with a sharp device that separates the tooth from the gum. It is then pulled out.

Next, the back molars will be addressed. Just like the front molars, the back molars can develop hooks or ramps that cause the jaws to be pushed out of alignment. In severe cases, these protrusions become large enough to actually dig into the gum on the opposite jaw. To correct this, the vet will eliminate the hooks or ramps using a hand-float or a power-driven dremel tool with a special guarded handle to prevent soft-tissue trauma in the horse's mouth. If the protrusions are large enough, they can even be cut using a molar-cutting device. FIGURE 14.6

After the front and the back of the horse's mouth are straightened out, the vet will focus his attention on the body of the molar arcade—the critical grinding surface that allows the horse to eat efficiently. A hand file or power tool will be used to flatten out any ridges, bumps, or other irregularities in the molar's surface that prevent proper grinding. At the same time, the sharp points that form on the outer edges of the upper molars and inner edges of the lower molars will be filed away to prevent trauma to the horse's cheeks or tongue. FIGURE 14.7

If the horse has canine teeth, they can become quite large and sharp, causing discomfort or even small wounds on the tongue. They will be cut off either using a sharp "diamond wheel" (a small, circular type of saw that's powered by a dremel) or by clipping them with a sharp pair of cutters. Then they can be smoothed and buffed using a hand file.

As a final step, the horse's incisors or front teeth will be balanced. It's critical that this step be performed last, because the incisors affect how the molars actually contact one another—and are the final determinants of the horse's ability to chew. If the horse's incisors are very long, they may prevent his molars from meeting one another at all—meaning that no matter how well balanced his molars are, they won't effectively do their job. And if the incisors are offset in any way, they'll cause the molars to grind unevenly. To reduce and straighten the horse's incisors, they'll be cut with a power-driven diamond wheel saw, then smoothed and adjusted with a small hand file. The end result is a balanced mouth that keeps the horse comfortable and allows him to chew efficiently.

TABLE 14.1

Basic Dental Imbalances Figures 14.8–14.17

IMBALANCE	WHAT IT IS	HOW IT HAPPENS	PROBLEMS CAUSED	SOLUTION
Hook	Protrusion from the front or back upper molars that hangs over the front or back lower molars (or from the front or back lower molars that extend up over the front or back upper molars).	Can result from a naturally occurring overbite or underbite, or secondary to other molar problems that push the jaw out of alignment.	Prevents the jaws from moving freely in a front/back direction. Can lead to excessive transverse ridges.	Rounding off with a hand file or power dremel tool.
Ramp	Molars take on a "ski jump" appearance. Occur at either front or back, upper or lower molars.	Can accompany hooks, or be secondary to other molar abnormalities that push the jaw out of alignment. Can occur if a hook is filed down on the top or bottom without a corresponding correction being made on the opposite molar.	Prevents the jaws from moving freely in a front/back direction. Can lead to excessive transverse ridges.	Rounding off with a hand file or power dremel tool. It's especially important that ramps be completely reduced to prevent abnormal wear on the opposite molar.
Step	A distinct bump in the molar arcade, where one tooth grows longer than its neighbors.	May occur when a deciduous cap is retained too long, preventing normal growth and allowing the molar on the opposite side to grow too long.	Prevents the molars from moving freely either front to back or side to side.	Reduce or flatten with a hand file or a power float.
Wave	The entire molar arcade becomes uneven and develops a wavelike appearance.	Often arises secondary to other factors, causing misalignment such as retained deciduous caps, missing teeth, or large hooks and ramps.	Prevents jaws from moving freely and inhibits effective grinding.	Can be partially corrected by reducing high areas with a hand file or power tool. Will improve when underlying factors are corrected. Likely to be a long-term management issue.

IMBALANCE	WHAT IT IS	HOW IT HAPPENS	PROBLEMS CAUSED	SOLUTION
Points	Sharp edges form on the outer edges of the upper molars and the inner edges of the lower molars.	Arise during normal wear because the wide upper jaw and narrow lower jaw configuration of the horse's mouth prevent these edges from being worn away.	Cause discomfort and if allowed to become sharp enough may even cause cuts to the cheeks or tongue.	Filing down the sharp edges usually with a hand file or power float. This constitutes the procedure known as floating.
Transverse ridges	A series of washboard-like side-to-side ridges that form along the molar arcades.	Arise when either the upper or lower jaw is shifted forward out of alignment, preventing even wear of the molar surface. Ridges form at the portion of the molar surface corresponding with the space between 2 molars on the opposite jaw.	Prevents the jaw from moving and grinding freely.	May be partially flattened using a hand float or power tool. Will improve when other factors causing poor alignment, such as ramps or hooks, are corrected.
Shear	Extreme angulation of the biting surface of the molar arcades. Angle between arcades should be between 10 and 15 degrees.	Forms when a horse has an unusually large difference in the width of the upper (wide) and lower (narrow) jaw. More common with an all-grain diet where vertical crushing stroke is diminished.	Prevents jaws from moving and grinding freely. Makes effective chewing difficult.	Difficult or impossible to correct completely, but angles can be prevented from becoming too extreme by regular filing of the outside of the upper jaw and inside of the lower molars using a hand file or power float.
Ventral curvature (smile)	The outer edges of the lower incisors grow long relative to the outer edges of the upper incisors.	May be a natural occurrence for your horse. Can occur when deciduous caps are retained on the upper corner incisors, preventing normal growth of permanent incisors. Can occur due to abnormal grinding patterns secondary to molar misalignments.	Inhibits normal side-to-side grinding.	Incisors are filed using a motorized or hand file to keep them level. In extreme cases, long outer edges of the lower incisors are cut using a motorized diamond wheel saw.

Continued on Page 248.

Continued from page 247

IMBALANCE	WHAT IT IS	HOW IT HAPPENS	PROBLEMS CAUSED	SOLUTION
Dorsal curvature (frown)	The outer edges of the upper incisors grow long relative to the outer edges of the lower incisors.	May be a natural occurrence for your horse. Can occur when deciduous caps are retained on the lower corner incisors, preventing normal growth of permanent incisors. Can occur due to abnormal grinding patterns secondary to molar misalignments.	Inhibits normal side-to-side grinding.	Incisors are filed using a motorized hand file to keep them level. In extreme cases, long outer edges of upper incisors are cut using a motorized diamond wheel saw.
Offset (diagonal bite)	Upper incisors on one side of the mouth are very long, and lower incisors on the opposite side are very long, causing the incisors to meet on a diagonal rather than on a straight line.	May develop over time if your horse has a tendency to chew in one direction only. May occur secondary to molar misalignments, or as a result of missing incisors.	Inhibits normal side-to-side grinding.	Incisors are filed using a motorized or hand file to keep them level. In extreme cases, long upper and long lower incisors are cut using a motorized diamond wheel saw.
Overbite	The upper incisors protrude over the front of the lower incisors.	Your horse may have been born with an overbite. Hooks or ramps on the front upper or back lower molars can also shift the upper jaw forward, resulting in an overbite.	Prevents the jaw from moving freely. The longer an overbite remains, the more severe it may become. Corresponding hooks, ramps, and transverse ridges will become more pronounced.	Correct corresponding molar abnormalities and reduce (cut) upper row of incisors using a motorized diamond wheel saw.
Underbite	The lower incisors protrude over the front of the upper incisors.	Your horse may have been born with an underbite. Hooks or ramps on the front lower or back upper molars can shift the lower jaw forward, resulting in an underbite.	Prevents the jaws from moving freely. The longer an underbite remains, the more severe it may become. Corresponding hooks, ramps, and transverse ridges will become more pronounced.	Correct corresponding molar abnormalities and reduce (cut) lower row of incisors using a motorized diamond wheel saw.

IMBALANCE	WHAT IT IS	HOW IT HAPPENS	PROBLEMS CAUSED	SOLUTION
Missing incisors	A front tooth is missing.	Teeth may be lost during a traumatic event, or may never erupt due to a congenital abnormality.	The corresponding tooth on the opposite jaw will overgrow, and eventually prevent the jaws from sliding freely side to side. Misalignment of the incisors themselves makes it difficult to grasp and tear pasture forage.	Keep the opposite row of incisors level by filing them regularly using a motorized or hand file. If opposite incisor has already overgrown excessively, it can be cut prior to filing.

TABLE 14.2

Dental Maintenance Schedule

Because the horse's teeth continually erupt throughout his life, proper balance and normal chewing stresses are critical for them to function properly. Once an imbalance begins, it can become worse and worse with time if it's not corrected and maintained. When the horse is young, he loses baby teeth on a regular basis as his mature teeth erupt. If these caps aren't lost at the right time, abnormal stresses can cause the uneven eruption of mature teeth, and imbalances will develop that will plague your horse for the rest of his life. The following schedule for dental examination and maintenance for the young horse will help ensure he has a balanced, healthy mouth as he grows old.

WHEN	WHAT	WHY
Weanling	Examination to evaluate jaw structure and balance.	If the foal is born with abnormal jaw structure, now is the time for orthodontic procedures to be planned.
Yearling	Examination, basic balancing, and removal of wolf teeth (small teeth that are situated just in front of the molars and can interfere with the bit).	Wolf teeth are easiest to remove now, before their roots are firmly set. Basic balancing will keep things developing properly.
2-year-old	Examination, basic balancing.	Basic balancing keeps jaws and teeth aligned.
3-year-old	Examination, basic balancing. Remove caps on front teeth and front of molars if needed.	Basic balancing keeps jaws and teeth aligned. Ensure caps are lost on schedule so mature teeth can develop properly.
3.5 years	Check and remove second set of caps.	Ensure caps are lost on schedule so mature teeth can develop properly.
4 years	Basic balancing. Check and remove third set of molar caps.	Basic balancing keeps jaws and teeth aligned. Ensure caps are lost on schedule so mature teeth can develop properly.
4.5 years	Check and remove final caps.	Ensure caps are lost on schedule so mature teeth can develop properly.
5 years	Examination, basic balancing.	Basic balancing keeps jaws and teeth aligned. Problems can be identified and treated before they progress.
Annually	Examination, basic balancing.	Basic balancing keeps jaws and teeth aligned. Problems can be identified and treated before they progress.

The following is a guide to problems that can arise within the horse's mouth beyond the basic imbalances that are corrected with routine dental care.

Periodontitis   FIGURES 14.18–14.19

WHAT IT IS. Periodontal disease, or periodontitis, is inflammation of the structures surrounding the horse's teeth, including the gums (gingiva), the ligaments that help hold his teeth in place (periodontal ligaments), the outer layer of the teeth (cementum), and even the underlying bone. These tissues become inflamed for a number of different reasons.

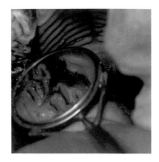

FIGURE 14.18. **Periodontal disease leads to the formation of deep pockets such as this in the tissues surrounding the horse's teeth. Left untreated, tooth loss is a likely result.** (Photo courtesy of David O. Klugh, DVM, FAVD, Equine)

- MALOCCLUSIONS: If the horse's teeth aren't lined up properly, they will experience abnormal stresses when he chews. These abnormal stresses may cause teeth to shift out of position even more, causing spaces between the teeth where deep pockets can easily form. The deeper these pockets get, the looser the attachments become, and the more the teeth will shift—creating a vicious cycle that will eventually result in tooth loss.

- SYSTEMIC DISEASE: Bacteria that colonize in the periodontal tissues contribute to the inflammation that causes problems to occur. Normal bacterial populations living in the mouth become altered, resulting in infection within the tissues surrounding the teeth. If the infection is allowed to increase in severity, it can spread to other sites. It's even possible that infections can occur in other organs, such as the heart or kidneys, secondary to an infection in the periodontal tissues. Certain diseases such as Cushing's disease (a common hormonal disease seen in older horses) can break down the horse's defenses, increasing the risk that bacteria will invade the area and cause significant periodontitis to develop.

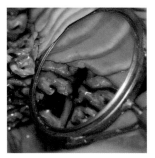

FIGURE 14.19. **With thorough cleaning and flushing to restore the health of the soft tissues, the horse's gums and associated soft tissues can be returned to good health.** (Photo courtesy of David O. Klugh, DVM, FAVD, Equine)

- HIGH-CONCENTRATE DIETS: A diet consisting of a lot of grain and little hay or pasture can contribute to periodontal disease in two different ways. First, it creates an environment where bacteria can flourish, invade the periodontal tissues, and result in calculus formation and inflammation. Second, it can affect your horse's normal chewing patterns, causing unbalanced stress on teeth and tissue loosening.

WHY IT MATTERS. The pockets that surround each of your horse's teeth (called the gingival sulcus) should be approximately 5 millimeters deep. If inflammation occurs, the pockets become deeper and ligaments loosen—putting your horse's teeth at risk for loosening or falling out. Some experts consider periodontal disease the number one cause of tooth loss in horses—as many as 60 percent of horses over 15 years old may be affected. If the horse loses a tooth, the balance of his mouth will become even more difficult to maintain. Other teeth will shift into the remaining space, causing more spaces between teeth to develop, and even more teeth can be lost. Tooth loss can make it difficult for the horse to chew properly, which can affect his overall health as he grows older.

THE TREATMENT. The first step to treating periodontal disease is to correct any imbalances in the horse's mouth. By doing this, the dental practitioner eliminates abnormal stresses that cause loosening of periodontal tissues. If the horse has pockets surrounding teeth that are deeper than they should be or are impacted with feed material, the vet will remove the impacted material and clean and flush out the pockets to remove all dead tissue. In severe cases, he may pack deep pockets with a special gel or other material to help them heal. But, in most cases, aggressive cleaning is the most important step. The horse's periodontal disease will improve with treatment, but may require ongoing monitoring and treatment to protect his teeth.

PREVENTION. Maintain a regular dental maintenance schedule with a special emphasis on the young and the old. When the horse is young, make sure he loses baby teeth on an appropriate schedule in order to ensure his mature teeth are properly aligned (see Table 14.2). The older horse is more at risk for a variety of reasons. As the teeth erupt, the diameter becomes gradually smaller. Normally, this decrease in size is compensated for by a crowding forward of all the teeth—a process known as "forward drift." This process keeps all of the teeth next to one another. If malocclusions are present, this normal forward movement is prevented and widened spaces will develop between the teeth. In addition, older horses are more likely to experience systemic diseases that can predispose to bacterial invasion of the periodontal tissues. At any age, schedule regular dental examination and balancing at least once each year, or more frequently if recommended by the vet. The horse should be maintained on a diet that's high in pasture whenever possible, and low on concentrate (grain). Not only will this keep him chewing properly, it will minimize bacterial growth to help protect his teeth.

Fillings   FIGURES 14.20–14.21

WHAT IT IS. The horse's teeth are composed of layers of three different calcified tissues: cementum, dentine, and enamel. Cementum is closely associated with periodontal tissues, and surrounds the entire tooth. It also fills deep enamel folds that extend into the center of the teeth. Dentine then makes up the bulk of the horse's tooth, and is closely associated with the very hard enamel folds that contribute to the strength required for grinding. A condition called cemental hypoplasia affects the cementum, causing it to weaken. This then leads to the formation of a cavity, or hole,

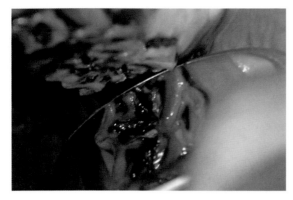

FIGURE 14.20. **This cavity or hole in the chewing surface of the tooth is likely to become more extensive over time, and may eventually weaken the tooth to the point of fracture.** (Photo courtesy of David O. Klugh, DVM, FAVD, Equine)

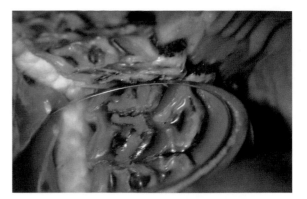

FIGURE 14.21. **By cleaning out the area, and filling it with a material similar to that used in human dentistry, the veterinarian protects the tooth from further decay.** (Photo courtesy of David O. Klugh, DVM, FAVD, Equine)

in the center of the tooth's grinding surface. If allowed to progress unchecked, these defects or cavities spread out through the layers of the tooth, from the cementum (stage 1), the enamel (stage 2), and eventually to the dentine (stage 3).

WHY IT MATTERS. If a cavity that's allowed to decay spreads out far enough across the surface of the horse's tooth it will compromise the strength of the tooth, eventually leading to a fracture and possible tooth loss. Just as with periodontal disease, once a tooth is lost it becomes much more difficult to maintain the balance of the horse's mouth. The horse may have difficulty chewing, uneven stresses during chewing may cause problems with other teeth, and overall health is compromised.

TREATMENT. If the veterinarian recognizes an area of cemental hypoplasia, or a cavity that's progressed into the enamel or dentine layers, he may recommend a filling to protect the area, just like fillings used in human dentistry. The dental practitioner will generally opt to fill stage 2 or stage 3 cavities. Because the horse's teeth continue to erupt over time, a filling can preserve and protect the tooth until a normal healthy chewing surface is restored. With proper chewing and basic dental care, the tooth will remain functional for a longer period of the horse's life.

PREVENTION. Just like periodontal disease, regular dental care to maintain proper balance in the horse's mouth can help minimize the incidence of cavities. A high-forage/low-concentrate diet helps maintain proper chewing stresses. Early recognition and treatment of cavities is especially important to protect the tooth from extensive decay and damage.

Orthodontics FIGURES 14.22–14.23

WHAT IT IS. An overbite, or "parrot mouth," in a youngster represents a disparity in growth between the upper and lower jaw. The upper jaw grows rapidly forward, while the lower jaw fails to keep up, resulting in a dental

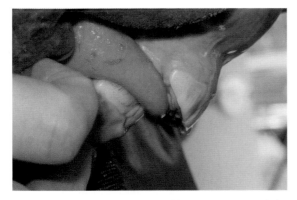

FIGURE 14.22. **This youngster's overbite, or "parrot mouth," is likely to result in significant dental imbalances as he grows and can lead to serious health problems if he can't eat and chew effectively.** (Photo courtesy of David O. Klugh, DVM, FAVD, Equine)

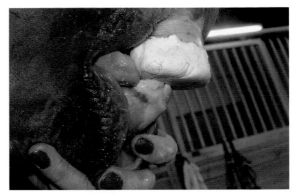

FIGURE 14.23. **A bite plate such as this over the upper incisors puts pressure on the lower jaw to help modify and direct its growth, minimizing, or even eliminating, this baby's overbite as he matures.** (Photo courtesy of David O. Klugh, DVM, FAVD, Equine)

misalignment that can cause problems for years to come. In a true parrot mouth, the upper jawbone may even begin to curve forward over the top of the lower because the normal pressures of the lower incisors against the uppers is absent.

WHY IT MATTERS. If an overbite is left untreated, it may become even more severe as a horse matures. Large hooks can form on the front of the upper molars and at the back of the lower molars because the teeth aren't lined up properly. This, combined with lack of contact between the incisors, means the upper jaw grows even more forward, while the lower jaw can't move. The overbite becomes more pronounced the longer these abnormal stresses exist.

TREATMENT. The upper incisors may need to be cut back to the level of the gums, and a bite plate can be placed over them. This solid plate is placed to allow contact from the lower incisors, which then allows the mandible (lower jaw) to grow and the lower incisors to move forward. As the lower jaw migrates forward (it actually grows from the back), it pushes against the upper incisors, slows forward growth, and helps straighten the curving of the upper jaw. If this treatment is applied early enough, the overbite can be completely corrected and the adult horse will have a normal mouth.

PREVENTION. The best tactic to avoid a parrot mouth is to treat it before the disparity in growth between the upper and lower jaw can progress to a significant overbite. Although it is widely believed to be genetic, some dental experts say no. A disparity in growth between the upper and lower jaws may begin in utero, however, and early recognition and treatment can prevent parrot mouth from becoming a serious problem.

Root Canals FIGURES 14.24–14.26

THE PROBLEM. There is an opening in the center of the tooth into the pulp chamber, or soft tissues within the center of the tooth. This defect can occur in incisors, canine teeth, or even molars. In a normal tooth, dentine is deposited in the pulp chamber as the tooth erupts, preventing exposure of the pulp.

WHY IT MATTERS. An open pulp chamber can be painful, causing the horse problems with chewing or discomfort in the bridle. If it's allowed to progress, death of tissues within the center of the tooth can compromise the health of the tooth, and eventually result in tooth loss.

THE TREATMENT. The dental practitioner will begin by taking radiographs to evaluate the pulp chamber and the tooth in question, status of the root, and depth of the hole. Based on what he sees, he'll then drill through the center of the tooth to clean out any necrotic (dead) tissue, chemically sterilize the canal, and insert a material to fill the hole. By protecting the exposed pulp and restoring health deep within the tooth, pain will be eliminated and the risk of tooth loss reduced.

PREVENTION. As with most dental problems, a proper diet high in forage and regular dental maintenance will reduce the risk of exposed pulp chambers. In addition, early recognition and treatment will prevent problems from becoming more severe.

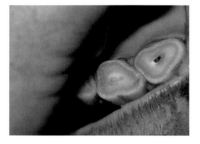

FIGURE 14.24. **A hole that forms in the center of the tooth can extend all the way into the pulp chamber, or soft tissues, within the center of the tooth, and compromise its health.** (Photo courtesy of David O. Klugh, DVM, FAVD, Equine)

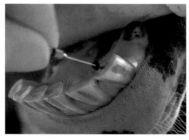

FIGURE 14.25. **To preserve the tooth, the veterinarian will perform a root canal procedure by drilling the hole in the tooth to clear away dead material.** (Photo courtesy of David O. Klugh, DVM, FAVD, Equine)

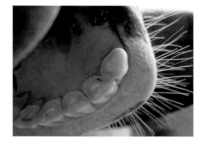

FIGURE 14.26. **The hole is then filled in with material to restore health.** (Photo courtesy of David O. Klugh, DVM, FAVD, Equine)

CHAPTER 15

The Immune System

THEN AND NOW

In 1796, Edward Jenner performed the first vaccination on a human in an effort to control the deadly smallpox virus. He took fluid from a cowpox cyst on the hand of a dairymaid and injected it into the arm of an 8-year-old child. The child developed cowpox symptoms immediately, but when injected with a smallpox two months later, he remained healthy. The success of this experiment led to the widespread vaccination of infants and less than 200 years later, the last reported case of smallpox was seen.

Manipulation of the immune system to protect against disease is now an essential part of human and equine life. Vaccinations are based on precisely the same mechanisms as that of the original smallpox vaccine. In the future, immunology may progress to where an animal's basic genetic makeup can be manipulated prior to birth to protect against disease.

THE IMMUNE SYSTEM IS RESPONSIBLE for protecting the horse's body against the constant threat of foreign attackers from his environment, including bacteria, viruses, and other microorganisms. This protection consists of physical barriers such as those provided by the skin and mucous membranes (gums, and linings of the respiratory, reproductive, and gastrointestinal tracts) and mechanical protection provided by the "small fingers" (called cilia) of the nasal passages and respiratory tract. In addition, mucous and oils released by protective cells line these barriers, trap invaders, and contain substances to kill them before they can wreak havoc in the horse's body.

Even so, large numbers of particularly strong invaders or other factors such as trauma can still allow penetration of these physical barriers. When this happens, the horse is dependent on internal mechanisms that involve cells and proteins circulating throughout the body that respond to threats. These internal mechanisms make up the immune system. FIGURE 15.1

The following structures are involved with immune system function.

Bone Marrow

This substance, which fills cavities within the bones of the horse, is where the white blood cells are produced. Different types of white blood cells, including macrophages, neutrophils, eosinophils, monocytes, and lymphocytes, are the body's primary defenders, and carry out most of the immune system functions.

Lymph Nodes

The lymph nodes are masses of lymphocytes that are distributed throughout the body. They multiply and produce antibodies in response to foreign invaders. They also filter fluids circulating throughout the body to help eliminate harmful substances.

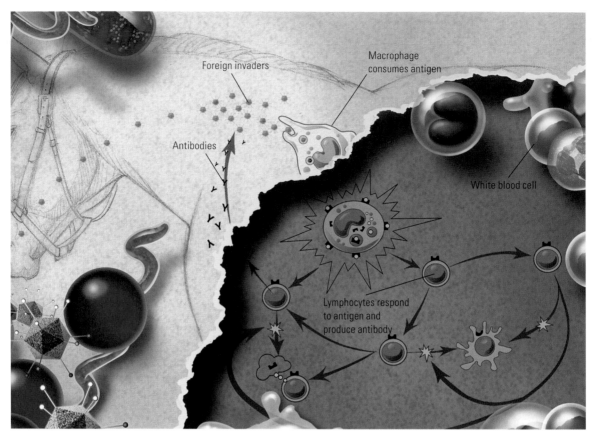

Antibodies

Foreign invaders

Macrophage
consumes antigen

White blood cell

Lymphocytes respond
to antigen and
produce antibody

FIGURE 15.1.
**The immune system.
Foreign invaders such as
bacteria and viruses
stimulate various arms of the
immune system.**

Liver

In the fetus, the liver is where most of the white blood cells are produced. As the body develops, this production shifts to the bone marrow. The liver also aids the immune system functions by helping to filter and clear debris and toxins that are produced within the body.

Spleen

Like the liver, the spleen participates in the production of white blood cells in the fetus until the bone marrow takes over this work. In the mature horse, the spleen acts as a reservoir where blood is stored, a filter to help clean substances from the blood, and a storage area for lymphocytes.

How the Horse Protects Himself

When a foreign invader breaches the physical barriers of the skin, cilia, mucous, and secretions that form the horse's first line of defense, internal defense mechanisms are activated. These mechanisms can be divided into two basic categories: humoral and cell-mediated immunity.

Humoral Immunity

This arm of the immune system involves a number of different cells and proteins that respond to a specific foreign invader (known as an antigen). Specific white blood cells known as plasma cells respond by releasing a type of protein called an antibody that's targeted against the foreign threat. These antibodies circulate throughout the horse's body, recognize the specific organism or cells infected with the organism, and destroy them. At the same time, the plasma cells multiply to produce even more antibodies (a process known as clonal expansion). The second part of the humoral immune system is the complement system. This system consists of a variety of different substances that are activated by a specific invader, and circulate throughout the body to break down infected or damaged cells.

In order for the humoral immune response to work, the horse must have been previously exposed to the antigen. This previous exposure primes the lymphocytes and complement system so that they will recognize the organism on subsequent exposures, and defend the horse as efficiently as possible. This is the system that supports the use of vaccination for protection against infectious diseases, as vaccination simply involves exposing the horse to potential threats to prime his immune system for a future response.

Cell-Mediated Immunity

This is the nonspecific arm of the immune system that responds whenever the horse is threatened, whether by a familiar or an unfamiliar attacker. White blood cells that respond in these conditions include macrophages, neutrophils, and monocytes. They protect in two primary ways. They travel to that area where protection is required and either "degranulate" (release substances that will help destroy the invaders), or "phagocytose" (eat and destroy the invaders directly). When this occurs, some of these white blood cells will die, producing pus in the tissues. This whitish, often smelly discharge is a common symptom that helps the veterinarian identify an infection.

Diagnostic Tests

The following diagnostic tests may be performed to evaluate the immune system.

Complete Blood Counts (CBC)

The vet will draw a blood sample to examine the numbers and types of different white blood cells—the cells primarily responsible for the immune response. As an example of information that might be obtained with this test, a very high white blood cell count may indicate that the immune system is responding to a bacterial infection. A very low white blood cell count, with large numbers of immature cells, may indicate that the immune system is being overwhelmed and unable to respond appropriately. In addition, greater numbers of different types of white blood cells might indicate a specific type of immune response.

Measurement of Immunoglobulins (Antibodies)

The vet draws a blood sample to look for specific antibodies that are circulating in the horse's system to protect him against a specific disease. This diagnostic test can be particularly helpful for determining whether a specific foreign invader is responsible. For example, if the vet is concerned about a certain viral cause of a disease, he'll measure antibodies against that virus when the horse first becomes ill, and then again 3 to 4 weeks into the recovery period. If the number of antibodies has increased dramatically (usually four times the original level), that's good evidence that the virus he's concerned about is really causing the problem. Specific antibodies might also be measured to determine whether a vaccine has had the desired effect of increasing antibody levels to protect the horse against that disease.

Overall immunoglobulins might also be measured to determine whether a horse has adequate levels in his system. Most commonly, a blood sample will be drawn on a foal following birth to determine whether he has gotten all of the antibodies he needs from his mother's milk. This indicates that his immune system is able to protect him in his early days of life.

Examination of Tissue

Sample of cells or small samples of tissues (biopsy) might help determine whether the immune system is involved with a disease. A skin sample, for instance, might contain white blood cells that would indicate an allergy-related problem.

Skin Testing

Skin testing is the most common method used for measuring the cell-mediated immune response involved with allergies. To perform this test, the veterinarian injects a small amount of different allergens (foreign materials) into the horse's skin. A small, fluid-filled, raised bump will appear at each injection site where the horse's immune system responds strongly enough to cause an allergic reaction. This testing can help identify substances that may cause allergies and aid the vet in formulating a specific treatment plan.

Diseases associated with the immune system can occur in a number of different circumstances: immune deficiency (the immune system isn't working properly, or at all), immune excess (the immune system is responding more strongly than necessary), or immune imbalance (the immune system is responding, but not how it should).

The following diseases are directly associated with the immune system and its ability to protect. (*Note: Because many problems associated with immune system function directly involve specific organ systems, those diseases have been discussed in detail in the appropriate chapters.*)

Failure of Passive Transfer

WHAT IT IS. Failure of passive transfer occurs if a newborn foal does not absorb adequate antibodies from the first milk (colostrum). During the first months of life, the newborn foal is dependent on these antibodies to protect it against infection, until its own immune system has had enough exposure to the outside world. Then it will be capable of producing enough of its own antibodies. Foals with failure of passive transfer are prone to infection, including life-threatening infection of the bloodstream (septicemia).

DIAGNOSIS. It is recommended that newborn foals be tested for antibodies 18 to 24 hours after birth. If antibodies are undetected or lower than normal, the foal is identified as having had a full or partial failure of passive transfer. If a foal is not tested as a part of a routine well-baby check, the same test will be recommended if signs of infection are observed, including depression, weakness, fever, hot swollen joints, or a hot swollen umbilical cord. A normal foal should have IgG levels (the antibody that's routinely measured) of greater than 800 mg/dl.

TREATMENT. If failure of passive transfer is a concern prior to birth because of leakage of milk or a prior history of the mare, the vet will administer antibodies through a nasogastric tube soon after birth. However, the foal is only capable of effectively absorbing antibodies for approximately 6 hours after birth. After that time, if low antibodies are detected as a part of a routine well-baby examination, or if the foal is already showing signs of infection, antibodies must be administered intravenously in the form of a plasma transfusion.

HOW SERIOUS IS IT? Failure of passive transfer can have extremely severe, even fatal consequences for a foal. It's best to identify this condition and provide treatment as early as possible to avoid complications.

POTENTIAL COMPLICATIONS. Infections that include septicemia, umbilical infections, joint infections, and pneumonia are common complications of low antibody levels.

Combined Immunodeficiency (CID)

WHAT IT IS. A failure of both arms of the immune system (humoral and cell-mediated immunity) seen in the Arabian breed. This is a genetic disease that requires two genes, one inherited from each parent (auto-somal recessive inheritance). Once a mare or stallion has produced a foal affected with CID, the horse has been identified as a carrier of the gene and should no longer be bred. Carrier horses have only one gene, and so will not be affected with the disease but will pass it on. A foal with CID will be unable to fight off infection and will often develop pneumonia.

DIAGNOSIS. Arabian foals with recurrent infections that do not respond well to treatment may be suspected to have CID. They will have low numbers of white blood cells. A diagnosis can be confirmed with examination of tissue taken from the lymph nodes. This is usually done after the death of the foal, and is useful for definite identification of carriers.

TREATMENT. There is no effective, practical treatment for this disease.

HOW SERIOUS IS IT? Death usually occurs due to overwhelming infections before an affected foal reaches 5 months of age. Identification of a mare or stallion as a carrier significantly impacts the horse's value for breeding.

POTENTIAL COMPLICATIONS. Overwhelming infection is the primary complication associated with CID, due to the immune system's inability to respond to foreign invaders.

Neonatal Isoerythrolysis (NI)

WHAT IT IS. Neonatal isoerythrolysis is a disease of newborn foals that occurs when the mother's milk contains antibodies that attack the foal's red blood cells. This can only occur if the mare has had previous foals that caused her immune system to respond by producing these antibodies. Foals with this disease are born normal, and then become weak and depressed within 1 to 3 days of birth. The foal's mucous membranes (gums, tissues around the eyes, and vulva in a filly) will become yellowed (jaundiced, or icteric).

DIAGNOSIS. NI should be suspected in any foal that appears normal at birth, then begins to show symptoms that include the yellowing of mucous membranes. Bilirubin levels in the blood will be increased, and the foal will be anemic. A test to examine compatibility between the mare's and foal's blood can confirm a diagnosis (called cross-matching).

TREATMENT. If NI is identified within the first 24 hours of life, the mare's milk should be withheld, and the foal fed a mare's milk replacer. After that time, antibodies have already been absorbed and there is minimal benefit to withholding milk. Then, supportive care and careful monitoring will be recommended. In severe cases, a blood transfusion will be necessary.

HOW SERIOUS IS IT? Many cases will result in death before the disease is even recognized. In foals where NI is recognized early and support is adequate, complete recovery is possible. It is best to avoid this problem altogether, which can be done by restricting all foals born to a mare known to have produced an NI foal from nursing during the first 24 to 48 hours of life, and providing colostrum from another source.

POTENTIAL COMPLICATIONS. A foal with NI will be more at risk for infections, and may have kidney damage because of the effects of breakdown products of the red blood cells that are eliminated through the kidneys.

Anaphylaxis

WHAT IT IS. A hypersensitivity reaction that results in a whole-body response. A foreign antigen interacts with antibodies (IgE type) that stimulate release of substances (histamines, prostaglandins, and others) from two primary types of immune system cells (basophils and mast cells). These substances create a response that includes sweating, difficulty breathing, alterations in the heart rhythm, and pooling of blood and fluids in various organs. The lung is the primary organ affected by anaphylaxis in the horse, and fluid accumulations in the lung can lead to respiratory distress and rapid death. An anaphylactic reaction can occur following exposure to any substance that the horse's immune system is sensitized to. Most commonly, it will occur following administration of a medication directly into the bloodstream.

DIAGNOSIS. An anaphylactic reaction will be suspected with a sudden onset of symptoms following exposure to a foreign substance—most commonly after the administration of a medication.

TREATMENT. Immediate treatment is necessary to stop the immune system response. The vet might administer epinephrine intravenously, which will constrict blood vessels to reduce blood and fluid pooling. Corticosteroids may also be given to help limit the release of inflammatory substances that play a part in the overall reaction. Although antihistamines are commonly used in humans, they are not as beneficial for managing anaphylaxis in horses because histamines play a smaller role in the overall response. They can be helpful used in combination with epinephrine and corticosteroids. In a severe anaphylactic reaction, a tracheostomy (opening in the trachea) may need to be performed in order for oxygen to be administered to the lungs.

HOW SERIOUS IS IT? A severe anaphylactic reaction is often fatal, even with immediate and aggressive treatment.

POTENTIAL COMPLICATIONS. Sudden death.

Allergies   FIGURES 15.2–15.4

WHAT IT IS. An allergy is a hypersensitivity reaction in which the immune system reacts excessively to a foreign substance or antigen (called an "allergen" when referring to an allergy-related problem). Many different types of allergies are common in horses (see Table 15.1). It is the same type of response as that seen with an anaphylactic reaction, except that the response is more localized to the site of exposure. Antibodies (IgE type) bind to white blood cells (primarily mast cells and basophils) to stimulate the release of histamines, prostaglandins, and other substances that cause symptoms to develop. Allergic reactions in horses commonly involve the lungs or skin (see related sections in chapters 7 and 10), and can lead to itching, hives, or fluid swelling in the skin layers or inflammation and mucous production in the airways.

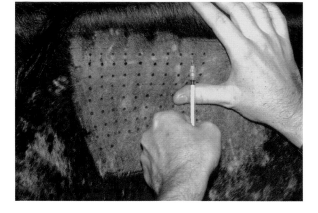

FIGURE 15.2. **To perform intradermal skin testing, the veterinarian injects a small amount of different foreign materials into the horse's skin.** (Photo courtesy of Anthony Yu, DVM, Diplomate ACVD)

DIAGNOSIS. Allergies are usually identified based on typical clinical signs and known exposure to common allergens. Specific information to support a diagnosis can be obtained through a skin biopsy if skin lesions are present, and collection of cells from the airways if the respiratory tract is involved.

Elimination strategies can be employed in an attempt to identify specific allergens affecting the horse. If an allergy to bedding or other substances in the environment is suspected, the horse can be removed to an environment where he has minimal exposure to potential allergens. For example, he can be put in a sand paddock, in an open area, with a single type of grass hay for feed. If his allergic symptoms disappear, new things such as bedding or different hays can be introduced one by one every 7 days. When the allergic symptoms reappear, an allergen has

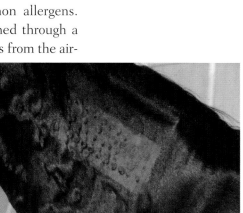

FIGURE 15.3. **A small fluid-filled raised bump can be seen at each injection site where the horse's immune system has responded strongly enough to cause an allergic reaction.** (Photo courtesy of Anthony Yu, DVM, Diplomate ACVD)

been identified. Unfortunately, this has a number of limitations. The first is simply the difficulty in arranging for such strict environmental controls. The second is that the majority of allergies involve a wide variety of allergens that all work together to overcome the "allergic threshold" and produce symptoms. The exception would be food allergies, where elimination trials are often essential for identifying foods that cause sensitivity.

In most cases, intradermal skin testing is the most accurate and practical method for identifying the full spectrum of specific allergens responsible for an allergic reaction. Blood tests that measure allergen-specific antibodies in the bloodstream are also available, although their accuracy is not as good as that obtained through skin testing.

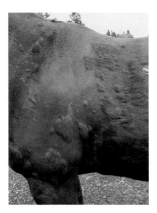

FIGURE 15.4. **These raised bumps and lines under the horse's skin, called urticaria or hives, are typical for an allergic reaction.** (Author photo)

TREATMENT. It is important for the owner of an allergic horse to recognize that allergy symptoms can be managed, but allergies cannot be completely eliminated. For successful management, a lifelong commitment to treatment is necessary. The most important component to management of an allergic horse is avoidance of potential allergens. This often involves changing the environment to minimize exposure to dust, insects, or other irritants (see page 265).

Medications play an important part in the management of an allergic horse. Antihistamines, corticosteroids, and dietary supplementation with fatty acids all help minimize the allergic response. Finally, hyposensitization through a series of injections with small amounts of allergen identified through intradermal skin testing can be very effective for minimizing symptoms in severely affected horses (see Table 15.2).

HOW SERIOUS IS IT? Equine allergies can be difficult to control and may result in severe symptoms if not controlled. Itching skin lesions can lead to self-trauma and severe skin damage. Respiratory allergies can be manifested as chronic obstructive pulmonary disease, a debilitating lung disease (see chapter 7).

POTENTIAL COMPLICATIONS.

Severe skin trauma, in-cluding secondary skin inf-ections. Heaves or chronic obstructive pulmonary disease can lead to pneumonia or respiratory failure.

TABLE 15.1

Common Equine Allergies   Figure 15.5–15.6

ALLERGY TYPE	TYPICAL SIGNS	MANAGEMENT TIPS
Insect hypersensitivity (Most commonly caused by *Culicoides* spp or no-see-um gnats, other insects as well)	Itching skin lesions. Commonly affects the mane, tail, belly, and back.	Fly control is essential. Bathing or topical medications to help control itching can minimize severity of signs. Usually 50% of affected horses will improve with hyposensitization.
Atopy (Allergy to inhaled substances such as pollen, molds, and dust)	Itching skin lesions. Commonly affects the face, ears, belly and legs. Hives over the entire body. Respiratory symptoms (COPD).	Avoidance of potential allergens. As many as 80% of horses will improve with hyposensitization.
Food allergy	Itching at the base of the tail. Hives or itching of the chest or flank area. Diarrhea, colic symptoms.	Eliminate exposure to food causing hypersensitivity, which can be difficult to identify. Requires elimination trials.
Contact allergy	Reddened skin, swelling, hair loss and erosions or ulcers of skin in contact with allergen.	Avoid contact with offending substance (specific bedding, leg bandages, etc.) once identified.

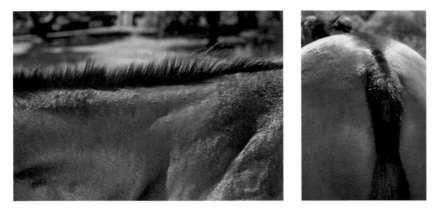

FIGURES 15.5–15.6. **This horse has rubbed his mane and tail, causing breakage of hairs and underlying skin damage. This is typical for an insect hypersensitivity.**

(Photo courtesy of Anthony Yu, DVM, Diplomate ACVD)

TABLE 15.2

Treatment Options for Equine Allergies

TREATMENT CLASS	SPECIFIC MEDICATIONS	WHY IT WORKS	COMMENTS
Antihistamines	Doxepin HCl. Hydroxyzine HCl. Diphenhydramine.	Prevents activity of histamine, the substance released by cells to produce allergy symptoms.	May cause mild sedation. Fewer side effects, but less effective than corticosteroids.
Corticosteroids	Dexamethasone. Prednisolone.	Counteracts effects of inflammation to eliminate swelling in airways or skin and minimizes allergy symptoms.	Dexamethasone, although very effective, can have significant side effects, including laminitis. Prednisolone is less effective, but also less risky.
Essential fatty acids (Omega-6 and/or omega-3)	Derm Caps (DVM pharmaceuticals). Omega Derm (Allerderm/Virbac). EicosaDerm (Dermapet).	Shifts the inflammatory process away from the release of substances that produce symptoms.	Feed supplements that modify the inflammatory response and have been shown to help minimize allergy symptoms with minimal side effects.
Hyposensitization	Customized allergy serums produced by equine allergist based on results of skin testing.	Desensitizes the immune system to allergens involved in the allergic response through repeated exposure of very low doses.	After initial induction phase, injections are administered every 7–28 days. Effective in many cases and eliminates need for ongoing medication.

The Horse's Body: Health and Disease

Allergy Management

FIGURE 15.7

To minimize symptoms, take the following steps:

- Keep the barn clean. Minimize your horse's exposure to dust and other potential irritants by sweeping, blowing or vacuuming the barn every day. Ideally, this is done when he is out in the field, away from the dust in the air when you clean.

- Turn him out as much as possible. An open field is a much better environment for an allergic horse than a closed-up barn. If turnout isn't possible, make sure the barn is well ventilated, and he is stabled as close to a door or window as possible.

- Keep your horse indoors if you'll be haying or mowing the lawn. Machinery stirs up pollen, insects, and mold spores that are close to the ground, and may stimulate his allergies.

- Try to turn out at mid-morning or late at night. Mid to late afternoon is when allergens are at their highest level in the environment because of the winds, smog, and movement of people.

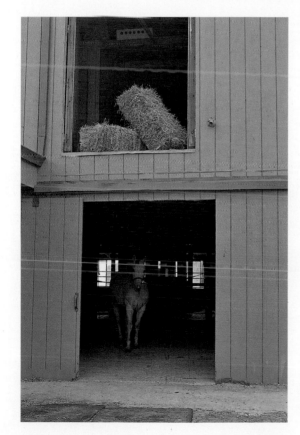

- Water-down feed. Hay is a huge potential source of allergens. By wetting hay before you feed, you minimize exposing your horse to feed or dust particles that may stimulate allergy symptoms.

- Avoid housing your horse in a barn attached to an arena. Because dust flies through the air when horses work, an attached arena barn can be problematic for an allergic horse. When you do ride inside, try to ensure that the arena has been watered for better dust control.

- Practice good insect control. Because insects play a role in many allergies, you'll minimize your horse's overall allergen load if you reduce his exposure to flies, mosquitoes, and other bugs.

FIGURE 15.7. **Environmental control is often an important part of minimizing exposure to dust and other potential irritants that cause allergies. Hay storage overhead, as seen here, should be discouraged.**

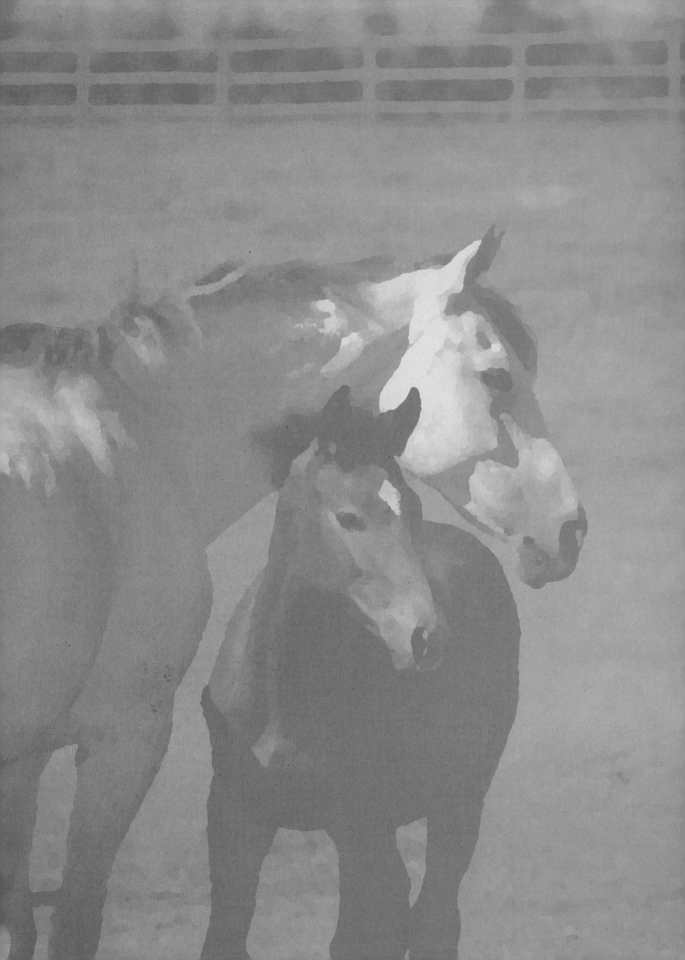

PART THREE

Special Horses

CHAPTER 16

The Broodmare

SHE'S PEACEFULLY GRAZING IN THE PASTURE with this year's foal at her side. Yet less than a month after giving birth, she's about to be bred again. She patiently tolerates the veterinarian's poking, prodding, and manipulations that this demand requires while dedicating her full attention to her current offspring. FIGURE 16.1

Such is the life of a professional broodmare. In this chapter we'll outline the steps involved with breeding, pregnancy, and successful foaling, as well as the problems that can arise during the breeding and foaling process.

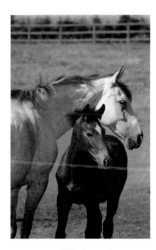

FIGURE 16.1. **The broodmare dedicates her full attention to her current offspring, even as she's supporting next year's foal.**

Getting the Mare in Foal

Before Breeding Begins

Before she's bred, the broodmare should be in optimal condition. She should be at a good weight, currently vaccinated for any infectious diseases, and have had routine dental work performed. Vaccination in the early months of pregnancy is not recommended, and any procedures that might be stressful or require medication should be avoided to minimize the potential for adverse effects on the developing fetus.

At least one month prior to the anticipated breeding date, the mare should undergo a pre-breeding examination to ensure that she is healthy and that her reproductive system is normal. This examination is likely to include rectal palpation and ultrasound, and uterine culture and cytology (examination of samples taken from the uterus for signs of infection or inflammation). Uterine biopsy may be recommended for older mares or mares with a history of reproductive problems. If abnormalities are detected with any of these diagnostic tests, the veterinarian will recommend treatment prior to beginning the breeding process.

The Breeding Process

Successful breeding requires that the mare be bred within an appropriate time frame around the release of an egg from the ovary during the estrous cycle. The most common methods likely to result in a pregnancy include live cover (the stallion physically breeds the mare), artificial insemination with fresh semen (recently collected semen is prepared and deposited into the uterus), and artificial insemination with frozen semen (semen that has been previously frozen and stored in liquid nitrogen is deposited into the uterus).

Live cover

With live cover, the mare's heat cycle is usually monitored through "teasing" or observation of her behavior when she's exposed to the stallion. When the mare exhibits signs of estrus (such as a winking vulva or squatting to urinate), she will be bred to the stallion every other day until she no longer accepts him, indicating that she has ovulated (released an egg).

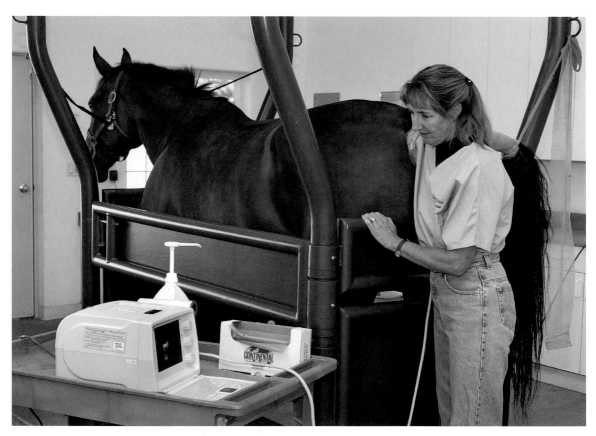

FIGURE 16.2. **Ultrasound examination allows the veterinarian to visualize the mare's uterus and ovaries to determine timing for insemination, detect pregnancy, or identify any abnormalities in her reproductive tract.**

Special Horses

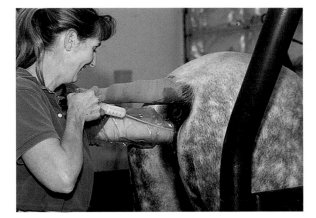

FIGURE 16.3. **For artificial insemination, the veterinarian deposits semen directly into the mare's uterus using a syringe and a long insemination pipette.**

Artificial insemination with fresh semen
FIGURES 16.2–16.3

Artificial insemination requires that the veterinarian closely monitor the mare's heat cycle, typically using daily palpations and ultrasounds, in order to determine the optimal time for insemination. The vet observes the growth of one or more follicles (fluid-filled structures on the ovary that mature and eventually release an egg), and changes that occur within the mare's uterus as the heat cycle progresses. Ideally, a single follicle will begin to dominate, and will eventually release a single egg.

If semen is being shipped from a stallion in a remote location, the vet will request semen when the follicle reaches a certain size. The goal is to have the semen in hand for insemination just before the mare ovulates, or releases the egg from her ovary.

As soon as the semen arrives, the mare will be inseminated. Semen is deposited directly into the mare's uterus using a long insemination pipette. Many stallion managers will send a second dose of semen for a subsequent insemination the following day. After the mare has been inseminated, a small sample of the semen will be examined under the microscope to assess its viability.

Ideally, the mare will ovulate within 24 hours of insemination, although many mares still conceive with transported semen even if ovulation does not occur until the 48-hour point. Much depends on the fertility of the stallion, and a very important factor in working with fresh, transported semen is maintaining good contact with the stallion manager.

Artificial insemination with frozen semen

Frozen semen offers the advantage that the semen is ready and waiting before the breeding process even begins. The disadvantage is that timing of insemination must be much closer than with fresh transported semen (usually within 6 hours of ovulation), and pregnancy rates are lower.

Because the timing is so critical, the mare may be examined with the ultrasound as often as 3 or 4 times a day during the final days of her heat cycle. The goal is to inseminate within 6 hours of ovulation. In some cases, the vet will inseminate both before and after ovulation for optimal results.

Post-Breeding Treatment

When the mare is inseminated, her uterus may become inflamed in response to the semen. This can cause fluid and inflammatory debris to accumulate within her uterus, which can be detrimental to the embryo and prevent a healthy pregnancy from being established. This problem is much more common with frozen semen because the natural protectants in the seminal fluid have usually been removed as part of the freezing process.

It takes approximately 6 days for the fertilized egg to travel down from the ovary into the uterus, giving the vet that amount of time to clean up the uterine environment. Post-breeding treatments may include the following:

- OXYTOCIN: An injection of this hormone stimulates uterine contractions that help push unwanted fluid and debris out of the uterus. It can be given as early as 4 to 6 hours after insemination, and may be repeated several times during the first day or so following insemination to help clear fluid.

- UTERINE INFUSION: A small volume of saline is placed into the uterus to help wash out unwanted fluid and debris. If the mare has a history of uterine infection, this infusion may include an antibiotic.

- UTERINE LAVAGE: If the mare accumulates a large volume of fluid, this procedure, which involves washing the inside of her uterus with several liters of saline, will be recommended. A large Y-shaped tube is inserted into the uterus, allowing fluid to be moved in and out.

Manipulation of the Estrous Cycle

In domesticated horses, an earlier breeding season is often imposed in order to produce foals born early in the year. Lighting adjustments during winter months may help to stimulate an earlier cycle. In addition, a wide variety of different hormonal treatments may be used throughout the breeding process at any time of year in order to facilitate timing for successful breeding. The following are the most common strategies used for manipulating the mare's estrous cycle:

Lights

In nature, daylight hours stimulate the mare to begin cycling by stimulating release of the gonadotropin-releasing hormone (GnRH) from the hypothalamus, which eventually leads to the onset of ovarian activity. To encourage this process to begin sooner, a mare can be placed under artificial lights during winter months. As a rule of thumb, 16 hours of light per day are required beginning sometime between November 15 and December 1 in order to stimulate cycling to begin around February 15.

Prostaglandin

This hormone injection, if given to the mare a minimum of 5 days after the end of her previous heat cycle, should stimulate a new heat cycle to begin within 3 or 4 days. It works by breaking down the corpus luteum, the structure that developed following ovulation of a follicle from the previous heat cycle, an event that must occur before a new follicle can develop.

When the mare is given a prostaglandin injection, she may sweat, cramp, or even act a little colicky for approximately 45 minutes. This is a normal reaction that should not be cause for concern.

Progesterone

This hormone can be used to regulate heat cycles. For example, the mare might be administered the oral synthetic progesterone Regu-Mate® (Intervet) daily for a period of 10 to 12 days. When the Regu-Mate® is discontinued, most mares will begin to cycle within 3 to 5 days.

Progesterone may also be administered as an injection either by itself or in combination with estrogen. Daily injections for 10 to 12 days or a single injection of a long-acting version of these hormones, similar to Regu-Mate®, will be given to prime the uterus for breeding. With either oral or injectable progesterone or progesterone/estrogen combinations, a prostaglandin injection may still be administered on day 10 of treatment to reliably stimulate a heat cycle.

Progesterone or progesterone/estrogen combinations may also be administered after breeding, or after pregnancy has been confirmed to help maintain the pregnancy.

Human chorionic gonadotropin (HCG)

This injectable hormone may be used to help stimulate ovulation. It assists with the timing of breeding by helping to coordinate the time of insemination with the time of ovulation. In most cases, HCG will stimulate ovulation within 48 hours of administration

Deslorelin

An alternative to HCG, this hormone may also be administered to stimulate ovulation. It is extremely reliable at inducing ovulation within 36 to 48 hours, and is especially useful for mares that have a tendency to develop very large follicles prior to ovulation.

Pregnancy

Detection of Pregnancy FIGURE 16.4

Pregnancy can be detected as early as 10 days using an ultrasound evaluation of the uterus. Most commonly, the veterinarian will recommend a first ultrasound at 15 to18 days following ovulation. During this ultrasound, a small fluid-filled sac will be seen in the uterus. If a pregnancy is confirmed at the first ultrasound, a second ultrasound is generally recommended just prior to 30 days following ovulation in order to look for a heartbeat and to make a final check for a twin that may have been too small to see during the first ultrasound. (See page 279 for information about twins.)

From this point forward, pregnancy checks may be required by the stallion owner at specific times. If a breeding contract doesn't specify

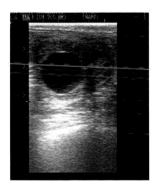

FIGURE 16.4. **The circular black area on this ultrasound image is the fluid-filled sac within the uterus that allows the veterinarian to diagnose an early pregnancy.**
(Author photo)

times for pregnancy confirmation, a palpation at 3 months and again at 5 months will usually be done. After this point, no monitoring should be required unless you have concerns.

Care of the Pregnant Mare

Feeding

The pregnant mare's feeding requirements do not change dramatically during the first 8 months of pregnancy. The developing foal is only gaining weight at the rate of approximately 0.2 pounds per day during this time. Good-quality hay with a balanced vitamin/mineral supplement is usually all that is necessary to maintain a good weight and provide necessary nutrients.

During the last months of pregnancy, the foal grows more rapidly, at a rate of approximately one pound per day. The mare will require more calories during this time, and her protein requirements may increase slightly to 14 percent of her total ration. Many veterinarians will recommend a supplement specifically balanced for pregnant mares during the end of pregnancy and into the lactation period, in addition to an increase in the hay ration.

Feeding recommendations will vary widely in different geographical areas depending on what feeds are available as well as possible deficiencies isolated to a specific place. For this reason, it's best to discuss a specific feeding plan for the pregnant mare with a local veterinarian or nutrition expert.

Regardless of the geographical area, it's best to avoid fescue hay and pastures. Fescue is often plagued by a fungus called endophyte (*Neotyphodium coenophialum*), which can cause mares to abort or hold pregnancies too long. It can also cause agalactia, or a failure to produce milk.

Vaccination

Vaccination during the first 3 to 4 months of pregnancy is generally discouraged, due to concerns about unnecessary stimulation of the mare's immune system that could have negative effects on the developing fetus. Following those critical early months, the mare's regular vaccination schedule should be maintained.

In addition, there are certain vaccinations that the mare should receive to help protect the pregnancy. She should be vaccinated against equine herpes virus-type 1 (EHV-1, or rhinopneumonitis) during months 5, 7, and 9 of her pregnancy in order to protect against the risk of abortion from this virus. Some veterinarians will also recommend this vaccination at month 3 in locations where risks are high.

Approximately 30 days prior to the anticipated foaling date, the mare should be administered a full set of basic vaccinations to stimulate the production of antibodies in the colostrum, or first milk. These antibodies help to protect the foal immediately following birth. These vaccinations generally include sleeping sickness (Eastern and Western equine encephalomyelitis), tetanus, influenza, rhinopneumonitis, and West Nile virus. Depending on disease prevalence, additional vaccinations may be recommended pre-foaling, including Potomac horse fever, botulism, or strangles. (*Note: Pre-foaling vaccinations should all be given intramuscularly, even for diseases where intranasal vaccines are available. Although very effective for preventing disease, intranasal vaccines stimulate a local immune response rather than the production of antibodies, so they won't help protect the foal.*)

Deworming

Pregnant mares should be maintained on a normal deworming schedule. Commonly used dewormers are safe in pregnant mares, including the benzimidazoles, ivermectin, pyrantel pamoate, and the daily dewormer, pyrantel tartrate, (See chapter 2 for more detailed information.)

The pregnant mare should also be administered a larvicidal deworming treatment with a double dose of fenbendazole given daily for 5 consecutive days as close to her actual foaling date as possible. This helps eliminate larvae migrating in her system, including those that can migrate through the mammary glands and increase the incidence of diarrhea in the foal following birth.

Exercise

For at least the first two-thirds of her pregnancy the mare can usually continue performing exercise at the same level of intensity she was performing prior to becoming pregnant. Common sense prevails when determining what amount of exercise is appropriate. Avoid introducing new, stressful activities, and pay attention to signals from the mare. If she becomes tired or uncomfortable, it's time to stop.

Foaling

The gestation period is 325 to 365 days, with an average of 345 days for normal foaling. (For a simple calculation, simply subtract 3 weeks from a year from the date of ovulation to estimate the mare's expected foaling date.)

Signs of Impending Foaling

Every mare is different, and close monitoring is essential to determine when foaling is imminent. The following are the most common indicators.

- Increase in mammary development (bagging up) as fluids start to accumulate in the udder as early as 6 weeks before foaling. Initially these fluids will be clear, and as foaling approaches they will become thick and sticky. During the days immediately prior to foaling, the mammary secretions will actually turn white, and drop down into the teats. Monitoring this change is one of the most reliable indicators to help predict foaling time. As the fluids turn to milk, the calcium levels begin to increase. These calcium levels can be measured using either a commercially available milk test kit, or simple chemical test strips. When calcium levels reach 200 ppm, chances are high that the mare will foal within the following 48 hours.

- Waxing, or accumulation of milk at the tip of the teats, may be detected in the day or two prior to foaling. If a mare is waxed, she should be closely monitored. FIGURE 16.5

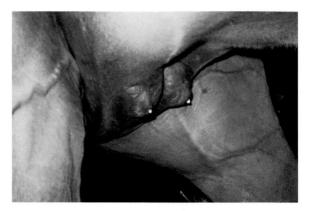

FIGURE 16.5. **This accumulation of fluid at the tip of the mare's teats, referred to as "waxing," is a sure sign that foaling time is near.** (Photo courtesy of Tina Gilmore)

- The mare's vulva will relax and elongate. This begins approximately 2 weeks prior to foaling. This relaxation may become especially apparent immediately before the onset of labor. FIGURE 16.6

- A softening of the muscles along either side of the mare's tail-head may be detectable during the 2 to 3 days prior to foaling.

- A mare will often evacuate her large intestines of fecal material in the hours before foaling.

The Foaling Environment

The mare should be introduced to the foaling environment at least 30 days prior to her expected delivery date. This allows her to be exposed to any potential infectious organisms in the environment, and produce antibodies that she can pass on to protect her foal.

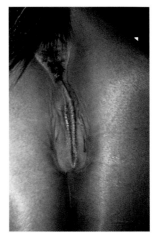

FIGURE 16.6. **The mare's vulva will relax and elongate as much as two weeks prior to foaling. (**Photo courtesy of Tina Gilmore)

A foaling stall for an average-sized mare should be at least 12×24' feet to allow plenty of room for her to get up and down without becoming cast during the foaling event. To prevent injury, walls should be solid and without gaps. Ideally, a foaling stall will have two doors that allow an attendant access to the stall even if the mare goes down in front of one door.

Stalls should be kept clean, and walls disinfected prior to foaling. Flooring should be a nonslip material, and straw is the first choice of bedding as it provides adequate cushioning and avoids small particles that can be a source of contamination or irritation to a newborn foal.

It's desirable that foaling be attended to minimize the risk of complications. Although the vast majority of mares will deliver successfully without assistance, potentially fatal complications can often be avoided if an attendant is present.

Many mare owners question whether foaling outside in a grass paddock is acceptable, and it is, under ideal circumstances. Grass is clean, air is fresh, and the foaling environment is as natural as possible. This situation, however, makes monitoring difficult, which puts the mare and foal

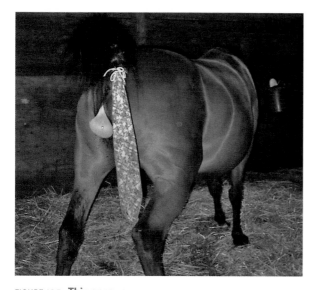

FIGURE 16.7. **This opaque membrane (the amnion) will appear at the mare's vulva after the water breaks. Second stage labor has begun.** (Photo courtesy of Tina Gilmore)

at risk for complications associated with an unattended foaling, such as an undetected dystocia (see page 281) or suffocation of the foal in the fetal membranes following birth.

Labor and Delivery

The majority of mares will foal during the hours between 10 PM and 4 AM. This may well relate to the horse's natural status as a prey animal, and the likelihood that the environment is most peaceful and nonthreatening during these late-night hours.

First stage labor

First stage labor usually lasts between 1 and 4 hours. During this time period the mare will begin to act restless or even colicky. She may sweat and bite at her sides, or stand stretched out in odd positions. These movements are believed to help position the foal for delivery. During first stage labor, the uterus begins to contract, the hormone oxytocin is released, and the cervix begins to open. At the end of first stage labor, the outer membrane of the placenta, called the chorioallantois, ruptures to release allantoic fluid—known as "breaking water."

Second stage labor FIGURES 16.7–16.11

After the allantoic fluid is released, strong uterine contractions cause the amnion, an opaque membrane that covers the foal's forelimbs, to appear at the vulva. The forelimbs should be visible within 5 minutes of the water breaking.

A normally presented foal appears with the two forelimbs slightly offset, followed by the nose. Once these structures are observed, it is

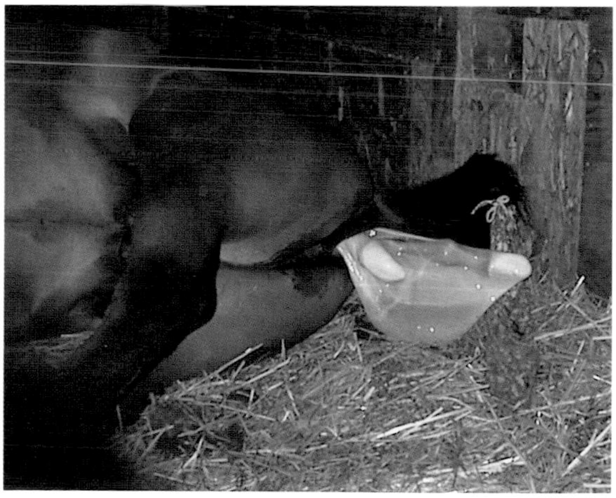

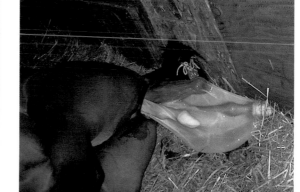

FIGURE 16.8. **The two front feet, slightly offset, should be seen within minutes of the appearance of the amnion.** (Photo courtesy of Tina Gilmore)

FIGURE 16.9. **A normally presented foal's nose will soon be seen resting on top of the forelimbs.** (Photo courtesy of Tina Gilmore)

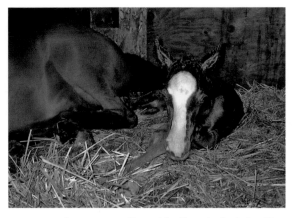

FIGURE 16.10. **In an uncomplicated foaling, the foal should be fully delivered within 15 to 20 minutes following the onset of second stage labor.** (Photo courtesy of Tina Gilmore)

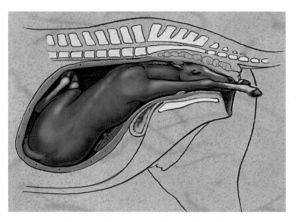

FIGURE 16.11. **A normally presented foal is delivered with his two front feet first, followed by his nose.**

likely that a normal delivery will follow. In an uncomplicated foaling, the foal should be delivered within 15 to 20 minutes following the onset of second stage labor. Fatal consequences can easily occur with prolonged delivery. The veterinarian should be called immediately if foaling is not progressing according to these guidelines.

Third stage labor   FIGURE 16.12

Third stage labor involves passage of the placenta and involution of the uterus. Following delivery of the foal, the mare will continue to have uterine contractions that may be quite intense and painful. In this case, the veterinarian may recommend administration of a nonsteroidal anti-inflammatory medication such as flunixin meglumine. The placenta should be passed within 3 hours of delivery. It may take up to a full month for the uterus to completely return to normal.

(Note: Monitoring and care of the foal following delivery will be covered in the following chapter.)

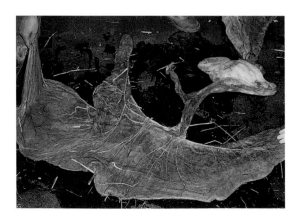

FIGURE 16.12. **This is an example of a normal placenta, which should be passed within three hours of delivery. The veterinarian will examine the placenta to make sure it's been passed intact.** (Photo courtesy of Jan Palmer, DVM, Diplomate ACVS)

The following are the most common complications likely to occur during breeding, pregnancy, and delivery.

Twins FIGURE 16.13

WHAT IT IS. A mare ovulates two eggs, and both become fertilized during the breeding process. Most mares will not carry a twin pregnancy to term because the placenta is unable to support both fetuses. For this reason, the veterinarian will recommend attempting to eliminate one embryo as early as possible to increase the chances that the second will survive.

DIAGNOSIS. Twins can be identified during an initial ultrasound as early as 12 days following conception. If a breeding is closely monitored and two ovulations are detected, ultrasound will usually be recommended prior to 15 days following ovulation, before the embryos become permanently fixed in position within the uterus. A second ultrasound between 28 and 30 days is recommended for all pregnancies in order to look for two heartbeats to accurately identify possible twins.

TREATMENT. If twins are identified prior to 15 days following conception, the vet can easily separate the embryos and crush one with his hand. Once the embryos become fixed in the uterus, they cannot be manipulated. In this case, one embryo can still be crushed prior to 30 days gestation if the embryos are located in separate horns, or widely separated in one horn. If embryos are located side by side, over 80 percent will "self-reduce," meaning only one will survive. The remaining 20 percent are difficult to manage, and may require termination of the entire pregnancy. Techniques to suck fluid out of one of the embryos by means of a specially designed probe may be attempted in order to eliminate one embryo, although the success rates of these techniques are not favorable.

HOW SERIOUS IS IT? Twins can have very serious consequences. If allowed to progress, they will often result in abortion during the final third of pregnancy when the uterus is no longer able to support both fetuses. If they do go to term, one twin may be very weak or dead, and the other may be compromised. Rarely do both twins survive.

POTENTIAL COMPLICATIONS. Risk to the mare delivering twin fetuses is significant, and could even be life threatening. As a general rule, it is not advisable to allow a twin pregnancy to progress.

Uterine Torsion

WHAT IT IS. The uterus twists within the abdominal cavity. This uncommon condition is most likely to occur during mid- to late-term pregnancy and,

FIGURE 16.13 **If a twin pregnancy is allowed to progress, it is likely to result in abortion during the final third of pregnancy when the uterus is no longer able to support both fetuses.** (Photo courtesy of Jan Palmer, DVM, Diplomate ACVS)

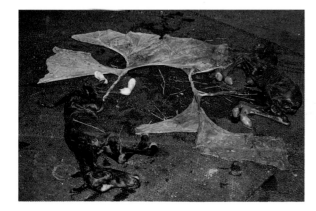

depending on the degree of torsion, can cause mild discomfort or severe colic symptoms.

DIAGNOSIS. A torsion will be identified by rectal palpation, usually performed when the mare is showing signs of colic.

TREATMENT. In some cases it may be possible to correct the torsion by anesthetizing the mare and rolling her with a board placed over her abdomen to hold the uterus in place. More commonly, surgery will be necessary to reposition the uterus.

HOW SERIOUS IS IT? Uterine torsion can cause severe colic symptoms, and surgery to correct the torsion can be risky to both the mare and the foal.

POTENTIAL COMPLICATIONS. Even when a torsion is corrected successfully, a compromised blood supply may result in loss of the pregnancy during or following surgery.

Placentitis   FIGURE 16.14

WHAT IT IS. Infection and inflammation of the placenta due to a variety of causes, including bacteria, viruses, or fungi.

DIAGNOSIS. A vaginal discharge may be observed in a pregnant mare. Ultrasound examination can show abnormal thickening of the placenta or abnormalities within the placental fluids. Culture of the vaginal discharge can help identify a cause to guide treatment.

TREATMENT. Antibiotics will be recommended if a specific organism can be identified. Progesterone may be administered to the mare to help maintain the pregnancy, as well as medications to minimize uterine contractions and decrease the chances of premature delivery.

HOW SERIOUS IS IT? Placentitis can have serious consequences, including abortion and severe illness or death of the newborn foal.

POTENTIAL COMPLICATIONS. Infection of the foal at birth. Abortion.

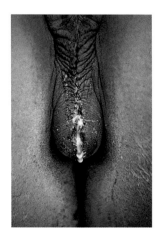

FIGURE 16.14. **A vaginal discharge, such as this, may indicate placentitis, or an infection of the placental membranes that could compromise the pregnancy.** (Photo courtesy of Lisa Metcalf, DVM, Diplomate ACVT)

Hydrallantois and Hydramnios

WHAT IT IS. An excessive accumulation of allantoic or amniotic fluid within the uterus due to a dysfunction of the placenta. Hydrallantois, which occurs during midgestation, is the more common occurrence , and generally appears over a period of approximately 2 weeks. Hydramnios occurs more gradually over the course of the pregnancy.

DIAGNOSIS. Large amounts of fluid can be palpated in the uterus of a mare that has an obviously overly distended abdomen for her stage of pregnancy.

TREATMENT. In most cases of excessive fluid accumulation the fetus is no longer alive, and termination of the pregnancy is recommended. The mare may need to be supported with intravenous fluids and corticosteroids during treatment to prevent shock due to excessive fluid losses.

HOW SERIOUS IS IT? In the majority of cases, these conditions result in loss of the pregnancy and are dangerous for the mare.

POTENTIAL COMPLICATIONS. Ruptured prepubic tendon.

Special Horses

Ruptured Prepubic Tendon

WHAT IT IS. The tendon that helps support the abdomen against the pelvis ruptures, resulting in a loss of support for the abdominal organs, pregnancy, and udder.

DIAGNOSIS. The typical physical appearance of the mare is usually sufficient to make a diagnosis. Palpation can help determine whether the tendon is simply stretched and at risk, or actually ruptured.

TREATMENT. In the case of rupture, the mare will be unable to support the developing fetus and termination of the pregnancy may be necessary to save the mare. In pregnancies that are close to term, support wraps and nursing care may make it possible to save the foal.

HOW SERIOUS IS IT? A ruptured prepubic tendon can be a serious risk to both the mare and foal, and will negatively impact the mare's ability to support future pregnancies. A mare with even a partially ruptured prepubic tendon should not be rebred.

POTENTIAL COMPLICATIONS. None.

Premature Placental Separation (Red Bag)

WHAT IT IS. The placenta separates from the wall of the uterus before the allantoic fluid is released (water breaks), resulting in loss of oxygen to the foal. This typically occurs at the end of gestation when labor begins, although the placenta can separate in midgestation with the death of a fetal twin or another cause of abortion.

DIAGNOSIS. A premature placental separation is identified by the appearance of a velvety, red mass ("red bag") at the vulva in a mare exhibiting signs of labor.

TREATMENT. The foaling attendant should immediately tear through the placenta if a "red bag" is observed in order to facilitate delivery of the foal before it suffocates from a lack of oxygen.

HOW SERIOUS IS IT? Premature placental separation can have fatal consequences if it is undetected or not corrected.

POTENTIAL COMPLICATIONS. A foal born under a condition of premature placental separation may have signs of oxygen deprivation, including neonatal maladjustment syndrome. (See chapter 17, "The Foal.")

Dystocia   FIGURES 16.15–16.16

WHAT IT IS. The mare is unable to deliver the foal unassisted due to factors such as abnormal positioning or an abnormally large fetus.

DIAGNOSIS. Delivery of a foal does not progress in a timely fashion following the water breaking. In the case of a malpositioned foal, the abnormal position will be identified by palpation and manipulation during attempts to assist delivery.

TREATMENT. The veterinarian will attempt to reposition the foal and assist delivery. This may involve sedating the mare, often to the point of general anesthesia, with the mare positioned with her head downhill to encourage the foal to move forward in the birth canal to make room for repositioning. If the foal cannot be repositioned or pulled following manipulation, a Cesarean section may be necessary.

HOW SERIOUS IS IT? A dystocia has life-threatening consequences for both the mare and foal. Rarely does a Cesarean section result in the birth of a live foal because of the time necessary to transport the mare to a surgical facility. Because timing is so critical, it is essential that foaling attendants call the veterinarian immediately if labor and delivery are not progressing normally.

POTENTIAL COMPLICATIONS. The mare is at risk for uterine infection or trauma to the uterus and birth canal, secondary to manipulation of the foal. Death of the foal is common.

Uterine Artery Rupture

WHAT IT IS. The large uterine artery that supplies blood to the uterus ruptures, most commonly during labor and delivery in older mares. The mare hemorrhages into the abdomen or the ligaments that support the uterus.

DIAGNOSIS. The mare will have a great deal of pain and exhibit colic symptoms which progress to shock, weakness, and collapse. A hematoma (accumulation of blood) may be palpated, or blood might be obtained from a belly tap to confirm a diagnosis.

TREATMENT. Supportive therapy may be attempted, including sedation and pain medications, but most cases there is no effective treatment.

HOW SERIOUS IS IT? The majority of mares that experience a uterine artery rupture will bleed to death.

POTENTIAL COMPLICATIONS. Death.

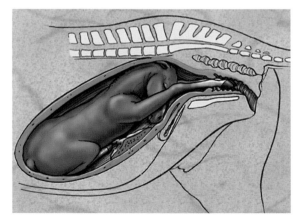

FIGURE 16.15. **A head-back presentation will require repositioning to pull the foal's nose forward in order for the foal to be successfully delivered.**

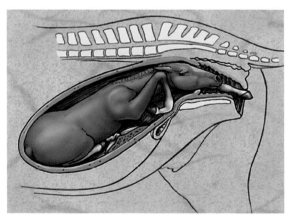

FIGURE 16.16. **A leg-back presentation is common, and the leg must be straightened before the foal can be delivered.**

Special Horses

Retained Placenta

WHAT IT IS. The mare fails to pass the placental membranes within 3 hours following birth.

DIAGNOSIS. A retained placenta will be obvious if placental membranes are still observed hanging from the vulva. During an examination of the placenta following birth, the veterinarian may detect that a piece of the placenta is missing and could have been retained. In this case, the vet will examine the uterus with a gloved hand and/or speculum.

TREATMENT. Initial treatment for a retained placenta is administration of the hormone oxytocin to stimulate contractions of the uterus. Injections of oxytocin may be repeated several times. If the placenta is not expelled, lavage of the uterus with large volumes of fluid will be recommended. Antibiotics and anti-inflammatory medications, such as flunixin meglumine, will usually be prescribed to help minimize complications.

HOW SERIOUS IS IT? A retained placenta can be easily managed with minimal consequences. However, an unrecognized or untreated retained placenta can lead to serious consequences.

POTENTIAL COMPLICATIONS. Endotoxemia with laminitis can result from a retained placenta if toxins are released into the mare's system. Uterine infection is a possible complication.

Perineal Lacerations   FIGURES 16.17–16.20

WHAT IT IS. Trauma and disruption to the perineum (tissues between the rectum and the birth canal) that occur during foaling. Lacerations can involve only the skin and outer layer of tissues (first degree), the middle layer of tissues (second degree), or can extend through all of the layers and penetrate the rectum (third degree).

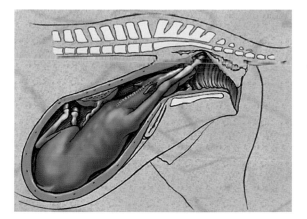

FIGURE 16.17. **This type of orientation of the foal can easily lead to a serious laceration at delivery if the hoof penetrates the rectal wall.**

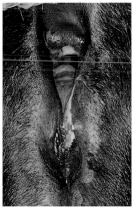

FIGURE 16.18. **Lacerations to the perineal area (tissues between the rectum and the birth canal) can occur.** (Photo courtesy of Jan Palmer, DVM, Diplomate ACVS)

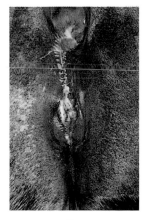

FIGURE 16.19. **Surgery to repair the laceration will usually allow the mare to be bred again.** (Photo courtesy of Jan Palmer, DVM, Diplomate ACVS)

DIAGNOSIS. Perineal lacerations can be identified and evaluated during a physical examination of the mare.

TREATMENT. First and second degree lacerations may require no treatment, whereas some second and all third degree lacerations will require surgical repair. The veterinarian will recommend delaying repair until inflammation of the tissues has had time to quiet down and tissues have healed. Antibiotics and anti-inflammatory medications are usually administered immediately after birth. Surgery will typically be performed to repair the laceration weeks or even months after it occurs.

HOW SERIOUS IS IT? Most perineal lacerations heal or can be repaired so the mare can be bred again, although one breeding season may be lost to allow for surgical repair and healing. Rarely, damage or contamination of the uterus can affect the mare's future fertility.

POTENTIAL COMPLICATIONS. Uterine damage.

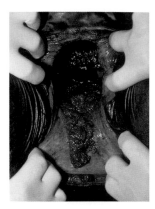

FIGURE 16.20. **Severe perineal lacerations can result in serious contamination of the mare's reproductive tract with fecal material, which can have lasting effects on future fertility.** (Photo courtesy of Lisa Metcalf, DVM Diplomate ACVT)

The Business of Breeding

Breeding Contracts

When breeding with live cover or fresh transported semen, the breeding contract usually has a "live foal guarantee," meaning that you can breed your mare on multiple heat cycles until she becomes pregnant and gives birth to a foal that stands and sucks. In general, contracts cover two or three breeding seasons, and may allow you to substitute mares if you have difficulty getting your mare pregnant. In most cases, you'll be required to pay collection and shipping fees after a certain point.

In many situations frozen semen is sold by the "breeding dose," meaning you'll be required to purchase an additional dose for each insemination. You may also be required to pay handling and shipping fees to obtain the semen. Frozen semen can also be sold with a live foal guarantee, similar to that of fresh transported semen.

Read the contract carefully and be aware of hidden costs. Collection and transport fees can add up over time, significantly adding to your breeding costs. Also pay close attention to the requirements for pregnancy monitoring. If your contract requires palpations or ultrasounds at specific times, you'll need to provide proof of these procedures for the contract to remain valid. If you don't, you could lose your right to another breeding should the pregnancy be lost between conception and foaling.

CHAPTER 17

The Foal

THEN AND NOW

Pliny the Elder, the first-century Roman writer, could determine the sex of a foal by simply turning the mare loose. The mare would either run north or south, depending on the sex of the foal she had conceived.

It's now possible to guarantee the sex of a foal before conception by inseminating the mare with sex-sorted semen. Or, if it's too late for that, the veterinarian can determine the sex with an ultrasound exam after development has begun.

H E'S JUST COME INTO THE WORLD, and his entire future lies ahead. He spends his days in the pasture, sacked out for a nap, nursing, or playing with his buddies. Little does he know that life won't always be so simple. For now, he just needs to grow up and learn the rules. FIGURE 17.1

The life of a foal. He has no worries. His well-being depends on you. In this chapter, we'll outline the important stages of a foal's life, beginning immediately after birth and continuing through his first year. You'll learn what to expect, what can go wrong, and how you should manage problems that should arise.

The First Critical Hours

Because the horse is a prey animal, even a newborn foal must rapidly become as strong and self-sufficient as possible. What follows are events you should plan for during the foal's first hours of life.

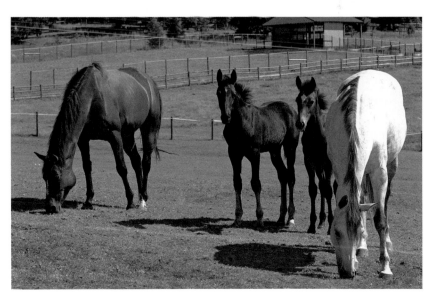

FIGURE 17.1. **These youngsters are growing up in an ideal environment where they can play together and romp in the pasture alongside their dams.**

285

What to Expect

When attending a foaling, it's important to monitor normal events closely, and take immediate action if the new foal's activities don't fall within normal guidelines. The interaction between the mare and foal in the first few hours of life is critical, and the foaling attendant should interfere as little as possible while taking the following necessary steps to insure the well-being of the foal:

- Remove fetal membranes that remain covering the foal's head immediately following birth. It's possible for a newborn foal to suffocate in these membranes if they don't come off naturally during the birth process.

- If the foal is born in cold conditions, he might begin to shiver immediately after birth. Dry him with a towel to help him warm up. An ideal foaling stall will have a heat source (such as a heat lamp) installed in one corner of the stall where the foal can go to keep warm once he's up and moving on his own. When he's first born, however, he'll be wet and unable to stand.   FIGURES 17.2–17.3

- Wait for the umbilical cord to break on its own, which usually happens when the mare stands up following birth. As soon as it breaks, dip the stump of the cord on the foal's belly with an antiseptic solution of either chlorhexadine or betadine. (*Note: Chlorhexadine has been suggested as the ideal choice for dipping the naval by veterinary researchers, although many practitioners still prefer betadine. Ask your vet for his or her preference. In any case, do not use a strong solution of iodine or tincture, which contains alcohol. These substances can scald the foal's sensitive tissues and cause more problems than they prevent.*)

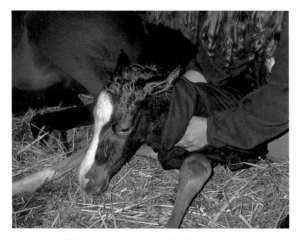

FIGURE 17.2. **If it's cold outside, the foaling attendant can dry the foal with a towel to help him stay warm.** (Photo courtesy of Tina Gilmore)

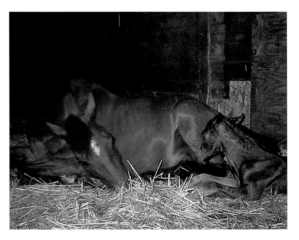

FIGURE 17.3. **The mare and foal may rest quietly for several minutes after birth.** (Photo courtesy of Tina Gilmore)

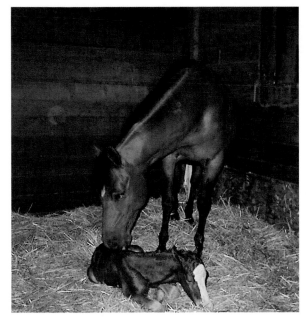

FIGURE 17.4. **Typically, the mare stands first, breaking the umbilical cord when she does. She'll then talk to her foal as the bonding process begins.** (Photo courtesy of Tina Gilmore)

- After the mare stands, her placenta may still be hanging from her vulva. Tie it up with a towel or piece of twine to prevent her from tearing away pieces as she walks around the stall. Once the placenta passes, collect it in a bucket and save it for the veterinarian to examine. If the placenta hasn't passed within three hours of birth, call the veterinarian for advice.

- Observe the mare's attitude toward the foal. A normal mare will whicker and show interest in her baby within minutes of birth—even as the foal is resting with his hind legs still within the birth canal. Once she stands, she'll go to the foal and begin licking and talking to him. If the mare appears disinterested or aggressive toward her baby, call the veterinarian for advice. FIGURE 17.4

- The foal should appear strong, and begin making attempts to stand after approximately 30 minutes. It's appropriate to help him stand the first time, especially if he's having trouble because of wet footing in the stall.

- The foal will begin looking for the udder and trying to nurse soon after he stands up. Make sure the mare will stand quietly and allow him to explore her hindquarters as he searches. Some new mothers will follow the foal in circles, and prevent him from nursing. If this happens, the foaling attendant should halter the mare and hold her still to help the foal get started. If the mare is agitated or aggressive and still won't stand for the foal to nurse, the veterinarian might recommend a tranquilizer to facilitate the process. Acepromazine is a good option because it has the side benefit of stimulating release of the hormone prolactin that also encourages milk letdown and maternal instincts.

- The foal should pass meconium, or the first fecal material, within several hours of birth. This is a black, tarry material that accumulates in the foal's rectum during the end of gestation. If meconium hasn't passed or the foal appears to be straining or uncomfortable, administer an enema to ease the process. A commercially available Fleet enema can be gently inserted into the rectum.

The foaling can be considered a success once the foal is up and nursing, the mare has passed her placenta, and the foal has passed meconium. If all is well, schedule a "well-baby check" with the veterinarian on the day following birth.

TABLE 17.1

The Normal Foal

This table outlines signposts to monitor during the first few hours of life.

SIGNPOST	TIMELINE	WHEN TO WORRY	WHAT TO DO
Suck reflex. The foal will make sucking movements with his mouth spontaneously, or when stimulated by a finger.	Immediately after birth.	If a such reflex isn't present after 15 minutes, especially if the foal seems dull or listless.	Call the vet. An examination is warranted.
Righting reflex The foal attempts to raise his head and rest in a sternal position (sitting up on his chest).	5–10 minutes after birth.	If the foal isn't raising his head attempting to sit up within 10 minutes, especially if a suck reflex is absent.	Call the vet. An examination is warranted.
Standing	The foal should make attempts to stand within 30 minutes of birth and should be able to stand unassisted within 2 hours.	If the foal isn't attempting to stand within 45 minutes, or standing unassisted within 2 hours.	Call the vet. If the foal is strong but struggling, help him to stand and look for the udder in order to begin nursing. Leg disorders such as contracted tendons may make it difficult for an otherwise healthy foal to stand without assistance.
Nursing	1–3 hours.	If attempts to nurse aren't observed by 2 hours, or the foal has not nursed by 3 hours.	Call the vet. The foal is only able to absorb essential antibodies from the colostrum within 6 hours of birth. The vet will want to prepare to administer colostrum, or a commercial colostrum replacement through a nasogastric tube before this critical time elapses.
Passed meconium (Tarry black material that is the first stool, and must be passed from the foal's rectum.)	1–3 hours.	If the foal is straining but not passing any material. If meconium is not observed after 3 hours. If pasty, yellowish stool is not being passed within 12 hours of birth.	Administer an enema. If the foal continues to strain or does not pass meconium within 1 hour, administer a second enema. If meconium still hasn't passed, call the vet.

The Well-Baby Check

A routine well-baby check to examine the mare and foal following birth is recommended by most veterinarians. This examination includes:

- Physical examination of the mare to check for tears or bruising that may have occurred during the birth process, presence of milk in the udders, and general physical condition.

- Physical examination of the foal to check for congenital abnormalities such as a cleft palate, heart murmur, or cataracts, as well as for signs of umbilical abnormalities, swollen joints, limb deformities, or other indications of problems.

- Examination of the placenta to ensure it has been passed in its entirety, and that it appears normal. Placental abnormalities may indicate potential risk factors for the foal that should be monitored.

- Collection of a blood sample to check for IgG or antibodies in the foal's blood, to insure the foal nursed effectively and received adequate protection from the colostrum. A foal that does not have adequate antibody levels is considered to have failure of passive transfer (FPT) and will be more at risk for significant problems such as septicemia. (See chapter 15 for more information on FPT.)

The First Year

After the foal has passed all of the important signposts that mark the first days of life, he enters a period of peaceful existence. He spends long days nursing, napping, and playing with his pasture mates. The ideal lifestyle for a foal during this first year is out in a green-grass pasture where he has room to roam and has shelter from adverse weather conditions. He'll live with his mother until weaning time, which usually occurs at around 6 months of age. Ideally, a group of compatible mares and foals can be kept together to provide companionship for the growing youngsters and a social structure where the foals can begin to learn important behavior skills. When weaning time comes, the foals can stay with their familiar group of friends—a situation that greatly reduces stress during this potentially worrisome event. The following section outlines basic care concerns for the foal during the first year of life.

Nutrition

For most foals nutrition comes from their mother's milk, until approximately 2½ months of age when they begin to rely more on solid food. It's crucial that the mare be fed a diet with adequate protein and balanced minerals to provide for the needs of the growing foal. As with any nutritional advice, specific feeding plans will necessarily vary widely depending on feed available in a given location. In general, however, veterinarians recommend feeding the mare a concentrate ration, in addition to her hay and pasture, that's specifically balanced for lactation, as well as being suitable as a creep feed for the foal when he begins experimenting with solid food. Usually, the foal can simply begin eating alongside his dam, sharing her ration as he makes the transition from milk to solid food. Increased calories will be needed as the foal grows, and should be adjusted based on the weight and condition of both the mare and foal.

Vaccination

The foal's protection against infectious diseases starts with vaccination of the mare. When the mare receives her pre-foaling vaccinations 30 days prior to her anticipated foaling date, her developing colostrum, or first milk, is loaded with antibodies to help her baby fight disease. The newborn foal must nurse within 6 hours of birth in order for the antibody-rich colostrum to be absorbed, and the antibodies he receives in that milk will protect him for his first months of life.

Scheduling of vaccinations in the months that follow birth is complicated by the fact that the maternal antibodies, those antibodies the foal received from the colostrum, will interfere with the ability of the foal's immune system to respond to the vaccine. These antibody levels must wane adequately in order for vaccination to be effective. An additional risk is that too-early vaccination can result in the foal's immune system recognizing the antigen administered as "self," meaning it will never mount an immune response to that specific substance.

To fall within these constraints, vaccination of the foal whose dam was properly vaccinated pre-foaling should begin at approximately 6 to 7 months of age. If the dam was not vaccinated pre-foaling, foal vaccinations should begin sooner in life, at approximately 3 to 4 months of age. A typical vaccination program for a foal born to a mare that was appropriately vaccinated prior to foaling is outlined in Table 17.2. (*Note: Additional vaccinations may be recommended depending on the geographical area. Adjustments in the vaccination program will also be recommended if the mare was not vaccinated pre-foaling. Consult your veterinarian. It has also been recently discovered that maternal antibody interference is not as significant a problem with West Nile virus as it is with other viruses. In areas of high risk, vaccination of foals against West Nile can begin as early as 3 months of age. In addition, the final West Nile vaccination should follow 10 to 12 weeks after the second of the series.*)

Deworming

Beginning at approximately 6 weeks of age, the foal should be dewormed on a regular schedule similar to that outlined for mature horses. (See chapter 2.) Most regularly used deworming medications, including ivermectin, benzimidazoles, and pyrantel pamoate, are safe for foals, and are

TABLE 17.2

A Typical Vaccination Program for a Foal

DISEASE	6 MONTHS	7 MONTHS	8 MONTHS	9 MONTHS	10 MONTHS	11 MONTHS	12 MONTHS
Tetanus	Yes.	Yes.	Yes.				Yes.
Sleeping sickness *(Eastern and Western equine encephalomyelitis, or EWEE)*	Yes.	Yes.	Yes.				Yes.
Influenza						Intranasal.	Yes.
Rhinopneumonitis	Optional.	Optional.	Optional.				Optional.
West Nile virus	Yes.	Yes.			Yes.		Yes.

effective against the major parasites. By the time the foal is 6 months old and reliably eating solid food, he can be started on a daily dewormer containing pyrantel tartrate.

Foot Care

The foal's feet should be trimmed every 6 to 8 weeks to ensure that they stay well balanced and in good condition. Regular trimming offers the additional advantage of regular handling, which will accustom the growing youngster to having his feet handled so that he will behave himself for the farrier in years to come.

Handling and Exercise

The foal should be introduced to the halter and lead within the first week of life. He can be taught basic rules of pressure and be led alongside his dam to facilitate his learning to lead. Once the foal wears the halter willingly and can be led without resistance, good behavior can usually be maintained with a short handling session 2 to 3 times each week. He'll get plenty of exercise living in the pasture. Exercise sessions including lungeing or other structured work are generally not needed or recommended during the first year of life.

Weaning

In a natural environment the foal will often live alongside his dam for a full year—until the birth of a new foal forces independence. With domestic horses, the foal is usually separated from his mother sometime between 4 and 6 months of age. Experts agree that weaning closer to the 6-month mark seems to be less stressful for both the mare and foal. When it's possible, the mare and foal can be separated gradually to reduce stress. For example, they may be kept in separate stalls with a half wall between them at night, and reunited during the day for a period of several weeks before they are completely separated. In many situations a gradual separation isn't practical. If that's the case, the mare will usually be removed from the pasture or paddock, leaving the foal behind in a familiar environment—ideally with his group of same-age playmates to keep him company. The mare and foal should be kept completely out of both sight and hearing during the weaning process. A complete weaning usually takes several weeks, although even after a separation of months a mare and foal can bond again if reunited. It's generally best if the mare and foal can be maintained separately once weaning is completed.

WHEN THINGS GO WRONG

The following are the most common problems seen in foals, up to the first year of life.

Septicemia

WHAT IT IS. Infection of the bloodstream with bacteria. Foals will be at risk for developing septicemia if they don't receive adequate antibodies from the colostrum following birth. In addition, any abnormalities of the pregnancy, such as placentitis, or at the time of birth, such as a dystocia, can put the foal at risk for septicemia. Septic foals will be lethargic and weak and may be unable to stand and nurse.

DIAGNOSIS. Septicemia will be suspected in a foal showing signs at birth, especially if IgG levels are low. A diagnosis may be confirmed with bacteria identified in the bloodstream following culture.

TREATMENT. Treatment requires an appropriate antibiotic targeted against the organisms involved with the infection. If IgG levels are low, plasma transfusions will be recommended to provide the foal with essential antibodies. Feeding through a nasogastric tube may be necessary for foals that are unable to nurse. Twenty-four-hour nursing care is usually necessary to prevent skin injuries in a foal unable to stand. Treatment of secondary problems, such as flushing infected joints, is also often necessary.

HOW SERIOUS IS IT? Septicemia is a very serious problem, one that is often life threatening. Early recognition and aggressive treatment are necessary if the foal is to have a chance at survival.

POTENTIAL COMPLICATIONS. Pneumonia, joint infections, and navel infections are all potential complications of septicemia that can have serious consequences.

Meconium Impaction

WHAT IT IS. The foal is unable to pass the meconium, or waste material, that has accumulated in the rectum during gestation.

DIAGNOSIS. A foal under 24 hours old that is straining to pass manure without success usually has a meconium impaction. The vet can palpate the meconium with a finger inserted into the rectum.

TREATMENT. A series of enemas is generally all that is needed to resolve a meconium impaction. In severe cases, intravenous fluids may be necessary. Rarely will an impacted foal require surgery.

HOW SERIOUS IS IT? Most meconium impactions will be easily resolved with minimal treatment. In the rare case that requires surgery, it becomes a much more serious condition with added risks.

POTENTIAL COMPLICATIONS. A meconium impaction that is not addressed can result in pressure buildup and rupture of intestines—a potentially life-threatening situation.

Patent Urachus

WHAT IT IS. The urachus, or tube within the umbilical cord where urine is eliminated by the fetus before birth, fails to retract and close normally at birth. Urine will continue to flow out of the umbilical stump of the foal and not be passed normally through the urethra.

DIAGNOSIS. A patent urachus can be identified when a foal is observed to have urine dripping from the umbilical stump.

TREATMENT. In mild cases, the urachus can be cauterized and closed using silver nitrate, strong iodine, or other caustic substances on the umbilical opening. If this is not successful, surgery can be performed to correct the problem.

HOW SERIOUS IS IT? Most cases of patent urachus can be resolved with minimal complications.

POTENTIAL COMPLICATIONS. Infection of the umbilicus can accompany a patent urachus.

Umbilical Infection

WHAT IT IS. The umbilical stump becomes infected with bacteria. This can occur if the umbilicus is not treated with an antimicrobial following birth, if the foal has low circulating antibody levels, or if there are other abnormalities of the umbilical stump, such as a patent urachus. The foal may become weak and develop a fever, and the stump may be swollen, hot, and painful.

DIAGNOSIS. An infected umbilicus will be suspected when typical signs are present. A sample taken from the area can help identify the bacteria involved, and ultrasound examination will be recommended to evaluate the depth and extent of infected tissues.

TREATMENT. Mild cases will resolve with antibiotic treatment. If tissues deep within the abdomen are involved, or an abscess (pocket of pus associated with the infection) is identified, surgery may be necessary.

HOW SERIOUS IS IT? A simple umbilical infection is likely to resolve without complications. However, if the foal has a compromised immune system, is lacking antibodies, or the infection is unrecognized until it becomes extensive, serious consequences, including death, can result.

POTENTIAL COMPLICATIONS. Septicemia can develop from an umbilical infection.

Umbilical Hernia FIGURE 17.5

WHAT IT IS. The abdominal muscles do not close properly around the umbilical stump, leaving an opening where intestinal material can protrude through the body wall into a sac of skin.

DIAGNOSIS. An umbilical hernia is easy to identify during a physical examination. The protruding sac will be visible, and it is possible to "reduce" the contents, or push them back into the abdomen through the defect in the body wall.

TREATMENT. Small umbilical hernias (less than 5 centimeters in diameter) will often resolve spontaneously as the foal grows. Surgery will be recommended for larger hernias or for those that do not appear to be resolving after 3 months of age.

HOW SERIOUS IS IT? Most umbilical hernias will be easily managed with minimal risk, even if surgery is required.

POTENTIAL COMPLICATIONS. Rarely, intestinal material can become trapped in the umbilical sac and become damaged.

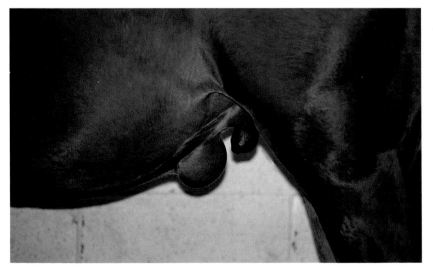

FIGURE 17.5. **This large umbilical hernia will require surgical repair to prevent intestinal material from becoming trapped within the sac of skin below the defect in the body wall.** (Photo courtesy of Jan Palmer, DVM, Diplomate ACVS)

Ruptured Bladder

WHAT IT IS. A tear in the bladder that occurs at birth, resulting in urine leaking out of the bladder into the foal's abdominal cavity. This condition is most common in colts and is believed to happen secondary to pressure during the birth process. The foal will act colicky and may strain to urinate repeatedly without producing a normal flow of urine. His abdomen will appear distended or enlarged.

DIAGNOSIS. A sample of fluid taken from the abdomen will have higher than normal creatinine levels, a component of normal urine. A contrast study—where contrast material is put into the bladder through a catheter, then identified in the abdomen on a radiograph—will confirm the diagnosis.

TREATMENT. Surgery will be recommended to repair the defect in the bladder.

HOW SERIOUS IS IT? A ruptured bladder can cause severe symptoms of colic and electrolyte imbalances that can be dangerous for the foal. If recognized early and taken to surgery, most cases of ruptured bladder will resolve without complications.

POTENTIAL COMPLICATIONS. High potassium levels in the blood can cause the heart rhythm to slow.

Diarrhea

WHAT IT IS. Inflammation of the intestinal tract results in soft or watery manure. Diarrhea can have a number of different causes in foals, including bacteria, viruses, parasites, or simply diet changes. Signs range from severe to mild, depending on the cause (see Table 7.3) and can include colic, fever, weakness, and depression in addition to changes in the consistency of the manure.

DIAGNOSIS. A diagnosis of diarrhea is based on the consistency of the manure. The specific cause may be identified through blood tests or examination and culture of the manure.

TREATMENT. If an underlying cause can be identified, treatments including antibiotics or deworming medications will be directed at the specific organism. Buildup of watery feces on the foal's hindquarters can cause hair loss and skin scalding. Gentle cleaning with warm soapy water and protection of this sensitive skin with a barrier ointment such as Desitin® will be recommended for all cases. If diarrhea is severe, supportive treatment with intravenous fluids may be necessary to help maintain hydration. Antidiarrheal medications such as Maalox® or probiotics may be recommended in all cases to help minimize symptoms.

HOW SERIOUS IS IT? Diarrhea can range from a mild, self-limiting problem to a life-threatening one depending on the underlying cause.

POTENTIAL COMPLICATIONS. Severe diarrhea can result in dehydration, toxicity, and even death.

TABLE 17.3

Causes of Foal Diarrhea

CAUSE	TYPICAL ONSET	SYMPTOMS	DIAGNOSIS	SPECIFIC TREATMENT
Foal heat diarrhea (Exact cause unknown)	Appears between 5 and 14 days of age.	Loose, watery manure with minimal other symptoms.	Assumed cause of diarrhea in foals at this age with no other signs.	None necessary.
Rotavirus	Observed in groups of foals up to 3 months of age.	Fever, depression, and watery diarrhea with a duration of up to 12 days.	Virus can be detected in manure in 1/3 of cases. Suspected in groups where virus is known to exist.	None necessary. Supportive care may be required.
Necrotizing enteritis (Clostridium perfringens type C)	Acute onset, often in very young foals. (Mare may be a carrier.)	Profuse, watery diarrhea may be bloody. Severe colic symptoms, depression. Foal may be unable to stand. Death is common.	Bacteria can be identified in manure.	Muzzle to prevent nursing to minimize exposure from mare. Supportive care necessary.
Parasites (Strongyloides westeri)	Appears between 8 and 12 days of age. (Passed to foal through mare's udder.)	Loose, watery manure with minimal other symptoms.	Parasite can be identified in feces.	Ivermectin treatment of the mare to reduce larvae in udder.
Protazoa (Cryptosporidium sp.)	Most commonly occurs in otherwise sick or compromised foals.	Loose, watery manure with minimal other symptoms. Duration 5 to 14 days.	Organism can be seen in feces of both normal and infected foals, so is not diagnostic.	Supportive care will be needed in addition to treatment of primary problem. (Organism can infect humans, so care should be taken when handling affected foals.)

Rhodococcus Equi Pneumonia

WHAT IT IS. An infection caused by the bacterial organism *Rhodococcus equi* that most commonly affects foals between the ages of 2 and 6 months. The organism lives in the GI tract of mature horses, and may be found in the environment after having been passed in the feces, where it can live for up to a year. It prefers hot, dusty conditions, making this type of environment the greatest risk. Foals receive antibodies against this organism from the colostrum, which generally protects them for the first 2 months of life at which time the maternal antibody levels decline. They then become susceptible to the organism, which can be concentrated in their GI tract as they ingest manure, or can enter through the lungs in dry, dusty conditions. Manure is the major source of contamination.

Foals with *Rhodococcus equi* infection may slowly develop signs that include coughing, abnormal breathing, and sometimes diarrhea. Some foals may also have swollen, painful joints due to inflammation that can accompany the disease. The organism causes large abscesses to form in the lungs as the disease develops. These abscesses develop very slowly, which is why signs may be insidious and not apparent until the disease becomes severe.

DIAGNOSIS. *Rhodococcus equi* may be suspected in foals showing typical signs, especially on farms where the organism is known to cause problems. Blood work will increase suspicion if there is a high white blood count indicative of infection, particularly if it is accompanied by a very high fibrinogen level—an indicator of inflammation that often elevates with the presence of abscesses. Diagnosis is confirmed if the organism can be cultured from samples taken from the respiratory tract. Radiographs or ultrasound of the lungs may help the vet to identify abscesses and the degree of lung involvement in order to determine the severity of the infection.

It is important to know that detection of antibodies against the organism in a blood test is not sufficient to make a diagnosis of the disease because many foals will have antibodies either from the colostrum, or due to exposure to the organism.

TREATMENT. Successful treatment of the disease depends on early diagnosis prior to the time when abscesses are firmly established. The most commonly recommended antibiotic regimen includes a combination of the antibiotics rifampin (5 mg/kg 2 to 3 times daily) and erythromycin estolate (25 mg/kg 2 to 4 times daily) for a period of 6 to 8 weeks. The long treatment time is necessary to ensure complete penetration and resolution of abscesses in the lungs. Very sick foals may require supportive treatment with intravenous fluids in the early stages of the disease. In addition, administration of plasma primed with large amounts of antibody against the *R. equi* organism has been recommended by some practitioners, and may be helpful in severe cases.

The key to successful treatment is prevention. Minimizing dust in the environment by maintaining grass pastures and removing manure will help greatly. The *R. equi* organism is everywhere. Veterinary researchers have isolated the organism from as many as 75 percent of farms investigated where mares and foals congregate. Farms that have problems with infection are likely to have a more virulent strain of the bacteria on the property, and management conditions may make disease a likely consequence of exposure. There is no vaccination currently available against this disease.

HOW SERIOUS IT? *Rhodococcus equi* can be a very serious disease. Mortality rates in one study were as high as 80 percent before treatment with rifampin and erythromycin was available. With treatment with these antibiotics, however, as many as 88 percent of foals in one study survived, even once pneumonia was established. If the disease can be recognized and treated early and appropriately, the outcome is most likely to be favorable.

POTENTIAL COMPLICATIONS. If severe disease develops and abscesses are well developed and accompanied by scarring, foals may experience lung damage that can affect their breathing ability, even after successful treatment. This can limit usefulness in some performance disciplines. In addition, treatment with erythromycin can cause severe diarrhea in some foals.

Developmental Orthopedic Disease (DOD)   FIGURES 17.6–17.9

WHAT IT IS. A variety of different conditions of the musculoskeletal system that affect young horses and are related to bone and joint development. The most common components of this disease complex are osteochondrosis, angular limb deformities, flexural limb deformities, and epiphysitis. (See Table 17.4.) These conditions are related in that they can all be linked to a variety of different causes, including genetics, nutrition, and environmental conditions.

DIAGNOSIS. Developmental orthopedic diseases will generally be identified based on the physical appearance of the foal, and specifically evaluated using radiographs.

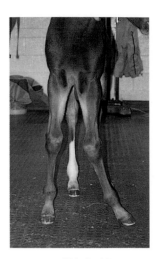

FIGURE 17.6. **This foal has a valgus-type angular limb deformity of the left front leg that is unlikely to correct itself with conservative treatment.** (Photo courtesy of Jan Palmer, DVM, Diplomate ACVS)

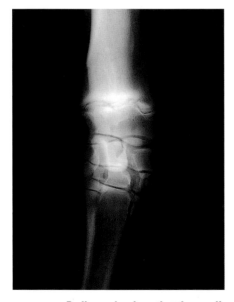

FIGURE 17.7. **Radiographs show that the small bones within the knee itself have developed normally, and the deformity originates primarily from the growth plate.** (Photo courtesy of Jan Palmer, DVM, Diplomate ACVS)

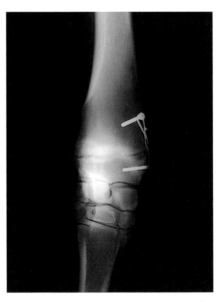

FIGURE 17.8. **Screws and wires surgically placed across the more rapidly growing side will slow growth and allow the limb to straighten.** (Photo courtesy of Jan Palmer, DVM, Diplomate ACVS)

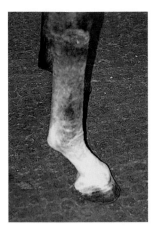

TREATMENT. Specific treatments vary for the different conditions. In all cases, a dietary evaluation will be recommended and adjustments made to balance trace minerals, calcium, phosphorus levels, and overall energy level.

HOW SERIOUS IS IT? The developmental orthopedic diseases can have serious implications on the future soundness of an affected foal.

POTENTIAL COMPLICATIONS. Permanent unsoundness can result from many of the conditions in the DOD complex.

FIGURE 17.9. **This upright foot conformation, or clubfoot, will be the end result if a flexural limb deformity (contracted tendon) can't be corrected.** (Photo courtesy of Jan Palmer, DVM, Diplomate ACVS)

TABLE 17.4

Summary of Developmental Orthopedic Disease in Foals

CONDITION	OSTEOCHONDROSIS	ANGULAR LIMB DEFORMITIES	FLEXURAL LIMB DEFORMITIES (CONTRACTED TENDONS)	EPIPHYSITIS
What it is	A defect that occurs during development of the joints, leading to cartilage abnormalities on the joint surface or development of cysts below the joint surface.	Deviations or crookedness of the legs, either knock-kneed (valgus deformity) or bow-legged (varus deformity).	Buckling forward of the front or hind limbs that can be present at birth (congenital) or develop over time (acquired). Contracted tendons can occur as a response to another painful condition of the limbs, such as osteochondrosis or epiphysitis.	Inflammation of the growth plates where growth of long bones occurs
Symptoms	A foal with osteochondrosis may have joint swelling and lameness associated with the involved joint. Radiographs will usually confirm a diagnosis.	Visual crookedness of the front or hind limbs. Radiographs can help determine where the defect is coming from, and identify cases where lack of development of the small bones in the knees and hocks is present.	Visual buckling forward of the limbs, usually involving the knees, fetlocks, and front feet of the forelimbs, or fetlocks and feet behind. If the foot is affected, radiographs can show whether there is an abnormal shape and orientation of the coffin bone (clubfoot).	Enlargement, heat, and pain during palpation of the affected growth plate will be observed. Lameness may be present. Radiographs will help determine the degree of growth plate inflammation.

Continued on Page 300.

Specific treatment	Recommendations will vary, depending on the joint involved, and severity of the lesions seen on radiographs. Surgery will be recommended in many cases. Anti-inflammatory treatments, injection of affected joints with anti-inflammatory medications, and medications that promote joint health may be recommended (e.g., Legend®, Adequan®).	Many cases respond well to restricted exercise with or without support wraps or splints. This takes stress off the growth plates and allows the limbs to straighten as they grow. Surgical corrections may be recommended, including periosteal transaction (periosteal stripping) to relieve tension on the shorter side of the deformity, or physeal bridging to restrict growth on the longer side of the deformity.	Congenital flexural limb deformities often respond well to physical therapy, restricted exercise, and support with bandages, splints, or casts during the first weeks of life. Regular trimming to lower the heels and protection against wear of the toe can help prevent the development of a clubfoot. In severe cases, surgery to cut a small supporting ligament of the lower limb, called the distal check ligament, may be recommended.	Epiphysitis is often associated with dietary imbalances, and adjustments in the ration will be recommended. Weight loss will be advised for an overweight youngster. Nonsteroidal anti-inflammatories will be recommended in the initial stages to decrease inflammation and pain.
Prognosis	Varies with the joint involved and severity of the lesion. Osteochondrosis can lead to development of arthritis due to instability of the affected joint, even when surgery is performed.	Many mild cases are self-limiting, and respond to conservative treatment with no complications. Surgery is usually successful at correcting more severe deformities.	Mild cases will often respond to conservative treatment with no long-term ill effects. If a clubfoot develops, permanent asymmetry will be present and lameness associated with the coffin bone, coffin joint, or deep digital flexor tendon is common.	Most cases of epiphysitis can be successfully managed if recognized and treated early.

CHAPTER 18

The Performance Horse

H E'S 10 YEARS OLD, and works hard for a living. For 6 days a week, he's groomed, tacked up, and worked—either in a training session or some form of conditioning. Day 7, although a day of rest, probably involves hand walking or maybe even a light trail ride. Twice a month during the season he's off to a competition. More hard work, long trailer rides, and an unfamiliar environment.

That's the life of a performance horse. And no matter what the discipline, these horses share one thing in common. Hard work. In this chapter, we'll outline what you should expect as the owner of an equine athlete, so you can meet his needs.   FIGURE 18.1

What to Expect

Is owning a performance horse just like owning any other horse? Not necessarily. These horses are kept in prime condition, and a couple of days of confinement without work is likely to produce a horse that's crawling out of his skin with excess energy. That's why attention must be paid to his exercise schedule and care, even during nontraining days.

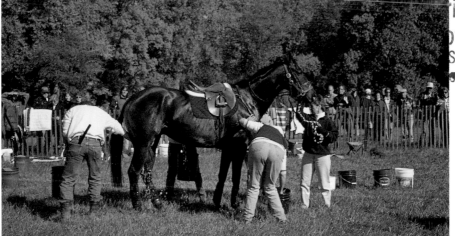

FIGURE 18.1. **The high-level performance horse leads a stressful life, often requiring a team of people to keep him healthy and performing at his best.** (Photo courtesy of Mark Revenaugh, DVM)

A performance horse also lives a high-stress lifestyle compared to his pleasure horse counterpart—both in terms of the physical demands of work and the emotional toll of travel and competition. Care must be taken to recognize these stressors and minimize their negative impact.

Special Needs

Nutrition

Monitoring the performance horse's feeding plan is vital. The following factors should be considered when formulating his ration.

Protein

The performance horse requires between 9 and 11 percent protein in his diet to ensure he has the necessary building blocks to keep his muscles functioning properly. This can be accomplished by feeding good-quality grass hay with a known protein content of at least 10 percent, perhaps with a small amount of alfalfa hay to increase protein levels slightly.

Forage

The performance horse should have plenty of hay or pasture to allow him to spend as much time eating as possible. More foraging time reduces risks for gastric ulcers, a common plague of high-level performance horses. In a stall-kept horse, hay should be fed at least 3 to 4 times per day.

Minimize carbohydrates

Grain really isn't needed in a horse's diet—even that of a hardworking horse. In fact, most studies agree that high-grain diets are detrimental.

Fat

Addition of fat to the diet has been shown to be beneficial, especially if a horse is prone to muscle disorders. Adding oil to a performance horse's ration is the simplest way to meet fat requirements, with the goal of 10 percent of the daily calories supplied as fat. Approximately 2 cups per day for a 1000-pound horse should accomplish this goal. In general, the type of oil is not significant, although horses seem to be more willing to eat corn oil or other vegetable-based oils than animal-based oil sources. Like all other feed changes, oil should be added to the ration gradually, beginning with ¼ cup per day, and by increments of ¼ cup per week until the goal of 2 cups is reached. If a horse won't eat oil provided on grain, rice bran or other high-fat supplements can be given. Studies have shown that horses fed fat-supplemented diets have better endurance.

Supplements

Supplements are often an important component of a performance horse's ration. Depending on the risks of the specific sport or problems the individual horse has experienced, these supplements may include chondroitin/glucosamine joint supplements, biotin supplements to help maintain hoof health, or electrolytes, to name just a few.

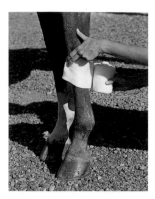

FIGURE 18.2. **Polo wraps are a popular method for leg protection, but must be applied properly to avoid injury. To begin, place the end of the bandage with its center even with the bottom of the horse's knee, at an angle that will allow you to spiral the bandage around the leg.**

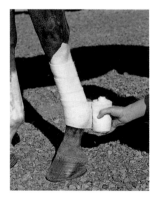

FIGURE 18.3. **Begin spiraling downward around the leg, overlapping each layer by half the width of the bandage. Apply just enough pressure so the bandage is snug, but not too tight, around the leg. You should just be able to slip one finger comfortably under the finished bandage.**

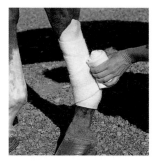

FIGURE 18.4. **When you reach the fetlock, pass the bandage behind this joint and begin angling upward on the other side. This will create a sling-like effect under the joint, at the same time allowing you to spiral back up the leg to finish the bandage.**

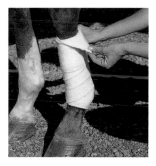

FIGURE 18.5. **When you reach the top, fold the small tab of bandage down over the top of your first layer of spirals. Then, wrap around it with the remainder of your bandage.**

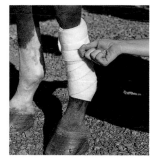

FIGURE 18.6. **Secure the bandage with the Velcro tab. The completed bandage should be smooth and snug around the horse's leg.**

Soundness

Not only is soundness critical for success, a performance horse is more at risk for both acute injury and chronic wear and tear from accumulated stress. The following strategies will help reduce those risks.

Shoeing

Regular shoeing by a competent farrier is one of the most important components to maintaining soundness. Most hard working horses will require regular farrier appointments every 4 to 6 weeks to ensure feet stay well balanced.

Various traction devices or other shoeing modifications might be recommended for specific athletic disciplines.

Footing

Good footing is essential for maintaining soundness—particularly for horses involved in disciplines where repetitive movement is an aspect (such as dressage) or where high impact plays a role (such as jumping). Although specific footing requirements will vary with the discipline, all footing where regular work is performed should be solid and consistent. A single step into an unexpected deep area or hole can be enough to cause an injury.

Conditioning

A prudent conditioning program helps maintain soundness by minimizing the effects of fatigue and ensuring that the horse has the strength he needs to perform what's asked of him. Most conditioning programs involve a certain amount of long, slow distance work—often accomplished with long walk sessions—to help strengthen without stress. Sport-specific exercises on hard work days help train the horse's muscles for the particular demands of his discipline. A typical schedule might include one day of conditioning work, a light training day, and a hard training day. This would be followed by a day of rest or light work, such as a trail ride. During competition season, schedules will also be adjusted over the weeks to ensure that the horse's training and conditioning peak at the appropriate times.

Leg protection FIGURES 18.2–18.6

Most horses in hard work should be outfitted in some type of leg protection during work sessions. Simple splint boots or polo wraps will help prevent interference injuries, while more supportive boots may be suggested under some conditions. Again, the leg protection used will depend on the demands of the specific sport, and vary widely.

Joint maintenance

Degenerative joint disease is one of the most common and career-threatening problems faced by the owner of a performance horse. And there is a huge selection of options to help prevent this problem. A schedule of joint maintenance supplementation may include any number of the following components.

The Performance Horse

HYALURONIC ACID (LEGEND®/BAYER). This FDA-approved medication consists of a polysaccharide present in normal joint fluid that helps protect and lubricate joint cartilage and soft tissues. It is normally secreted by both synoviocytes (cells that make up the joint lining or synovium) and chondrocytes (cells that make up the cartilage at the joint surface). The medication is administered intravenously, and is a well-documented, effective treatment for diagnosed joint disease that helps stop acute damage before it becomes chronic.

Although the efficacy of IV hyaluronic acid administered for the prevention of joint disease is not completely established, it's commonly accepted that this medication can help prevent joint damage by maintaining adequate levels of hyaluronic acid within the joints to prevent acute injuries from causing long-term damage. Many high-level performance horses receive this medication at regular intervals, on average every 4 to 8 weeks.

POLYSULFATED GLYCOSAMINOGLYCAN (ADEQUAN®/LUITPOLD). This FDA-approved medication has anti-inflammatory effects that minimize the heat, swelling, and pain associated with joint damage. When inflammation occurs, it blocks the destructive enzymes released during the inflammatory process—halting inflammation in its tracks and minimizing the breakdown of joint fluid and cartilage that occurs following injury. It also stimulates the joint lining to produce new, thick joint fluid for lubrication and nutrition. Studies show that Adequan® reaches the joint fluid within 2 hours of intramuscular injection.

Like hyaluronic acid, the efficacy of PSGAGs administered to prevent joint disease is not completely established. However, it's reasonable to believe this medication would be beneficial for prevention, and many high-level performance horses receive it at intervals of 4 to 8 weeks, often timed just prior to a competitive event when anti-inflammatory effects may be most beneficial.

ORAL SUPPLEMENTS (CHONDROITIN SULFATE AND GLUCOSAMINE SULFATE/HYDROCHLORIDE). These large molecules make up components of healthy joint cartilage and are available as supplements purported to help prevent degenerative joint disease. It is important to recognize a number of facts when it comes to these supplements.

- They are not FDA-approved medications, meaning there has been no solid research supporting their efficacy, proper dosing, or potential toxicity. In addition, there is no regulation regarding their manufacture or labeling. Instead, they are marketed as "nutriceuticals" in the United States, with no guarantee of their effectiveness for treating or preventing joint disease.

- Although there are studies that document absorption from the GI tract in both dogs and humans, there is uncertainty about the ability of the horse to absorb these substances. That means it's not clear how much of these supplements—or if any—actually reaches the joints in order to have an effect. In fact, estimates are that as little as 10 percent of chondroitin sulfate is absorbed from the horse's intestines. Glucosamine (two forms exist, glucosamine hydrochloride and glucosamine sulfate) is a smaller molecule, so absorption of this substance is likely to be better. However, glucosamine is broken down into its component sugars in the liver unless a large enough dose is administered. It's estimated that a dose of 10 grams or more of glucosamine will allow 30 percent of this substance to pass through the liver without breakdown in order to reach the cartilage. In addition, chondroitin sulfate may be broken down into smaller molecules prior to absorption, contributing to the number of molecules that may be able to reach the joints.

- In spite of questions about absorption, efficacy, and labeling, joint supplements containing chondroitin sulfate and glucosamine appear to have some benefit for horses that is supported by clinical field trials and anecdotal reports. Although FDA-approved medications such as Legend® and Adequan® have more proven benefits, oral supplements are a common component of many performance horse programs. In summary, supplements containing a combination of chondroitin sulfate and glucosamine have the best chance of being effective, and a dose of at least 10 grams of glucosamine should be administered.

Alternative Therapies

It takes a team to keep a performance horse at his peak. Depending on his needs, this would include rider, trainer, veterinarian, farrier, as well as sport horse therapists. Regular therapy sessions ranging from chiropractic manipulations, acupuncture, and massage therapy or bodywork are often part of the working horse's life—particularly if he suffers from physical problems that might limit his performance without ongoing maintenance.

WHEN THINGS GO WRONG

There are a number of diseases most likely to affect the performance horse. The following will refer you to appropriate sections of the preceding chapters for detailed information.

- Degenerative joint disease (musculoskeletal system, page 81).
- Tendonitis/desmitis (musculoskeletal system, pages 87 and 88).
- Equine gastric ulcer syndrome (gastrointestinal tract, page 107).
- Pneumonia/pleuritis (respiratory tract, page 149).
- Viral respiratory disease(respiratory tract, pages 152 and 153).

TABLE 18.1

On the Road

Transport ranks high in the number of causes of stress in the performance horse. Many horses travel multiple times each week, or over periods of many days, to reach distant competitive destinations. Most horses are transported either by trailer or airplane. This Table outlines sources of stress during trailering and gives tips to reduce transport risks.

STRESSOR	PROBLEMS CAUSED	STRESS-REDUCTION TIPS
Poor ventilation	Respiratory problems, both inflammatory (allergic) and infectious (viral or bacterial). Overheating if lack of ventilation causes the trailer to become too hot.	Open all possible windows and vents. Avoid bedding the trailer floor. Bedding only creates additional dust that can act as a respiratory irritant. (Not only that, if left on a wood floor it can contribute to floorboard rotting.) Maintain current vaccination against common respiratory illnesses such as influenza to reduce risk of contracting a virus. Ask the vet about administration of an immune system–stimulating medication prior to transport that can help reduce risk of contracting an infectious disease.
Overheating	Heat stress in extreme conditions. Dehydration leading to colic or other problems.	Don't blanket the horse in the horse trailer. Even if it's cold outside, he'll stay warm enough. Open all vents and windows to allow airflow and maintain cool temperature.
Dehydration	Colic due to impaction if dried feed material balls up in the intestines. Susceptibility to other diseases such as infections due to physical imbalances.	Offer water every 2–3 hours when on the road. Add a tablespoon of powdered lemonade or Kool-Aid to at-home water sources, then continue when you're on the road. This will help maintain a familiar flavor in the water to encourage the horse to drink. Feed soaked hay or bran mashes at rest stops along the way. If you know your horse won't drink and he'll be transported during hot weather, ask your vet whether it would be advisable to tube him with water and electrolytes before you depart.
Trauma	Lacerations, abrasions, or other injuries.	Outfit the horse in protective leg bandages whenever you are hauling. Most injuries occur during loading and unloading, so bandages or boots should be used even for short distances. If the horse doesn't tie well outside of the trailer, don't tie him when you're hauling. Most horses can be safely transported untied. Outfit your horse in a head bumper to protect his poll area from trauma. Drive safely and slowly. Perform regular trailer maintenance, including checking floors, brakes, and wheel bearings to minimize risk of accidents.

CHAPTER 19

The Geriatric

THEN AND NOW

Geriatric medicine was unheard of in years past. The teenage horse was often no longer able to perform the duties required of him and when the end of life approached, euthanasia might have been performed. However, barbiturate injections were considered too expensive for use in the horse. Magnesium sulfate was a less expensive and in his *Veterinary Pharmacology and Therapeutics* text, Iowa State professor L. Meyer Jones suggests that it could be obtained from the household of the client during an emergency call. Not a likely request from a veterinarian today.

As the horse transitioned from working animal to family pet, attention to conditions affecting the older horse became important. With the introduction of senior feeds, advanced dental care, and more sophisticated diagnostic tools and treatments, a horse can live well into his thirties. And when it's time to make the end-of-life decision, the veterinarian will come with his own supply of medications.

H E'S 27, AND HAS EARNED HIS RETIREMENT. He lives in a big green pasture with a loafing shed for shelter. Most days he's just expected to hang out and enjoy life, but a couple of times a week he takes the grandkids for a trail ride.

That's the life of the geriatric horse. Some may work a little harder, and some may simply be retired. But most of these deserving old-timers still require a little extra care to keep them healthy. In general, a horse can be considered geriatric when he reaches age 16. In this chapter we'll outline the special needs of the geriatric horse, including basic management requirements and strategies to meet them.

What to Expect   FIGURE 19.1

The older horse will begin to show his age in a number of different ways. Just like people, some horses show their age a little sooner than others—often depending on the care they receive. Look for the following physical changes that indicate your horse is aging:

- **GRAYING HAIR.** Older horses will begin to show gray hairs—first over the eyes and around the muzzle, and later over other parts of the body.

- **LONGER HAIR-COAT.** Many horses begin to grow a longer, thicker hair-coat as they age. Although they still shed during warmer months, even their summer coat is heavier than that of their younger counterparts. If this long hair-coat is excessive, begins to curl, or fails to shed, the old-timer could be developing Cushing's disease, a hormonal abnormality that's common in older horses.

- **LOSS OF MUSCLE TONE.** An older horse may begin to lose muscling over his back and hindquarters, often accompanied by a swaying back and pendulous belly. This can be a completely normal physical change, but it might indicate the need for changes in his care. Confirm that he's getting enough protein in his diet. A horse won't use protein as efficiently as he ages, which can cause him to look more swaybacked and potbellied than he should. A loss of muscle tone is another possible sign of Cushing's disease, so ask your vet if this change in physique is extreme.

Behavior changes are another part of the aging process, and a horse is likely to become more settled as he ages. He's less likely to spook or resist requests from handlers because he's "seen it all." It's this maturity that makes an older horse the ideal mount for children or beginning riders.

However, physical problems can cause an older horse to become more difficult. For example, a horse with Cushing's disease may become aggressive, and a horse with arthritis may become resistant to work. If you detect behavior changes, such as depression, schedule an examination by your vet to ensure there's nothing physically amiss. In fact, an annual geriatric examination is something to consider once a horse reaches 16.

Special Needs

Even a healthy older horse will face physical challenges, and may require special care. The following are some areas of particular concern in caring for an aging horse.

Nutrition

Old age brings on a number of changes in the horse's nutritional requirements. Most important, his intestinal tract will not function as efficiently, making it more difficult for him to digest his feed to make use of energy and protein. His ability to absorb and process vitamins and minerals also changes. Specifically, the aged horse will experience reduced digestion of fiber, protein and phosphorus.

To accommodate his nutritional needs, he should be fed a diet that consists of 12 to 14 percent protein, 0.3 to 0.4 percent phosphorus, and 0.6 to 0.8 percent calcium. In addition, the feed supplied should be in a highly digestible form, such as good-quality hay with minimal stems or in a processed pellet. If weight management becomes difficult, up to 2 cups of vegetable oil can be added to his daily ration.

The simplest way to achieve good nutrition in an older horse is by providing a commercial feed or "senior diet" designed to meet his needs. These products can either be fed in addition to hay and pasture, or as a complete feed if the old-timer can no longer chew effectively.

Dentistry

As the horse matures, his teeth continue to erupt to permit the grinding necessary to process feed. Eventually, the "reserve crown," or portion of the tooth buried under the gum, is expired or "used up." Although this generally doesn't occur until the mid to late 20s, it will affect the horse's ability to chew. In addition, the exposed teeth become smaller in diameter as they erupt, resulting in spaces between the teeth that are prone to

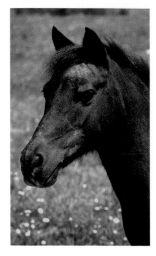

FIGURE 19.1. **These gray hairs over the eyes are a part of the aging process, as is the wisdom that accompanies them.**

Special Horses

infection. Finally, tooth loss is more likely to occur as a horse ages, compromising his dental balance and his ability to chew.

To identify and correct problems an annual or biannual dental examination is advisable. Eventually, problems may not be correctable, making it important to know when feeding should consist entirely of a moistened, pelleted ration that can be easily digested without excessive chewing.

Musculoskeletal Disorders

Many horses will experience problems with bones and joints as they age and become arthritic. In addition, laminitis is more common especially if the horse suffers from a metabolic abnormality such as Cushing's disease.

To keep an older horse comfortable if he's no longer working, it's critical that he get regular daily exercise. He should be maintained on a regular trimming schedule with the farrier every 6 to10 weeks. Corrective shoeing to manage specific problems may be neccessary.

Dietary supplements—those containing glucosamine and condroitin sulfate and MSM—focused on maintaining joint health may help manage arthritic conditions. The veterinarian may recommend regular treatment with intravenous hyaluronic acid (Legend®), polysulfated glycosaminoglycans (Adequan®) for managing conditions of degenerative joint disease, or even nonsteroidal anti-inflammatories such as phenylbutazone to help keep the horse comfortable.

Basic Care

Even if the older horse is no longer being used, his basic health care program must be maintained. He should be checked on daily, even if he's retired to pasture. He should continue on a regular vaccination and deworming program, and should have adequate shelter. These factors may become even more important as the horse ages and his immune system becomes compromised, putting him more at risk for contracting diseases or falling victim to internal parasites.

WHEN THINGS GO WRONG

There are a number of diseases most likely to affect the geriatric horse. The following will refer you to appropriate sections of the preceding chapters for detailed information.

- Degenerative joint disease, pages 4 and 81.
- GI neoplasia, pages 5 and 118.
- Cushing's disease, page 12, 223, and 224.
- Periodontal disease, pages 14 and 250.
- Colic due to strangulating lipoma, pages 108 and 113.

The End of Life

Every owner of an older horse wonders when the end will come. It's natural to worry about how it will happen, and what steps should be taken to make it as peaceful as possible for a faithful companion. Of course, it's always easiest if a horse, well along in years, dies on his own and is found resting peacefully in a pasture. Sadly, that rarely happens. Instead, the owner of an older horse is likely to be faced with the tough decision of when it's time to have the veterinarian perform a euthanasia. The following are some common scenarios that might mean the end is near.

- The horse is down and unable to rise. Many older horses will begin having difficulty getting up and down—until the day when it's no long possible for the horse to stand. If a geriatric horse is unable to get up with urging from family members and the veterinarian, euthanasia is usually the most humane choice.

- Surgical colic. If an older horse experiences a colic that doesn't respond to medical treatment, surgery may not be an option. Of course, an older horse in good physical condition may still be a surgical candidate. However, if the horse is very old and has other significant health conditions, euthanasia may be recommended.

- Laminitis that's not responding well to treatment. This extremely painful condition can be impossible to manage, especially if it's complicated by other diseases such as Cushing's. In these cases, the horse will live in pain for the rest of his life. Once it has progressed to the point where the horse can no longer be kept comfortable, euthanasia is often the most humane decision.

Once the difficult decision to schedule euthanasia is reached, arrangements must be made for the body. In some areas, it's possible to bury a horse on country property, and many owners choose this option. Private cremation is also becoming more available, although this option is expensive and may be difficult to arrange. By far, the most common choice is to have the horse's body picked up by a rendering company that will process it to produce products.

The decision is made, arrangements coordinated, and an appointment set with the veterinarian. What's next? When the veterinarian arrives, he may decide to sedate the horse if he feels it will make things easier. Then he will administer an overdose of a general anesthetic (usually sodium pentobarbital) directly into the horse's bloodstream. The anesthetic works quickly. Within seconds, the horse's eyes will glaze over and he'll no longer be aware of his surroundings. It may be a minute or more before he drops to the ground, and even longer before his heart stops beating. The veterinarian will monitor the process, and tell you when the heart has stopped. It's a quick and painless procedure that can be the kindest thing you'll do to help protect your beloved companion from pain and suffering.

Appendices

◆

Glossary

Abduction. Moving away from the body.

Abrasion. An injury to the skin or mucous membranes that has been rubbed or scraped but does not completely penetrate to deeper tissues.

Acquired. Describes a condition that develops after birth (not inherited).

Acute. Describes condition that occurs suddenly and often has severe symptoms.

Adduction. Moving toward the body.

Adjuvant. A substance that's given with a drug or medication to increase its effectiveness. Adjuvants are commonly used in the preparation of vaccines.

Agonist. When referring to muscle action, a muscle that contracts to move a body part and is countered by the activity of another muscle (the antagonist). When referring to medications, a drug that has an affinity for specific receptors in the body to exert its effect.

Anaphylaxis. A reaction of the immune system to a foreign substance that results in the release of substances that cause exaggerated responses ranging from localized swelling to sudden shock, difficulty breathing, or even death.

Antimicrobial. Suppressing or destroying microorganisms which can include bacteria, fungi, or viruses. Specific substances having antimicrobial activity may be referred to as antibacterials, antivirals, or antifungals.

Antibody. A molecule that is produced by the immune system in response to a foreign substance (including viruses and bacteria). Antibodies attach themselves to these foreign proteins and help the body destroy them to rid the body of disease.

Antigen. Any substance that stimulates an immune system response. Antigens can be toxins, bacteria, or viruses.

Ataxia. Loss of coordination and the awareness of the position of the limbs. The ataxic horse will stagger, stumble, and may even fall when asked to move.

Auscultation. Listening, usually with a stethoscope, to sounds within the body, such as the heart beating or movement of the gastrointestinal tract.

Autosomal. Relates to the non–sex determining chromosomes, or genetic material inherited from the parents.

Bacterial. Describes a condition that involves bacterial organisms.

Biopsy. A sample taken from a tissue in the body for microscopic evaluation.

Bursa. A fluid-filled sac that is present in areas of the body where cushioning or a reduction of friction between structures is needed.

Caudal. At or near the tail-end of the body.

Chronic. Describes condition that has persisted for a long period of time.

Colic. Abdominal pain that can arise from any structure within the abdomen including the gastrointestinal tract, kidneys, liver, or urinary bladder. Commonly used to refer to conditions of the intestines in the horse.

Congenital. Describes condition that is present at the time of birth.

Contamination. Invasion of any location by dirt, debris, microbes, or other undesirable substances. Often used to refer to a wound or other injury.

Cranial. Toward the head.

Creep feed. Feed provided to foals prior to weaning.

Culture. Cultivation or growth of a microorganism to determine a specific cause of disease. For example, a sample taken from a diseased area of the body (such as a wound) would be cultured in a laboratory to determine what specific organism is present, and what medications would be most effective for treatment.

Cytology. Evaluation of cells under a microscope. Cytology is performed on samples taken from the body in order to help make a diagnosis of a specific abnormality.

Degenerative. Describes condition that deteriorates over time.

Desmitis. Inflammation or injury to a ligament.

Developmental. Describes condition that occurs during stages of growth.

Diagnosis. Determination of the nature or cause of a disease.

Distal. Farthest away from the central axis of the body.

Dorsal. Near the back or vertebral side of the body.

Efficacy. The ability, usually of a medication or other treatment, to produce the desired result.

Effusion. A release of fluid into a body structure. Often used to refer to excess fluid accumulation within a joint, tendon sheath, or other fluid-filled structure.

Endoscopy. Examination of structures by means of flexible tube (called an endoscope) that allows enclosed structures to be seen through the use of either fiber-optic or video technology.

Endotoxemia. A condition that occurs in response to toxins released from the death of bacteria in the body and results in a serious reaction that includes fever and shock symptoms.

Extension. The opening or increasing the angle of a joint.

Fasiculation. Contraction of tiny, individual muscle fibers in a specific area of the body.

Fibrous. Containing fibers, or thin, threadlike structures.

Flexion. The bending of a joint or decreasing its angle.

Foal heat. The mare's first estrous cycle following foaling.

Foal heat diarrhea. Mild, self-limiting diarrhea that often occurs in foals. Although typically timed with the foal heat, it is actually unrelated except by coincidence.

Forage. Food source containing a high fiber content, such as hay or pasture grass.

Foreign body. An object found in a wound, or another structure that is not normally found within the body. For example, a sliver of wood within a wound would be a foreign body.

Generalized. Describes reaction that involves the whole body, rather than being isolated to a specific location.

Hematoma. A localized collection of blood, such as a bruise or blood clot in an organ or body tissue.

Hydration. State of fluid balance within the body. If fluids are lacking, the horse is said to be dehydrated.

Iatrogenic. Describes condition that occurs due to activities of the veterinarian or caretaker of the horse. For example, a common iatrogenic injury would be damage to a tendon or ligament from an incorrectly applied bandage.

Idiopathic. Describes condition that develops with no identifiable cause.

Infection. A condition that occurs due to invasion or multiplication of microorganisms within the body. (Unlike contamination, which applies if microorganisms are simply present but not invading the tissues or multiplying.)

Infectious. Describes disease that can be transmitted from horse to horse.

Inflammation. A condition of the body in response to injury that helps to ward off or minimize damage. The classic signs of inflammation include pain, heat, redness, swelling, and loss of function.

Intramuscular. Within the muscles. Describes a medication administered through injection directly into the muscles.

Intranasal. Within the nasal passages. Describes a medication administered through a spray into the nasal passages.

Intravenous. Within the veins. Describes a medication administered through injection directly into the bloodstream through a vein.

Laceration. A wound that involves tearing of the skin or other structures.

Lactation. Secretion of milk from the mammary glands or udder.

Lateral. Away from the midline of the body. For example, the outside of the horse's lower leg is referred to as the lateral side.

Localized. Describes condition that is restricted to a specific area or location within the body.

Medial. Toward the midline of the body. For example, the inside of the horse's lower leg is referred to as the medial side.

Neoplastic. Describes a process of abnormal growth that often involves uncontrollable multiplication and spread. A neoplastic process is commonly referred to as a tumor or cancer.

Palpate. To feel portions of the body with the hand or fingers to determine the condition of underlying structures as an aid in making a diagnosis. In a rectal palpation, the veterinarian inserts his or her arm into the rectum in order to feel structures within the abdomen.

Palmar. The lower surface of the forelimb below the knee (or the back of the lower foreleg).

Parasite. An organism that lives on or in another organism at the expense of its host. For example, worms living within the intestinal tract of the horse feed from the horse's blood and tissues, causing damage and disease.

Peripheral. Outside or away from central structures or parts. For example, peripheral nerves are found in the legs, distant from the central structures of the nervous system.

Plantar. The lower surface of the hind limb, below the hock (or the back of the lower hind limb).

Prognosis A forecast about the likely progression and outcome of a disease or injury.

Proximal. Toward the central axis of the body.

Puncture. A wound that most likely occurs when a sharp object pierces or penetrates the body. Puncture-type wounds can also occur following a blow, such as a kick from another horse, that creates a deep tract within the tissues.

Radiograph. An image produced by exposing a special type of film to X rays passed through the tissues. Radiographs are most useful for the examination of skeletal structures.

Range of motion. Amount of movement in a joint between full flexion and full extension.

Rostral. When referring to the head, located toward the nose.

Septicemia. A condition of the bloodstream caused by an invasion of microorganisms.

Sesamoid. A small, usually rounded bone embedded within soft tissues around a joint that helps to distribute stress from tendons or ligaments. The distal sesamoid bone in the foot of the horse is referred to as the navicular bone.

Sheath. A tubular case of soft tissue that surrounds another structure.

Sterile. Free of microorganisms.

Syndrome. A set of symptoms that occur together characterizing a specific disease or condition.

Systemic. Affecting the whole body.

Thromboembolic. Describes condition that occurs when a blood clot obstructs blood flow through a vessel, resulting in tissue death due to a loss of blood supply.

Traumatic. Describes condition that occurs due to a wound or injury.

Ultrasound. A imaging modality that allows for visualization of structures within the body by detection of sound waves passed through the tissues. Best used for evaluating soft-tissue structures such as tendons and ligaments.

Ventral. On or near the belly, or underside of the body.

Virulence. A measure of the ability of a microorganism to cause disease, and the severity of symptoms it causes.

APPENDIX B

Guide to Drugs and Medications

A VARIETY OF DRUGS AND MEDICATIONS are likely to be prescribed to treat the wide range of problems a horse may experience. The following guide outlines dosing options and calculation, drug handling information, basic facts about categories of medications, and details about the most common specific medications used in horses. (*Note: Dosages listed are guidelines only, and may vary. Consult with your veterinarian if you have questions about specific dosage recommendations for your horse.*)

Routes of Administration

TOPICAL. Medications are applied to the body surface and may include ointments or salves to treat wounds, ophthalmic ointments placed in the eye, and liniments applied to the legs. In most cases, topical medications only affect the location where they are applied. Rarely, topical medications may pass through the skin to be absorbed into the horse's system.

PARENTERAL. Medications are given through the mouth or via injection for a whole-body, or systemic, effect.

ORAL (PO). Medications administered orally are absorbed through the horse's gastrointestinal tract and delivered to the appropriate tissues through the bloodstream. Oral medications are desirable due to ease of administration, particularly when they can be given on the feed.

INTRAMUSCULAR (IM). Medications are injected deep into the muscles using a sterile needle and syringe and are absorbed from the muscles into the bloodstream to have their effect. IM medications will take effect faster than orally administered medications, but not quite as quickly as intravenous medications. Some medications should not be given IM due to their irritating effects on tissues, which can lead to swelling or even sloughing of skin or underlying tissues.

INTRAVENOUS (IV). Medications are injected directly into the bloodstream through a vein using a sterile needle and syringe. The route of administration allows the medication to take effect quickly and efficiently. Medications that can be administered through any parenteral route (PO, IM, or IV) will have a faster, more profound effect with a smaller total dose when given IV.

INTRA-ARTICULAR (IA). Medications are administered directly into a joint, and are used to treat a problem in the specific joint that is affected. Due to the risk of joint infections, administration of IA medications requires careful preparation, sterile equipment and sterile technique to perform an injection.

OTHER. Rarely, medications may be administered through alternative routes. Examples include laxative substances placed directly into the stomach through a nasogastric tube, and some antibiotics that may be placed in the rectum where they are absorbed into the horse's system.

Frequency of Administration

The dosing schedule for a specific medication is determined by how the body processes, or metabolizes, the drug. The efficacy of some medications is determined by their peak levels (the point where they are at their highest concentration in the tissues), whereas others depend more on achieving a steady level. Usually, medications are administered once daily (SID), twice daily (BID), three times daily (TID), or four times daily (QID). The interval between dosages should remain the same. For example, a BID medication should be given at 12-hour intervals, while a QID medication should be given at 6-hour intervals.

Calculating Dosages

Medications are prescribed in an amount or dose according to the horse's weight, and the amount of drug required to have the desired effect. Most medications are measured in milligrams, and doses are determined according to milligrams per kilogram of body weight (expressed mg/kg). A kilogram is equal to approximately 2.2 pounds, meaning that the 1000-pound horse weighs approximately 450 kilograms.

To confuse matters further, medications that are in liquid form will have a concentration that's usually expressed in milligrams per milliliter (mg/ml). This means that the volume of liquid to be administered depends on this concentration. For example, if the dose of the drug is 10 mg/kg, the 450 kg horse would need 4500 mg per dose. If the medication is provided in a liquid form with a concentration of 100 mg/ml, the horse would be administered 45 ml per dose.

Finally, different units of measurement may be used for certain medications. These include micrograms (µg), which are equal to 1/1000 of a gram; grams (gm), which are equal to 1000 milligrams; international units (IU), which are units determined for certain individual substances (such as penicillin and vitamin E) based on their clinical effect; and grains, which are equal to 64.8 milligrams.

Nonsteroidal Anti-inflammatory Drug (NSAIDS)

NSAIDS are medications that inhibit the production of these substances. When a horse is ill or injured, its body produces substances to create an inflammatory response. Different NSAIDS may affect different branches of the inflammatory response, thereby having variable effects. The veterinarian will select a NSAID based on a number of different variables. These include onset and duration of effects as well as the specific condition requiring treatment. Most NSAIDS have potential side effects that include ulceration of the gastrointestinal tract and kidney damage if administered when the horse is dehydrated. Therefore, they should be used with care, and their use in combination with one another should be limited unless specifically directed by the veterinarian.

DRUG	WHAT IT DOES	DOSAGE	ROUTE OF ADMINISTRATION	COMMONLY USED FOR	COMMENTS
Aspirin	Prevents blood clots. Anti-inflammatory. Pain relief. Fever reducer.	15–100 mg/kg SID–BID.	Oral.	Laminitis. Eye problems.	Very short duration of action. Can increase risk of stomach ulcers.
Flunixin meglumine (Banamine®)	Anti-inflammatory. Pain relief. Fever reducer. Anti-endotoxic.	0.25–1.1 mg/kg SID–QID.	Oral. Intravenous.	Colic. Musculoskeletal pain. Fever reduction. To combat endotoxemia Eye problems.	Can cause stomach ulcers and kidney damage. Irritating to tissues if injected in the muscle.
Ketoprofen (Ketofen™)	Anti-inflammatory Pain relief. Fever reducer. Anti-endotoxic .	2.2 mg/kg SID.	Intravenous.	Colic. Musculoskeletal pain. Fever reduction. To combat endotoxemia.	Can cause stomach ulcers and kidney damage but less toxic than flunixin meglumine or phenylbutazone.
Meclofenamic Acid (Arquel™)	Anti-inflammatory. Pain relief. Fever reducer.	2.2 mg/kg SID–BID.	Oral.	Musculoskeletal pain	May take 2–3 days for full effect. Can cause stomach ulcers and kidney damage.
Naproxen	Anti-inflammatory. Pain relief.	10 mg/kg SID–BID.	Oral.	Musculoskeletal pain.	May take 5–7 days for full effect. Can cause stomach ulcers and kidney damage.
Phenylbutazone	Anti-inflammatory. Pain relief. Fever reducer.	2.2–4.4 mg/kg BID.	Oral. Intravenous.	Musculoskeletal injury. Fever reducer.	Can cause stomach ulcers and kidney damage. Never inject intramuscularly due to severe tissue damage.

Antimicrobial Drugs

Antimicrobials are medications used to combat infection from microbial agents, including bacteria (antibiotics), fungi (antifungals) and protazoa (antiprotazoals). Antimicrobial medications are selected based on the location of the infection and type of organism involved. In some cases, the veterinarian will select an antimicrobial medication based on the most likely organism causing the infection. In other situations, samples will be taken from the infected area for identification of the specific organism and to determine the most effective medication against the organism identified (called culture and sensitivity testing). In addition, the medication selected must be able to reach the location of the infection. For example, some antibiotics are able to penetrate abscesses while others are less effective for this purpose. Finally, antimicrobial drugs may be administered prophylactically in order to prevent infection in situations of risk.

DRUG	WHAT IT DOES	DOSAGE	ROUTE OF ADMINISTRATION	COMMONLY USED FOR	COMMENTS
Amikacin	Combats gram negative bacteria.	15 mg/kg SID. 125–250mg per joint.	Intravenous. Intramuscular. Intra-articular.	Susceptible infections. Foal septicemia. Prophylactic in joint injections.	May cause kidney damage.
Ceftiofur sodium (Naxcel®)	Combats a broad spectrum of bacterial organisms.	1.1–4.4 mg/kg SID–BID.	Intravenous. Intramuscular.	Respiratory infections. Other infections requiring broad-spectrum activity.	Can cause severe diarrhea. May be irritating to tissues with intramuscular injection.
Chloramphenicol	Combats a broad spectrum of bacterial organisms.	10–50 mg/kg QID.	Oral. Intravenous.	Eye problems. Joint infections. Other infections requiring broad spectrum activity.	Risk of aplastic anemia to humans administering medication.
Enrofloxacin (Baytril®)	Combats a broad spectrum of bacterial organisms.	2.5 mg/kg BID.	Oral. Intravenous.	Serious infections resistant to other antibiotics.	Not used in young horses due to effect on growth plates.
Erythromycin	Combats *Rhodococcus equi* bacteria.	25 mg/kg BID.	Oral.	*Rhodococcus equi* infections.	Used with rifampin.
Gentamicin	Combats gram negative bacteria.	6.6–8.8 mg/kg SID.	Intravenous. Intramuscular.	Susceptible infections.	More resistant bacteria likely compared with Amikacin. Can cause kidney damage.
Griseofulvin	Combats fungi.	10 mg/kg SID.	Oral.	Ringworm. Other fungal infections.	Metabolized in liver and should not be used in horses with liver problems. Dosages not well established.

DRUG	WHAT IT DOES	DOSAGE	ROUTE OF ADMINISTRATION	COMMONLY USED FOR	COMMENTS
Metronidazole	Combats anaerobic bacteria.	7.5–15.0 mg/kg QID.	Oral. Well absorbed if placed in rectum.	Susceptible infections. Dental problems. Foot problems.	Bad taste may put horse off feed. Can cause increase in liver enzymes.
Oxytetracycline	Combats rickettsial organisms and other bacterial infections.	5–20 mg/kg SID.	Intravenous	Potomac Horse Fever. Susceptible bacterial infections.	Can cause diarrhea.
Miconazole	Combats fungi.	1–2% solution.	Topical.	Ringworm. Other localized fungal infections	None.
Penicillin	Combats gram-positive bacteria and anaerobic bacteria.	10,000–50,000 IU/kg QID IV. 25,000–50,000 IU/kg BID IM.	Intravenous (potassium or sodium penicillin). Intramuscular (procaine penicillin).	Susceptible infections.	Often used with gentocin or amikacin for broad-spectrum activity.
Ponazuril (Marquis™)	Combats protazoa.	5.5 mg/kg SID for 28 days.	Oral.	Equine protazoal myelitis (EPM).*	Crosses blood-brain barrier to reach high levels in CSF.*
Pyrimethamine	Combats protazoa.	0.2–2.0 mg/kg SID–BID for up to 4 months.	Oral.	Equine protazoal myelitis (EPM).*	Combine with sulfa antibiotic for best effect in treating EPM.** May cause anemia.
Rifampin	Combats *Rhodococcus equi* bacteria.	5.0–20.0 mg/kg SID or BID.	Oral.	*Rhodococcus equi* infections.	Must be used with another antibiotic to avoid resistance. Combine with erythromycin for *R. equi* infections.
Trimethoprim sulfadiazine (Uniprim® Tucoprim®)	Combats a broad spectrum of bacteria.	25 mg/kg sulfadiazine SID.	Oral.	Susceptible bacterial infections.	May be more effective at twice daily dosing.
Trimethoprim sulfamethoxazole	Combats broad spectrum of bacteria.	20–30 mg/kg BID.	Oral.	Susceptible bacterial infections.	Most common antibiotic prescribed. Can cause severe diarrhea.

* CSF: Cerebrospinal fluid. The fluid that surrounds the brain and spinal cord.

** EPM: Equine Protazoal Myelencephalitis. A neurologic disease caused by parasites migrating through the brain and spinal cord.

Corticosteroids

DRUG	WHAT IT DOES	DOSAGE	ROUTE OF ADMINISTRATION	COMMONLY USED FOR	COMMENTS
Betamethasone	Combats inflammation.	Varies with joint and condition.	Intra-articular.	Joint trauma or degenerative joint disease.	No FDA-approved product is available.
Dexamethasone	Combats inflammation. Modifies immune system response.	0.02–0.2 mg/kg SID.	Oral. Intravenous. Intramuscular.	Allergic reactions. Auto-immune disease.	Can cause laminitis. Depresses immune system.
Isoflupredone acetate (Predef® 2X)	Combats inflammation.	Varies with joint and condition. 0.02 mg/kg SID for intramuscular use.	Intra-articular. Intramuscular.	Joint injection COPD*	Decrease dose to effect when using to treat COPD.*
Methyl-prednisolone (Depo-Medrol®)	Combats inflammation.	Varies with joint and condition.	Intra-articular.	Joint trauma or degenerative joint disease.	Crystalline structure may damage joints.
Prednisolone	Combats inflammation. Modifies immune response.	0.2–4.4 mg/kg SID	Oral.	Allergic reactions. Auto-immune disease.	More effectively metabolized than prednisone.
Triamcinolone (Vetalog®)	Combats inflammation.	Varies with joint and condition.	Intra-articular.	Joint trauma or degenerative joint disease.	In small dosages may actually protect joints by minimizing negative effects of inflammation.

COPD: Chronic obstructive pulmonary disease or heaves. An obstructive airway disease with underlying allergic cause.

TABLE B.4

Antihistamines

Antihistamine medications may be prescribed to combat allergic reactions, most commonly those resulting in hives or other itchy skin reactions. Although antihistamines may not be as effective as corticosteroids such as prednisolone or dexamethasone for treating allergic problems, they are generally considered safer for long-term use, with very limited side effects at lower dosages. Just like humans, horses respond differently to the antihistamines and trial and error may be necessary to determine the most effective medication for the individual horse.

DRUG	WHAT IT DOES	DOSAGE	ROUTE OF ADMINISTRATION	COMMONLY USED FOR	COMMENTS
Diphenhydramine hydrochloride (Benadryl ®)	Blocks histamine activity.	0.75–1.0 mg/kg TID.	Oral.	Allergic reactions (hives).	Can cause sedation or excitement with tremors at high dosages.
Doxepin hydrochloride	Blocks histamine activity.	0.5–0.75 mg/kg BID.	Oral.	Allergic reactions (hives).	Can cause sedation or excitement with tremors at high dosages.
Hydroxyzine hydrochloride	Blocks histamine activity.	1.0–1.5 mg/kg TID.	Oral.	Allergic reactions (hives).	Can cause sedation or excitement with tremors in high dosages.

TABLE B.5

Joint treatments

DRUG	WHAT IT DOES	DOSAGE	ROUTE OF ADMINISTRATION	COMMONLY USED FOR	COMMENTS
Hyaluronic acid (HA) (Legend ® Hylartin ® Hyalovet ® Hycoat ® Hyvisc ®)	Reduces inflammation and combats joint damage.	40 mg IV, repeated at weekly intervals for 3 weeks, 10–40 mg per joint .	Intravenous (Legend ® only). Intra-articular.	Acute and chronic joint damage.	IV HA is commonly used to protect the joints in performance horses.
Polysulfated glycosamin- oglycan (PSGAG) (Adequan ®)	Reduces inflammation, protects cartilage, and slows progression of arthritis.	500 mg IM, repeated at 4-day intervals for 7 injections, 250 mg per joint.	Intramuscular. Intra-articular.	Acute and chronic joint damage.	IM PSGAG is commonly used to protect the joints in performance horses.

Tranquilizers, Sedatives, and Anesthetics

DRUG	WHAT IT DOES	DOSAGE	ROUTE OF ADMINISTRATION	COMMONLY USED FOR	COMMENTS
Acepromazine	Sedative.	0.03–0.1 mg/kg. Single dose.	Oral. Intravenous. Intramuscular.	Routine sedation.	Variable efficacy. Must wait until full effect before stimulating.
Butorphanol	Sedative. Pain reliever.	0.02–0.05 mg/kg. Single dose.	Intravenous. Intramuscular.	Sedation and pain relief.	FDA-regulated narcotic.
Mepivacaine (Carbocaine®)	Deadens skin and tissues.	Varies with area blocked.	Subcutaneous.	Deadening skin for procedures. Nerve blocks.	Longer duration of effect than lidocaine.
Detomidine	Sedative. Pain reliever.	0.005–0.02 mg/kg. Single dose.	Intravenous. Intramuscular.	Sedation when profound effect required. Pain relief.	More profound sedation than xylazine and longer duration of effect.
Diazepam	Sedative. Anti-convulsant.	0.05–0.4 mg/kg. Single dose.	Intravenous. Intramuscular.	Sedation of foals, young horses. Controlling seizures.	Safe medication. Can be repeated at 30-minute intervals if needed.
Fluphenazine	Long-acting sedation.	Consult your veterinarian.	Intramuscular.	Long-term sedation for layups. Behavior modification in show horses.	Safe dosages and use not well established.
Ketamine	Dissociative agent.	2.2 mg/kg. Single dose.	Intravenous.	Procedures requiring short anesthesia, such as castration.	Commonly used for routine castration with xylazine or detomidine.
Lidocaine	Deadens skin and tissues.	Varies with area blocked.	Subcutaneous.	Deadening skin for procedures. Nerve blocks.	Shorter acting than mepivicaine.
Reserpine	Long-acting sedation.	Consult your veterinarian.	Oral. Intravenous.	Long-term sedation for layups. Behavior modification in show horses.	May cause gastrointestinal upset, including colic and severe diarrhea. Safe dosages not well established.
Sarapin®	Deadens skin and tissues.	Varies with area blocked.	Subcutaneous. Intramuscular.	Relief of pain with long duration.	None.
Xylazine	Sedative. Pain reliever.	0.2–1.1 mg/kg. Single dose.	Intravenous. Intramuscular.	Routine sedation. Pain relief.	May cause aggressive behavior. Horse can react unpredictably.

Reproductive Hormones

DRUG	WHAT IT DOES	DOSAGE	ROUTE OF ADMINISTRATION	COMMONLY USED FOR	COMMENTS
Cloprostinol (Estrumate®)	Breaks down the corpus luteum on the ovary to allow follicle development.	0.5–1.0 µg/kg. Single dose.	Intramuscular.	Stimulating estrous cycle. Clearing uterine fluid.	Causes sweating and cramping following administration.
Deslorelin	Stimulates ovulation.	1.5–300µg. Single dose.	Intramuscular.	Assists with timing of insemination.	Overdose may prolong interval between ovulations.
Domperidone	Blocks dopamine receptors to stimulate milk production when suppressed.	1.0–2.0 mg/kg SID for 7–10 days.	Oral.	Fescue toxicosis in pregnant mares.	Can be used preventatively if fescue exposure is suspected.
Human chorionic gonadotropin (HCG)	Stimulates ovulation.	2,000–3,000 IU per horse. Single dose.	Intravenous. Intramuscular.	Assists with timing of insemination.	Not as reliable as deslorelin.
Progesterone (Regu-Mate®)	Hormone produced by ovary and placenta to regulate heat cycles and maintain pregnancy.	0.44 mg/kg SID.	Oral.	To synchronize estrus and help maintain pregnancy. Used to modify behavior in show horses.	When administering medication, avoid skin contact.

Miscellaneous

DRUG	WHAT IT DOES	DOSAGE	ROUTE OF ADMINISTRATION	COMMONLY USED FOR	COMMENTS
Acetazolamide	Increases potassium excretion. Regulates glucose metabolism.	2.0–4.0 mg/kg BID–TID	Oral.	Hyperkalemic periodic paralysis.	None.
Albuteral	Dilates airways.	1.0–2.0 µg/kg.	Inhaled.	COPD (heaves).*	Administered to open airways prior to administration of inhaled corticosteroids.
N-butylscopol-ammonium bromide (Buscopan®)	Relieves intestinal spasms.	0.3 mg/kg. Single dose.	Intravenous.	Colic.	30-minute duration of effect. Elevates heart rate.
Cimetidine (Tagamet)	Blocks production of stomach acid.	15.0–25.0 mg/kg TID.	Oral.	Gastric ulcers. Melanomas.	Marginal efficacy for healing ulcers. May reduce clinical signs.
Clenbuteral (Ventipulmin®)	Dilates airways.	0.8–3.2 µg/kg BID.	Oral.	COPD (heaves).*	May develop resistance after a period of treatment and lose efficacy.
Cyproheptadine	Blocks the neurotransmitter serotonin. Blocks histamine.	0.25–0.5 mg/kg SID–BID.	Oral.	Cushing's disease. Headshaking.	Generally thought to be less effective than pergolide for treating Cushing's disease.
Furosemide	Diuretic.	0.25–3.0 mg/kg SID–BID.	Intravenous.	Exercise-induced pulmonary hemorrhage. Heart failure. Collection of urine sample.	Commonly used prerace to prevent bleeding.
Imipramine	Blocks uptake of serotonin and norepinephrine and suppresses REM sleep.	0.5–1.5 mg/kg BID–TID.	Intravenous. Intramuscular.	Narcolepsy.	May be impractical for long-term use.

DRUG	WHAT IT DOES	DOSAGE	ROUTE OF ADMINISTRATION	COMMONLY USED FOR	COMMENTS
Isoxsuprine hydrochloride	Dilates blood vesels.	0.5 mg/kg BID.	Oral.	Laminitis. Navicular disease.	Minimal side effects.
Methocarbamol (Robaxin®)	Muscle relaxant.	5.0–55 mg/kg BID–QID.	Oral. Intravenous.	Musculoskeletal disorders. Back pain.	May cause sedation.
Omeprazole (GastroGard®)	Stops production of stomach acids.	4.0 mg/kg SID for 4 weeks to treat. 2.0 mg/kg SID for prevention.	Oral.	Gastric ulcers.	Most effective ulcer treatment.
Pergolide mesylate	Binds dopamine receptors in brain.	0.5–1.5 mg/day SID.	Oral.	Cushing's disease.	Drug may lose efficacy over time.
Phenobarbital	Blocks neurotransmitters in brain. Anticonvulsant.	2.0–12.0 mg/kg SID.	Oral.	Seizure disorders.	Can cause increase in liver enzymes. Blood levels should be monitored for determination of dosage.
Potassium iodide	Expectorant.	2.0–20 grams/day SID	Oral.	COPD.* Inflammatory airway disease.	Can be irritating to respiratory tissues.
Ranitidine (Zantac®)	Counteracts effects of stomach acid.	6.6 mg/kg BID oral. 2.2 mg/kh BID intravenous.	Oral. Intravenous.	Gastric ulcers.	Marginal efficacy for healing ulcers. May relieve clinical signs.
Sucralfate (Carafate)	Protects lining of gastrointestinal tract.	2.0 mg/kg TID.	Oral.	Gastric ulcers. Colonic ulcers.	None.

COPD: Chronic obstructive pulmonary disease or heaves. An obstructive airway disease with underlying allergic cause.

The New Horse Owner

So You Want to Buy a Horse?

CONSIDER THIS: The horse you purchase may well be a part of your family for the next 30 years. He has to be fed at least twice each day and needs a safe place to live and regular exercise. He'll wear out his shoes in less than 2 months and has to see the dentist at least once a year. His clothes will get dirty every day, and he'll probably need different outfits for sleeping, playtime, and exercise. The vet will become like an old family friend, and vacations will require a full-time babysitter. Have kids? If not, you're about to. And if so, you can only hope they're old enough to help out with the new addition.

When you consider the commitment required to care for a horse, you'll realize it's not a decision to be taken lightly. And finding the right match can be as difficult as finding a suitable spouse. With that in mind, it's good advice to prepare carefully before you take the plunge. The following guide will not only help you understand just what horse ownership is all about, but also will help you make the right choices as you make the move to becoming a "horsehold."

Learn First

If you're not a rider, and are just exploring the horse world for the first time, it makes sense to gain some experience before you take on ownership.

- **TAKE LESSONS.** By establishing yourself with a knowledgeable trainer and mentor, you'll learn how to handle a horse safely, how to care for a horse, and how to ride. Perhaps most important, you'll discover what type of riding you especially like and what kind of horse would best suit your needs.

- **TAKE A CLASS.** Many community colleges and adult education programs offer courses on basic horse care, taught either by veterinarians or established horse professionals in the area. If you take the time to learn the essentials of caring for your horse before you buy, you'll be much better prepared. You'll also make connections with other horse owners, and you might find a good mentor in your instructor.

THEN AND NOW

Horse trading during the 16th century was a tricky business. Owners learned how to alter their horse's teeth by grinding them into a shape characteristic of a much younger horse in order to deceive potential purchasers about the horse's age. Creative tooth grinding was so widespread that it actually became a punishable crime.

These days, it still pays to be careful when purchasing a horse. The veterinary prepurchase examination helps potential buyers learn whether there might be secrets about the horse they're considering. And a thorough dental exam is still an important part of that evaluation.

- **SUBSCRIBE TO MAGAZINES.** There are many good horse magazines out there that can help you learn about horse care and management. Select a general magazine and perhaps one targeted toward the specific discipline you find most interesting. Books, videos, and other sources of information—such as seminars and clinics—can help you round out your horse knowledge so you'll be ready when the time finally comes to buy a horse for yourself or your child.

- **CONSIDER A LEASE.** If you've never owned a horse, leasing one might be a good option. A lease generally involves your taking on the expense and care of a horse in exchange for riding privileges. In effect, you will enjoy all of the benefits of horse ownership without many of the risks.

Prepare, Prepare, Prepare

If you've decided that you want to own rather than lease a horse, it's best to have basics in place before you actually begin your search. Will you board your horse at a boarding stable or keep him at home? What kind of equipment will you need? Will you work with a trainer, or do you just want to trail ride? These questions are best answered *before* you find the horse of your dreams and plan to bring him home.

Where Will He Live?

Your first decision when making arrangements for your horse is where he'll live. In general, options range from a full-service boarding stable, where care, including multiple daily feedings, stall cleaning, turnout, blanketing, and 24-hour surveillance are provided, to at-home care where you do all the work. The advantages of the full-care option are obvious: you'll have the expertise of an experienced barn owner or manager to help you care for your horse, you'll enjoy socializing with friends at the barn (as well as learning from other horse owners), and you can rest assured your horse is looked after whether you make it to the barn on a particular day or not. Of course, cost is a major factor and can be a disadvantage. Paying for all of that expertise and care can be expensive. Even so, some horse owners may prefer to have their horse at home, enjoying the interaction and bonding that goes along with providing daily care. If you do decide not to board but to bring your new horse home, you must have adequate facilities to insure his safety and comfort. At minimum this means good shelter and a pasture or paddock for turnout. And be aware that horses are social animals, who aren't likely to be happy living alone. If two at-home horses aren't part of your plan, consider a companion such as a goat to keep your horse company.

For most new horse owners, the boarding option is preferable—at least during the first several months of ownership. Even though you hope to bring your horse home eventually, you might consider boarding to begin with so you can find out just what kind of at-home care is necessary.

Choose a Vet and Farrier

Just like a new parent selecting the pediatrician before the baby's born, as a new horse owner you would be wise to locate a veterinarian and farrier who will help care for your horse. If you plan to board at a stable where a good vet and farrier already provide the necessary care, this decision has been already made for you. If you need to make the choice yourself, however, be sure to ask other horse owners for recommendations and ask for references as well. Usually veterinarians will be happy to talk to you about your new horse's needs, and may even have a preventative health care plan in place that can help you cope with health-care requirements such as vaccinations, deworming, and dentistry. The veterinarian you select is likely to know who the competent, reliable farriers in your area are and can give you a solid reference.

Budget Carefully

There's no doubt about it. Horses are expensive. And with ownership comes the responsibility of providing proper care. When you calculate your horse budget, consider costs for boarding, feed, the farrier, the vet, and any additional equipment you might find necessary. In addition, you should plan to set up an emergency fund that can be used should disaster strike, or consider purchasing major medical insurance. (See page335.) A serious injury or surgery could cost thousands of dollars—a stressful reality once that horse becomes a part of your family.

Beyond what you'll have to spend on ongoing care, you'll need to consider how much money you'll need to actually make the purchase. First, costs associated with traveling to see potential prospects can range from as little as the gas required to drive to barns in your area, to as much as airfares and hotels if you'll be traveling out of town. Next, you should consider whether you'll pay a trainer or other expert to help you locate prospective horses and evaluate their suitability. If you'll be paying a commission on an eventual purchase, make sure you have a written agreement before you begin your search. Commissions typically range between 10 and 15 percent of the purchase price. Some horse professionals prefer to work on an hourly or service-by-service basis, charging for the assistance they provide. Ideally, a written contract will outline how you'll pay expenses and commissions associated with your purchase.

You'll also need to budget for the cost of a veterinary prepurchase examination on the horse you choose. This expense can range from hundreds to thousands of dollars, depending on the extent of the examination, and any necessary tests. Of course, you have to recognize the possibility that the first horse you select will have problems, requiring that you begin your search all over again before you ultimately make your purchase. Finally, once you've found a suitable horse with a clean bill of health, you'll have the expense of bringing him home. This can be as simple as trailering from one barn to another or as complicated as shipping him across the country or even flying him from abroad.

The Search Is On

Ready to buy? You've done your homework, have reservations at the boarding stable, and your bank account is stocked. Now it's time to start your search.

Know What You're Looking For

Before you start looking at horses, know exactly what you're looking for. If you're new to horses, an older, predictable animal is the best place to start. Make a checklist of the attributes you hope to find, such as breed, sex, age range, and level of training. Determine how much you can afford to pay. Then, know in what ways you might be willing to compromise versus what you won't give up. For example, if you find the perfect 15-year-old horse that meets all of your requirements but he's a little older than your ideal 6 to 10 age range, it's probably wise to make that compromise. However, if the horse meets every requirement except that he tried to kick you when you approached his hindquarters, you'll probably want to walk away. As a new owner, the horse's training and temperament should be your first priorities. Breed, beauty, and size (within reason) should just be happy extras if you happen to get lucky.

Hit the Road

Don't buy the first horse you've been shown. In fact, if you think you want to make an offer and you've just started looking, check out a few more horses first. At the very least, it will give you a basis for comparison if you ultimately decide to buy the first horse you looked at. At best you'll prevent yourself from falling in love with the wrong partner, and may find a much better match is out there waiting to be found.

The Prepurchase Examination

The veterinary prepurchase examination is an important step you'll need to take before finalizing your purchase decision. Prior to scheduling this exam, request a release of medical records from the buyer. You can obtain records of routine health care such as vaccinations and dentistry, and also learn about any previous medical problems. Your vet will want to focus on reported problem areas during the exam. Try to have all information available, including radiographs that may have been taken in the past, and copies of lab work.

When you do schedule the exam, both you and the seller should be present. The seller can answer questions that might arise, and both of you will have a better understanding of any concerns your vet raises. Your veterinarian will then perform a thorough examination to identify all possible health issues or potential risks. This exam may include the following steps.

Clinical exam

This overall physical examination includes an evaluation of the eyes, teeth, heart, lungs, neurologic system, and musculoskeletal system. The musculoskeletal portion of the exam is often the most extensive, and involves the evaluation of movement and stress tests performed on joints. If you intend to use the horse for riding, be prepared to ride the horse during the examination. Your vet may also have comments on the horse's temperament based on his behavior and willingness to submit to tests performed during the examination. Pay attention to what the vet has to say— especially if you're buying your first horse and don't have a lot of experience. Veterinarians work with a lot of horses, and they may be able to detect behavior issues that could be quite significant.

Radiographs

Many prepurchase examinations include radiographs. If the vet detects any sign of irregularity in the horse's gait, is concerned about responses to stress tests, or sees any other red flags that could indicate a soundness issue, he's likely to recommend radiographs to evaluate the areas in question if you still intend to pursue purchase of the horse. If everything looks good on the clinical examination, routine radiographs may also be recommended as a screening test to identify any existing abnormalities that could increase future risk.

Blood tests

If the vet has any concerns about the horse's overall physical condition, he may recommend a comprehensive blood test that looks at the white and red blood cells, as well as indicators of organic disease such as liver- or kidney-related enzymes. It's also possible to look for traces of medications such as tranquilizers or NSAIDS (nonsteroidal anti-inflammatory medications that could provide pain relief) in the horse's blood if there is any suspicion the horse might have been given drugs prior to the exam. It's sad but true that not every person with a horse to sell is ethical, and your vet will do what is necessary to protect you from a bad first purchase experience. Finally, if you'll be transporting the horse across state lines or importing him from another country, he may need to undergo testing for infectious diseases. Most commonly, a Coggins test that looks for antibodies against equine infectious anemia may be required. Your veterinarian can advise you if additional testing will be required.

Other diagnostics

The vet may recommend additional diagnostics such as an endoscopic examination if he has concerns about the horse's respiratory tract, or ultrasound if he has a question about a soft-tissue structure. Each individual situation will determine which tests the vet will ask for.

Paperwork

Usually veterinarians will provide you with a written report of findings from the prepurchase examination that you can maintain in the horse's records. And again, if all looks good on the exam and you intend to purchase the horse, make sure you obtain paperwork you'll need for transport. These include health certificates, a verification of Coggins testing, as well as insurance company forms if you plan to insure the horse. It's also advisable to have a formal, written bill-of-sale from the seller that describes the horse in detail and includes any agreements made regarding the sale, such as a trial period or return option.

The Break-in Period

You've found your perfect horse, finalized the purchase, and brought him home. A bit like adopting an older child—it may take weeks or even months to work out your new relationship. Don't be dismayed if you discover quirky behaviors or have some difficulties with your horse during this initial period. Seek help, and work on getting to know one another. Rarely is the road to a solid relationship without a bump or two.

Insurance

As a new horse owner, costs may seem overwhelming—especially if you're faced with a veterinary emergency. One way to protect yourself from the devastation of a colic surgery or severe injury is to buy major medical insurance. In order to obtain this coverage, you'll first need to insure your horse against mortality, usually for a minimum value of $5,000. Costs for mortality insurance vary, but generally average around 3 percent of the horse's value. With this coverage you'll have the option of adding major medical or surgical insurance for just a couple of hundred dollars a year. With a major medical policy, you can rest easy knowing that the bulk of veterinary bills incurred during a health crisis will be covered. Your only worry need be what's best for your horse.

You might also ask your veterinarian about programs offered through his or her veterinary practice that can help cover veterinary costs. For example, several pharmaceutical companies offer colic surgery coverage for horses maintained on daily deworming medications.

TABLE C.1
The Horse's Daily Schedule

Think it can't be that much work? This is a typical schedule for care in a well-run boarding stable.

6 am	Breakfast. Check and fill water.		**4 pm**	Groom. Tack up. Ride.
8 am	Clean stall. Turn out to pasture.		**6 pm**	Dinner. Pick out stall. Scrub and fill water buckets.
12 pm	In from pasture. Lunch. Check and fill water.		**10 pm**	Evening snack. Lights out.

TABLE C.2
Basic Care Calendar

MONTH	VACCINATIONS	DEWORMING*	SHOEING	DENTISTRY	OTHER
January		5-day fenbendazole larvicidal treatment.	Trim/shoe.		Body clipping if necessary.
February				Basic dental balancing.	
March	Tetanus. Sleeping sickness. West Nile virus. Influenza.	Ivermectin.	Trim/shoe.		
April					
May		Ivermectin/praziquantal combination.	Trim/shoe.		
June	Potomac Horse Fever.				
July			Trim/shoe.		
August		Moxidectin.			
September	West Nile virus. Influenza.		Trim/shoe.		
October		Ivermectin.			
November			Trim/shoe.		
December		Ivermectin.			

* Assuming an interval deworming plan. If horse is maintained on a daily dewormer, ivermectin should be administered in the spring and fall. (See preventative care chapter on deworming.)

INDEX

◆